Advanced Techniques in Image-Guided Brain and Spine Surgery

Advanced Techniques in Image-Guided Brain and Spine Surgery

Isabelle M. Germano, M.D., F.A.C.S.
Associate Professor of Neurosurgery and Neurology
Director of Functional and Stereotaxy
Department of Neurosurgery
Mount Sinai School of Medicine
New York, New York

Thieme
New York • Stuttgart

Thieme Medical Publishers, Inc.
333 Seventh Ave.
New York, NY 10001

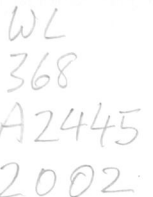

Editor: Felicity Edge
Editorial Assistant: Diane Sardini
Director, Production and Manufacturing: Anne Vinnicombe
Production Editor: Becky Dille
Marketing Director: Phyllis Gold
Sales Manager: Ross Lumpkin
Chief Financial Officer: Peter van Woerden
President: Brian D. Scanlan
Compositor: Compset, Inc.
Printer: Maple-Vail Book Manufacturing Group
Library of Congress Cataloging-in-Publication Data is available from the publisher.

Copyright © 2002 by Thieme Medical Publishers, Inc. This book, including all parts thereof, is legally protected by copyright. Any use, exploitation or commercialization outside the narrow limits set by copyright legislation, without the publisher's consent, is illegal and liable to prosecution. This applies in particular to Photostat reproduction, copying, mimeographing or duplication of any kind, translating, preparation of microfilms, and electronic data processing and storage.

Important note: Medical knowledge is ever-changing. As new research and clinical experience broaden our knowledge, changes in treatment and drug therapy may be required. The authors and editors of the material herein have consulted sources believed to be reliable in their efforts to provide information that is complete and in accord with the standards accepted at the time of publication. However, in the view of the possibility of human error by the authors, editors, or publisher, of the work herein, or changes in medical knowledge, neither the authors, editors, or publisher, nor any other party who has been involved in the preparation of this work, warrants that the information contained herein is in every respect accurate or complete, and they are not responsible for any errors or omissions or for the results obtained from use of such information. Readers are encouraged to confirm the information contained herein with other sources. For example, readers are advised to check the product information sheet included in the package of each drug they plan to administer to be certain that the information contained in this publication is accurate and that changes have not been made in the recommended dose or in the contraindications for administration. This recommendation is of particular importance in connection with new or infrequently used drugs.

Some of the product names, patents, and registered designs referred to in this book are in fact registered trademarks or proprietary names even though specific reference to this fact is not always made in the text. Therefore, the appearance of a name without designation as proprietary is not to be construed as a representation by the publisher that it is in the public domain.

Printed in the United States of America
5 4 3 2 1
TMP ISBN 1-58890-067-3
GTV ISBN 3 13 131521 0

Contents

Contributors	vii
Preface	xi
Dedication	xii
Acknowledgments	xiii

PART I   PRINCIPLES AND TECHNOLOGY

1. Historical Perspective of Image-Guided Neurosurgery	2
2. Sources of Error in Image Registration for Cranial Image-Guided Neurosurgery	10
3. Spinal Registration Accuracy and Error	37
4. The Optical Digitizer	45
5. The Mechanical Arm System	54
6. The Magnetic System	60
7. The Passive Navigational System	68
8. Image-Guided Neurosurgery Combining Mechanical Arm and Optical Digitizer	73
9. Videotactic Surgery	80
10. Endoscopic Image-Guided Surgery	87
11. Robotic Microscopes	98
12. Image-Guided Robotic Radiosurgery	107

PART IIA   CRANIAL APPLICATIONS

13. Image-Guided Brain Biopsy	116
14. Cerebrovascular Applications of Image-Guided Surgery	121
15. Image-Guided Brain Tumor Resection	132
16. Intraoperative Image Update by Interface with Ultrasound	141
17. Intraoperative Image Update by Magnetic Resonance Imaging	146
18. Image-Guided Epilepsy Surgery	156
19. New Directions in Atlas-Assisted Stereotactic Functional Neurosurgery	162

PART IIB   SPINAL APPLICATIONS

20. Image-Guided Cervical Instrumentation	176
21. Thoracic Instrumentation: Stereotactic Navigation for Placement of Pedicle Screws in the Thoracic Spine	182

22.	Image Guidance for Scoliosis	191
23.	Image-Guided Lumbar Instrumentation	197
24.	Computer-Assisted Image-Guided Fluoroscopy (Virtual Fluoroscopy)	207
25.	Controversies in Image-Guided Spine Surgery	218

Index 224

Contributors

John R. Adler, Jr., M.D.
Professor of Neurosurgery
Department of Neurosurgery
Stanford University School of Medicine
Stanford, California

Gene H. Barnett, M.D.
Department of Neurosurgery
Cleveland Clinic Foundation
Cleveland, Ohio

Christopher J. Barry, M.D.
Resident
Department of Neurosurgery
The University of Iowa Hospitals and Clinics
Iowa City, Iowa

Joshua B. Bederson, M.D.
Professor and Vice Chairman
Department of Neurosurgery
Mount Sinai School of Medicine
New York, New York

Alim-Louis Benabid, M.D.
Department of Clinical
  and Biological Neurosciences
Joseph Fourier University of Grenoble
Hopital A. Michallon
Grenoble, France

Mitchel S. Berger, M.D.
Professor and Chairman
Department of Neurosurgery
University of California at San Francisco
San Francisco, California

William E. Bingaman, Jr., M.D.
Head–Section of Epilepsy Surgery
Cleveland Clinic Foundation
Cleveland, Ohio

Richard Bucholz, M.D.
Professor of Neurosurgery
Division of Neurosurgery
Saint Louis University School of Medicine
Saint Louis, Missouri

Steven D. Chang, M.D.
Assistant Professor of Neurosurgery
Department of Neurosurgery
Stanford University School of Medicine
Stanford, California

Gordon Dandie, M.D., B.S., F.R.A.C.S.
Division of Neurosurgery
Toronto Western Hospital
Toronto, Ontario
Canada

David Dean, Ph. D.
Assistant Professor of Neurosurgery
Case Western Reserve University
University Hospitals of Cleveland
Cleveland, Ohio

Harel Deutsch, M.D.
Neurosurgery Resident
Department of Neurosurgery
Mount Sinai School of Medicine
New York, New York

Rudolf Fahlbusch, M.D.
Professor and Chairman
Department of Neurosurgery
University Erlangen-Nuremberg
Erlangen, Germany

Michael G. Fehlings, M.D., Ph.D., F.R.C.S.C.
Professor of Neurosurgery
Division of Neurosurgery
Toronto Western Hospital
Toronto, Ontario
Canada

Kevin T. Foley, M.D.
Associate Professor of Neurosurgery
Department of Neurosurgery
University of Tennessee, Memphis
Memphis, Tennessee

Oliver Ganslandt, M.D.
Department of Neurosurgery
University Erlangen-Nuremberg
Erlangen, Germany

Isabelle M. Germano, M.D., F.A.C.S.
Associate Professor of Neurosurgery and Neurology
Department of Neurosurgery
Mount Sinai School of Medicine
New York, New York

Iris C. Gibbs, M.D.
Assistant Professor of Radiation Oncology
Department of Radiation Oncology
Stanford University Hospital
Stanford, California

Philip L. Gildenberg, M.D., Ph.D.
Clinical Professor
Departments of Neurosurgery
 and Radiation Oncology
Baylor Medical College
Houston, Texas

Elad J. Hadar, M.D.
Assistant Professor
Head, Section of Epilepsy Surgery
Division of Neurosurgery
University of North Carolina
Chapel Hill, North Carolina

Peter Heilbrun, M.D.
Professor of Neurosurgery
Department of Neurosurgery
Stanford University
Stanford, California

Charles Joseph Hodge, Jr., M.D.
Department of Neurosurgery
SUNY Health Science Center at Syracuse
Syracuse, New York

J. Patrick Johnson, M.D.
Co-director
Cedars Sinai Institute for Spinal Disorders
Los Angeles, California

Iain H. Kalfas, M.D.
Head, Section of Spinal Surgery
Department of Neurosurgery
Cleveland Clinic Foundation
Cleveland, Ohio

Dean Karahalios
Assistant Professor of Neurosurgery
Department of Neurosurgery
Evanston Northwest Hospital
Evanston, Illinois

G. Evren Keles, M.D.
Assistant Professor of Neurosurgery
Department of Neurosurgery
University of California at San Francisco
San Francisco, California

Kee D. Kim, M.D.
Assistant Professor Neurosurgery
Department of Neurosurgery
University of California–Davis School of Medicine
Sacramento, California

Wesley A. King, M.D.
Associate Professor
Department of Neurosurgery
Mount Sinai School of Medicine
New York, New York

Seiji Kondo, M.D.
Assistant Professor of Neurosurgery
Department of Neurosurgery
Mount Sinai School of Medicine
New York, New York

Eric L. Lapresto, M.S.
Department of Neurosurgery
Cleveland Clinic Foundation
Cleveland, Ohio

Michael A. Lefkowitz, M.D.
Fellow
Department of Neurosurgery
University of Tennessee, Memphis
Memphis, Tennessee

Jae Y. Lim, M.D.
Sacred Heart Medical Center
Spokane, Washington

Robert J. Maciunas, M.D.
Professor of Neurosurgery
Department of Neurosurgery
Case Western Reserve University
University Hospitals of Cleveland
Cleveland, Ohio

David P. Martin, M.D.
Clinical Associate Professor of Neurosurgery
Department of Neurosurgery
Stanford University School of Medicine
Stanford, California

Christopher R. Mascott, M.D., F.R.C.S.
Professor of Neurosurgery
Paul-Sabatier University
CHU-Toulouse/Rangueil
Toulouse, France

Calvin R. Maurer, Jr., Ph. D.
Assistant Professor of Neurosurgery
Stanford University
Stanford, California

Kensaku Mori, Ph. D.
Associate Professor
Department of Computational Science
 and Engineering
Nagoya University
Nagoya, Aichi
Japan

Christopher Nimsky, M.D.
Assistant Professor of Neurosurgery
Department of Neurosurgery
University Erlangen-Nuremberg
Erlangen, Germany

Wieslaw L. Nowinski, D.Sc., Ph.D.
Director
Biomedical Imaging Lab
Kent Ridge Digital Labs
Singapore, Japan

Stephen L. Ondra, M.D.
Assistant Professor of Neurosurgery
Department of Neurosurgery
Northwestern University School of Medicine
Chicago, Illinois

Stephen M. Papadopulos, M.D.
Department of Neurosurgery
Barrow Neurosurgical Associates
Phoenix, Arizona

Naresh P. Patel, M.D.
Department of Neurosurgery
Mayo Clinic-Arizona
Scottsdale, Arizona

Torsten Rohlfing, Ph. D.
Postdoctoral Research Fellow
Department of Neurosurgery
Stanford University
Stanford, California

Daniel Rueckert, Ph.D.
Lecturer
Department of Computing
Imperial College
London, England

Timothy C. Ryken, M.D.
Assistant Professor of Neurosurgery
Department of Neurosurgery
The University of Iowa College of Medecine
Iowa City, Iowa

Amit Y. Schwartz, M.D.
Neurosurgery Resident
Department of Neurosurgery
Mount Sinai School of Medicine
New York, New York

Ramin Shahidi, Ph. D.
Assistant Professor
Department of Neurosurgery
Stanford University
Stanford, California

Adnan H. Siddiqui, M.D.
Neurosurgery Resident
Department of Neurosurgery
SUNY Health Science Center at Syracuse
Syracuse, New York

Lisa Tansey, M.D.
Image-Guidance Engineer
Department of Neurological Surgery
Case Western Reserve University
University Hospitals of Cleveland
Cleveland, Ohio

William D. Tobler, M.D.
Associate Professor of Neurosurgery
Department of Neurosurgery
The Christ Hospital
Cincinnati, Ohio

Vincent C. Traynelis, M.D.
Professor of Neurosurgery
Division of Neurosurgery
The University of Iowa Hospitals
    and Clinics
Iowa City, Iowa

Eiju Watanabe, M.D., Ph.D.
Department of Neurosurgery
Tokyo Metropolitan Police Hospital
Tokyo, Japan

Jay B. West, Ph. D.
Staff Scientist
Department of Engineering
CBYON, Inc.
Mountain View, California

Andrew S. Youkilis, M.D.
Neurosurgery Resident
Department of Neurosurgery
University of Michigan Medical Center
Ann Arbor, Michigan

Preface

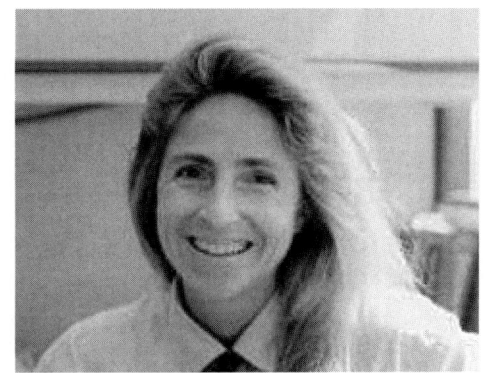

"Nel mezzo del cammin di nostra vita
entrai per una selva oscura
che la dritta via era smarrita"

"Midway upon the journey of our life
I found myself in a forest dark
For the straightforward pathway had been lost"

Dante Alighieri (1265–1351), Divina Commedia, Inferno, Canto I, I

The number of neurosurgeons practicing image-guided techniques is growing rapidly. Image-guided stereotactic neurosurgery has evolved into a discipline that every neurosurgeon should know as the concept of "minimally invasive surgery" is endorsed by most practicing surgeons.

Although image-guidance allows surgeons to maintain the *"straightforward pathway"*, there is increasing evidence that the use of this technique offers several other advantages. Image-guided brain and spine surgery can make neurosurgical procedures more efficient, minimize the size of the exposure and the invasiveness of the surgery, allow an approach through the least eloquent path, define resection boundaries that may not be apparent to the surgeon's eye, optimize placement of hardware in spinal surgery, and decrease the manipulation of nervous tissue outside the pathological process in both cranial and spinal cases. Thus, it is not surprising to envision image-guided neurosurgery being used by the majority of neurosurgeons and considered the "standard of care."

This book represents the fruit of the effort of several neurosurgeons that have significantly contributed to the evolution of the field of image-guided surgery. The intention of this text is to review the current state-of-the-art techniques of image-guided brain and spine surgery. The current and future applicability of the current available systems is reviewed. This book provides neurosurgeons with modern concepts and serves as an exceptional resource for basic, practical, and advanced information on this field. For the residents in training, this publication can supplement areas that might not be covered in depth in the training program.

This book is divided into three sections. The first section is an overview of the principles and technology of image-guided neurosurgery, including description of the instrumentation. Each chapter contains an individual perspective of a different technology used for image-guided neurosurgery. The second section contains seven chapters on different applications of image-guided cranial procedures. These chapters describe the use of the image-guided technology for intracranial procedures, such as cerebrovascular, tumor, epilepsy, and movement disorders. The authors of each chapter share with the reader their experience with this technology, outlining benefits and limitations. The third section describes, in six chapters, the clinical applications of image-guided technology for spine surgery. The reader will find that each chapter contains the best, current assessment of the covered topic.

I would like to express my deepest appreciation to each contributor for the work involved in compiling these chapters and for their willingness to share their experience with the reader.

Isabelle M. Germano, M.D., F.A.C.S.

Dedication

To all our patients who have benefited
or will benefit from image-guided neurosurgery.

Acknowledgment

The editor wishes to acknowledge Jennifer Fable for her valuable contribution to the preparation of this book.

PART I

Principles and Technology

1

Historical Perspective of the Components of Image-Guided Neurosurgery

RICHARD D. BUCHOLZ AND ISABELLE M. GERMANO

It is an essential aspect of neurosurgery that every cranial procedure must be conducted with the utmost precision. The brain, as opposed to any other organ in the body, is highly organized into structures that serve specific and irreplaceable functions. Collateral damage to these structures in the surgical pursuit of a deep target carries obligatory neurological deficits that are often permanent, and inexcusable. Further the external appearance of the brain gives little in the way of clues to the function subserved within, providing neurosurgeons with a formidable challenge to achieve intraoperative localization. The duration of training of every neurosurgeon is testimony to the challenge of achieving a sense of precise cranial navigation that is based in a firm comprehension of the three-dimensional (3-D) organization of the human brain. However even a perfect and encyclopedic knowledge of the normal functional anatomy of the brain is inadequate when confronted by the need to operate upon a brain altered either through normal variation or the presence of a disease process. Given the ability of the brain to compress, shift, and distort in the presence of disease it follows that neurosurgeons rely upon preoperative imaging more than any other surgical subspecialty in preparation for a procedure upon the brain to contort their concept of normal anatomy to match the distorted anatomy of the patient.

Neurosurgeons have been the beneficiaries of a rich variety of choices in the imaging of the brain. Computed tomography (CT), followed by magnetic resonance imaging (MRI), has most recently provided detailed 3-D images to guide cranial procedures. Even before the advent of these inherently three-dimensional techniques, neurosurgeons developed and were the first to use contrast techniques that improved the ability of two-dimensional radiographs to depict the position of the brain. Dandy's use of pneumoencephalography, and Muniz's development of cerebral angiography serve as testimony to the dependence of even veteran and experienced neurosurgeons to alter their well-developed visualization of the brain to match the actuality of a specific patient. In a very real sense neurosurgeons have always sought, and even striven, to be guided by images as they take on the challenges of operating on the brain. Indeed the apparent novelty of the concept of image guidance is a non sequitur, in that all surgery is image guided as surgeons operate guided by images of the surgical field formed on their retinas. It would therefore appear to be presumptuous to suggest that the history of image guidance is somehow distinct from the history of neurosurgery itself, as the two are essentially inseparable and likely synonymous. However, as recent developments in diagnostic imaging offer the potential of extending the vision of the surgeon far beyond the surface of the surgical field, the true power of image guidance will become increasingly apparent.

If a distinction can be made between the histories of image guidance and neurosurgery it can be found within the technology underlying image guidance, and the individuals who adapted said technology to fit the environment of an operating room. Given the challenges of neurosurgical procedures, it is to be expected that neurosurgeons, in addition to the ability to think in three dimensions, have strong personalities. Only individuals confident in their own abilities could enter the brain, address a problem within this most complex and least understood structure known in the universe, and tolerate horrific and disabling complications that would strip less confident individuals of any desire to take on such a challenge again. Given the confidence and self-reliance integral to their personalities it is common for many veteran neurosurgeons to dismiss intraoperative technological advances as being the unreliable infrastructure required by less confident, and perhaps less talented, surgeons to bolster their attempts to perform cranial surgery. Just as the microscope was seen as an unneeded operative toy when it was first employed intraoperatively, the proponents of image guidance and its predecessor stereotactic surgery were ostracized from the mainstream of neurosurgical history. This phenomenon was perhaps most notable in Europe, where entire departments of stereotactic surgery were founded outside existing departments within neurosurgery. Therefore, if image guidance has a history separate from that of neurosurgery, it is one created by the enmity of the majority of the neurosurgical community toward individuals who, rather than being uncertain of their surgical skills were beholden to the tremendous responsibility of operating on the seat of a patient's psyche.

The history of image guidance consists of the stories of individuals confident not only in their surgical capabilities but in their ability to apply technological advances to reliably assist in navigation through the brain. These individuals could see beyond the limitations of existing techniques and apply untested technology to remove these limitations. As a result, neurosurgical procedures became more complex as new techniques and instrumentation supplanted preexisting technology. This increased complexity of cranial procedures, albeit a drawback, diminishes the discomfort and complications of conventional surgery and therefore is justified by the improved outcome for patients. Indeed, the majority of neurosurgeons have adopted these techniques. Just as any contemporary neurosurgeon would reject replacement of modern and complex powered drills by the simple trephines of yesteryear, so will the neurosurgeon of the future refuse to operate without the presence of an operative computer. (As all recent advances of new imaging technologies are based on the use of computers, the computer has become a new instrument in the operating room. Thus, an alternative name for the field could be computer-assisted surgery, although this appellation stresses the means over the benefits of this technique.) As minimally invasive procedures are more broadly adopted, there will be less opportunity for conventional orientation during surgery and a greater reliance on guiding technology and its inherent complexity.

This chapter defines the processes unique to image guidance—periprocedural information acquisition, information registration, and intraprocedural tracking—and uses this structure to recount the history of their development and provide a brief indication of the probable future of each process.

■ Periprocedural Information Acquisition

The name *image-guided surgery* implies the coupling of some form of imaging to the surgical act and is the first essential component of such procedures. The history of image guidance is therefore inherently intertwined in the history of radiology as successive imaging advances underwent modifications to allow their use either prior to or during surgery. A history of radiology is beyond the scope of this chapter; but these modifications of imaging technology are central to the history of the topic.

It is important to note that the term *image-guided surgery* is at best a misnomer. Surgeons are not necessarily guided by images themselves, but rather by the information contained therein. Therefore, a more appropriate term for the field would be *information-guided therapy*, acknowledging not only the role of information but also the fact that many therapies that would benefit from such a coupling are not surgical in nature. Because these techniques can be used broadly with any invasive therapy that produces local effects with minimal collateral damage, newer forms of radiation therapy, such as particle beam therapy, can benefit by the use of identical visualization techniques. Further, the nature of the information employed can be quite diverse. The customary means of acquiring information is to subject the patient to a process that extracts the information from the anatomy of the patient. Usually the information extracted is organized in a 3-D virtual structure matched as precisely as possible to the anatomy of the patient, such as a CT or MRI scan. In other less demanding situations it is sufficient to employ two-dimensional information obtained by projecting the anatomy of the patient onto a single plane. In either situation, the resultant information can be categorized as an information data set, emphasizing the fact that the extraction process renders data that are an incomplete representation of the reality of the patient. The fidelity of the extraction process largely determines the utility of the resultant information to guide therapy. Given these considerations the term *information-guided therapy* will be used throughout the rest of this chapter to describe this field.

An important alternative to the extraction of data from the patient is to match the patient to a preexisting source of information obtained through the study of prior individuals. This preexisting repository of information is usually organized three-dimensionally and is termed an atlas. Atlas-based interventions suffer inaccuracy due to improper matching of the patient to the atlas or to inherent variability between individuals that diminishes the resolution of the atlas-based information. As our ability to extract information from patients improves, it can be anticipated that atlas-based interventions will be replaced; but in the early history of the field, atlases were the only source of information available. Because atlas-based interventions do not employ any data extraction from the patient, the history of the field actually predates the invention of imaging as we currently use the term.

The history of atlas-based interventions starts in 1889 with Dr. Zernov, a Russian surgeon who proposed the first device that superimposed a coordinate system on the patient's head for localization of brain structures.[1] It is of great interest that the information employed consisted of a phrenological atlas relating the contour of the patient's head to prior patients with known psychological conditions. Dr. Zernov hoped to employ this matching process to guide the production of lesions within the brain to resolve the psychological condition implied by this matching process. Although his confidence in the technology did not allow him to employ the device clinically, his use of contour matching was the first instance of a registration technique that is enjoying a resurgence of interest in contemporary systems. In 1873, another early investigator, Dr. Dittmar, created the first device designed to develop a stereotactic atlas.[2] He proposed investigating the function of the spinal cord in the rat by using his apparatus to insert a blade into the structure and recording the subsequent neurological deficit. Once again it was hoped that by matching the patient's anatomy to the resultant atlas, information about the deficit experienced by the patient could be obtained, with essentially no concept of imaging being employed in the process. Atlas-based technology reached its zenith after 1952 when Spiegel and Wycis published the first stereotactic brain atlas for operative use.[3] Subsequently numerous other stereotactic brain atlases have been produced since the early days of stereotactic neurosurgery. This topic is reviewed in Chapter 19 of this book.

As imaging techniques became available and progressively refined, neurosurgeons employed them to lessen the inherent inaccuracies of atlas-based interventions. All imaging technologies tend to be cumbersome and expensive in their first incarnations prior to advances that allow miniaturization. In early applications the act of imaging would therefore traditionally be employed in a suite that contained the necessary equipment, and surgery would be performed afterward in a setting less demanding in terms of capital outlay and more consistent with the demands of surgical asepsis. Hence a significant number of procedures employed information obtained preoperatively and were matched to the anatomy of the patient through a process of registration, which will be discussed subsequently. However, as the underlying assumption that the therapeutic process does not alter the anatomy of the patient is obviously untenable in the majority of cases, there will always be a need to perform information extraction during the delivery of therapy, as exemplified in the use of intraoperative MRI. Further, as an individual patient's outcome can itself be a source of information, postoperative information extraction, if carefully preserved and organized into a highly resolved data set, could be employed as an atlas for subsequent patients. The history of information guidance has been determined in part by the timing, and adoption, of imaging techniques to make them usable within the operating room.

Just as the timing of information extraction has evolved over the history of the field, the nature of the information extracted is also undergoing intense development. Given the difficulty in determining the position of specific functions within the brain, surgeons assumed function to be consistent between individuals and would therefore assume in the development of early systems that anatomy would precisely depict function. By tracking the deformation of anatomy, as depicted by structural imaging such as CT or MRI, it was assumed that function would be deformed in a lockstep fashion. Once again, atlases of function, assembled by experience with prior patients, were employed in these deformation attempts to depict the location of function within the patient. This assumption is rendered imprecise once again to the variability between patients, and to lack of specific knowledge as to how a particular deformation was produced. It would be expected that deformations caused by an intrinsic malignant glioma or a meningioma that appear structurally similar would have quite disparate effects on the eventual location of function, as one process consists of invasion of tissue, as opposed to pushing tissue away. Technologies currently becoming available that provide information about the location of function in a specific patient are now being employed to guide therapeutic interventions. Many of these technologies, such as magnetoencephalography, do not result in the production of images, emphasizing once again that information, and not imaging, is the key to new advances in the field.

Kelly was a true pioneer in the effort to use a variety of information sources during the performance of cranial surgery.[4] He was the first to describe the use of CT images, computer-generated stereotactic atlases, and, subsequently, MRI for tumor and functional procedures. Subsequently, Berger[5] and Zamorano et al[6] reported the use of intraoperative ultrasound and endoscopic images used in conjunction with frame-based stereotactic equipment.

■ Information Registration

The advent of digital scanning techniques has resulted in medical images of exquisite detail and has revolutionized the planning of neurosurgical operations. Although these images are compelling, it must be stressed that they are only representations, or pictures, of the relevant anatomy. Without a frame of reference by which one can register this image space to the physical space of the patient's anatomy, the use of such images to guide surgery employs their subjective interpretation by a clinically experienced neurosurgeon. Superimposing a frame of reference or coordinate system upon the preoperative images and using the same frame of reference during the therapeutic procedure can apply the full advantage of the fidelity of these sophisticated pictures to the real-time guidance of neurosurgical procedures. The use of a coordinate system during information extraction and therapy delivery is the second essential component of information-guided therapy.

Given the distortion and time constraints of early imaging technologies it was key to establish a rigid coordinate system that could mechanically survive both the imaging and the surgical process. The construction of most stereotactic frames is based on a system of rectilinear coordinates for determining a specific target point in the human brain. This coordinate system was devised by a French mathematician, René Descartes, in the seventeenth century and is known as the Cartesian coordinate system. Descartes stated and proved that any point in 3-D space can be defined by its relationship with three intersecting planes, designated as x, y, and z coordinates, that are oriented at 90 degree angles to each other. This superimposition of a Cartesian coordinate system onto human anatomy was first accomplished by the application of an external frame of reference to the patient's cranium and is known as "frame-based" stereotactic neurosurgery. In 1947, Spiegel and Wycis introduced the first stereotactic frame to be used clinically for humans.[7] In addition to the challenge of localizing intracerebral structures based on skull landmarks, calcified pineal gland, and ventriculography, the other problem facing neurosurgeons was the variability of the human brain.

Given advances in imaging technology as well as the availability of more powerful computer software and hardware, frame-based registration methods have been supplanted by less invasive "frameless" techniques. Conventional frame-based registration is perceived to be more accurate than frameless techniques by many surgeons and is therefore used by the vast majority of neurosurgeons performing procedures designed to restore function. These procedures can be categorized by their requirements for extreme accuracy because the therapeutic target is usually quite small. Most conventional neurosurgical procedures have relatively large targets and are well served by frameless technology that is less invasive for the patient. Given the lower risk and demands of other surgical subspecialties it can be contemplated that frameless registration techniques will be utilized by all of the nonneurosurgical surgical specialties.

■ Intraprocedural Tracking

The third essential component of information guidance is the technique by which the surgeon either visualizes the specific relation of information to the anatomy of the patient or is confined to a specific location within the patient. Either function can be accomplished by tracking the surgeon; that is, determining the exact location of the surgical instruments within the body of the patient employing a reference system that can be related to that of the information data set. As this need to track the movement of an operating surgeon is relatively unique to information-guided therapy, the history of these technical advances is unique to the field and not paralleled by the history of other medical fields.

As would be expected, early devices confined the surgeon to a specific surgical path rather than taking on the more complex task of locating a surgeon moving freely. In 1908, Horsley and Clarke introduced the first linear stereotactic apparatus for use in animal experimental surgery.[8] This mechanical device was used to introduce a lesion probe into the cerebellar nuclei of a monkey. Direct electrical current, producing electrolysis at the anode made the lesions.

Mussen, a Canadian surgeon, conceived the first stereotactic instrument designed for human use at the beginning of the twentieth century (Fig. 1–1).[9] However, he could never convince other neurosurgeons to use it clinically. Subsequent stereotactic systems place the target at the center of a semicircular arc, and the coordinates are entered by adjusting mechanical knobs attached to the frame on the patient's head. There are basically four types of stereotactic apparatuses that can be categorized by how the tool carrier (such as an electrode holder or guide tube) is mounted on the frame. These systems are called translational, arc, and burr hole systems. A fourth type, known as an interlocking arc system, was developed following the advent of CT. In a translational system the tool carrier is held vertically and moved by a translational stage system in two dimensions, with a microdriver employed to advance the electrode in the third dimension. Examples of this system include the original Spiegel–Wycis apparatus,[7] along with its six modifications, and the Talairach[10] system. In contrast, the arc system consists of an arc or polar coordinate system employing a tool carrier fitted to an arc in such a way that it always points to the center of the arc. Examples include the Leksell[11] system and the Todd–Wells apparatus.[12] Burr hole mounted systems consist of a fulcrum attached to a burr hole made in the skull, to which is fixed a tool carrier with angular adjustments to

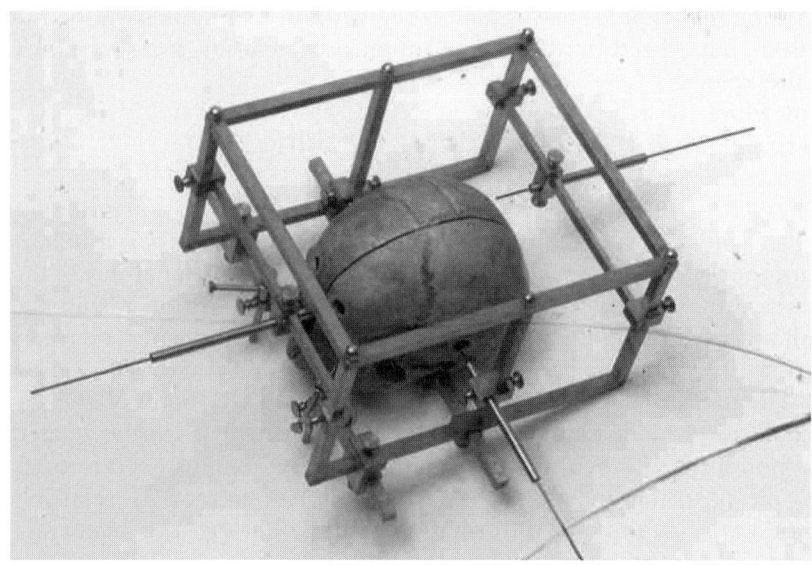

FIGURE 1–1. Dr. Mussen's stereotactic frame. (Courtesy of Dr. André Olivier, Montreal Neurological Institute, Montreal, Canada.)

point to the target and a microdrive to advance the tool. The interlocking arc system, such as the Brown–Roberts–Wells (BRW)[13] and Cosman–Robert–Wells (CRW)[14] frames, position the tool holder using multiple arcs. Due to the complexity of adjusting the individual arcs of these systems, a computer is necessary to define the coordinates of the target point and the adjustment necessary to reach the target.

The advantages of mechanically based stereotactic systems are their accuracy, simplicity of use, and stability. A distinct disadvantage of a rigid system is lack of flexibility. The more rigid the frame and the tool holder, and the greater the precision of the positional adjustments used in setting the device coordinates, the greater the accuracy of the device in positioning the tool. However, those very properties make changing the settings to move a tool holder to a second site difficult and tedious. Therefore a mechanical stereotactic system is optimally suited to confining a surgeon to a preselected path, but is very poor at determining where a surgeon's instrument is during freehand surgery. In addition, the hardware partially obscures the surgical field, and the determination of tools positioned intraoperatively usually requires a phantom pointing device and manual entry of coordinates into a computer system. These considerable limitations have relegated mechanical systems to use in functional procedures and needle biopsies of deeply seated small lesions.

To overcome some of the limitations of frame-based stereotaxy, in the 1980s several neurosurgeons investigated electronic alternatives to mechanical devices to determine intraoperative position while maintaining reasonable accuracy. All of these systems can be categorized as three-dimensional digitizers, devices that are capable of reading out position accurately in three dimensions using some sort of electromagnetic or resistive information. Because these devices were developed while improvements in CT and MRI scanning removed the need for framed imaging, they were called "frameless" stereotactic systems. Developments in this area followed two paths, one in which the virtual "eye" of the surgeon was tracked, such as systems that followed the movements of endoscopes or microscopes, and another in which the position of surgical instruments was related to the position of the body part undergoing surgery.

In 1986, Roberts et al replaced the mechanical localization of a microscope with a sonically based digitizer thereby fabricating the first freely adjustable "neuronavigational" device.[15] The digitizer embedded in their system consisted of sonic emitters mounted on an operating microscope with a detector array consisting of microphones mounted on the operating room walls. The location of sound emission was calculated by determining the time of flight of sound from the emitters to the detectors. By using a multiplicity of sound emitters the position and orientation of the microscope could be precisely determined and coupled to an image display system to guide intracranial procedures. Additional work using the operating microscope as a navigational tool stemmed from the work by Kwoh et al,[16] who described an alternative technique to position a microscope using a PUMA industrial robot (Westinghouse Electric, Pittsburgh, PA) for CT-directed framed-based stereotactic surgery. Drake et al published clinical results describing the use of this technology in 1991.[17] Although several advantages of using this technique were outlined in the paper, the bulk of the robotic arm was felt to be restrictive in the surgical setting. Subsequently, the Zeiss Corporation (Thornwood, NY) coupled a robotic arm within the surgical optic microscope, eliminating some of the drawbacks. In 1992, Heilbrun et al[18] described the use of the "machine vision" whereby cameras placed above the surgical field were able to determine the position of any object in the surgical work space, including surgical instruments. Finally, the use of a robot to improve conventional stereotactic neurosurgery by Young[19] in 1987 should be mentioned.

Within the area of neuronavigation using a digitizer, two different concepts were pursued: a digitizer using a mechanically linked arm and a digitizer using a nonmechanically linked device. The latter are based upon magnetic field detection or triangulation of sound or light. It is important to notice that advances in all of these areas gave birth to numerous sophisticated devices currently still used in neurosurgical practice and described in great detail throughout this book.

The first description of a "frameless," nonmicroscope-based tool for frameless neurosurgery was in 1987 by Watanabe.[20] He described the use of an intraoperative device other than the microscope for intracranial procedures. This device consisted of an articulated arm with six joints, a personal computer, and an image-display monitor. The position of the tip of the arm was determined by digitizing the angles at each of the arm joints. In 1992, Olivier and Germano[21] participated in the preclinical testing of the Viewing Wand System (ISG Technologies, Toronto, Ontario, Canada) subsequently used by numerous surgeons.[22] This system consists of a mechanical arm and utilizes custom-designed computer hardware and software for surgical planning and intraoperative localization. In 1992, Maciunas et al[23] reported on the use of high-resolution optical encoders for extreme accuracy of the mechanical arm. During the same period, Guthrie and Adler[24] reported on a series of localization arms with counterbalancing of the joints.

Although the use of an articulate arm was shown to add significant advantages to intraoperative localization, several neurosurgeons investigated devices that were not dependent upon a mechanically linked localizer. In particular, the use of digitizers based on magnetic field, sound, and light were explored. Magnetic field deflection was introduced by Kato and colleagues in 1991.[25] This was subsequently used by other neurosurgeons.[26] In 1993 Barnett et al[27] reported on the use of a sonic digitizing wand for intracranial procedures. In 1993 Bucholz et al[28,29] introduced the use of the optical digitizer. This technology uses light emitting diodes (LED) on surgical instruments and on fixed references constantly emitting infrared light that is being triangulated by linear-charged cameras arrays. After its creation at St. Louis University, Michigan, this technology was released for experimental clinical work and first used in the United States by Germano (Fig. 1–2).[30,31] Over the past 10 years, this methodology has been proven to have significant advantages as shown by the fact that most commercially available image-guided systems are currently based on LEDs.

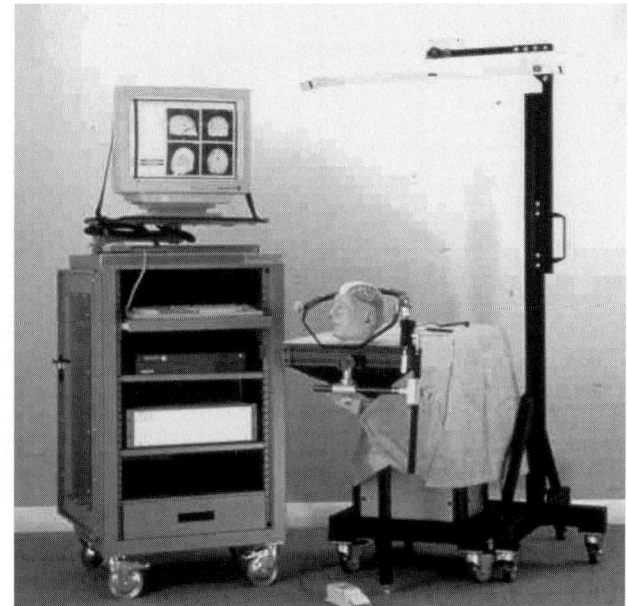

FIGURE 1–2. Early version of the optical digitizer station in 1993 (Stealth, Medtronic SNT, Louisville, CO).

In essence the field of image-guided neurosurgery had a phenomenal explosion of ideas and technologies in the past decade. At the present time, this armamentarium is no longer an experimental device, and it is considered standard of practice by most neurosurgeons.

■ The Future of Information-Guided Therapy

When writing about the past it is inevitable to speculate about the future. At the beginning of the twentieth century, technology was considered magic by most people, including physicians, as expressed by Dr. Arthur Clark: "Sufficiently advanced technology is indistinguishable from magic." Nowadays, however, the advances in technology are understandable to most neurosurgeons and not confused with magic. Industry, engineers, and surgeons are working together to elevate the standard of current care. The use of computers, micro-engineering, and molecular biology technology most likely will lead the continued development of image-guided neurosurgery in the next decade.

Computers are currently used as a widespread means of communication. In particular the Internet is and will be used in more ways and by more individuals. It is not inconceivable to think that neurosurgeons could share intraoperative information in real time and "consult" with each other during surgery by computer. At the time

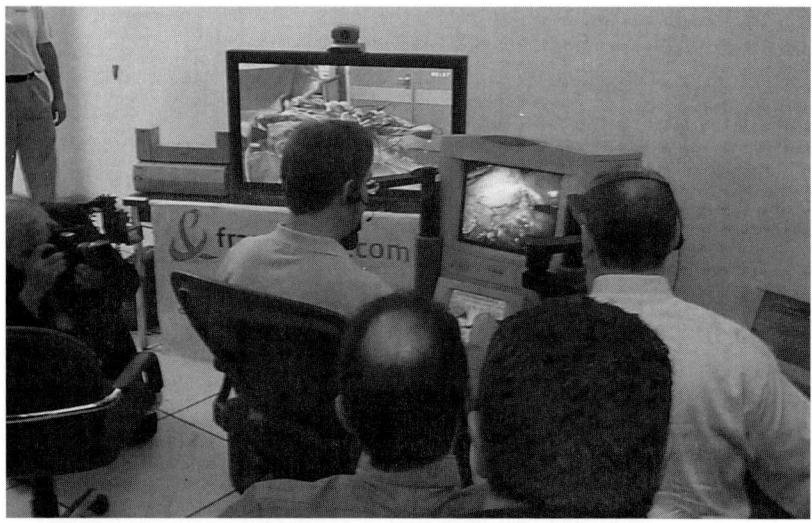

FIGURE 1–3. Transatlantic telesurgery performed by the laparoscopic surgeons at Mount Sinai Medical Center in New York on a patient in Strasbourg, France. (Courtesy of Dr. Michele Gagner, Mount Sinai Medical Center, New York, New York.)

of preparation of this chapter telesurgery is being performed. At Mount Sinai Medical Center in New York, a 68-year-old patient underwent gallbladder surgery in Strasbourg, France, by a team of laparoscopic surgeons in Manhattan, New York. The surgeons used specialized equipment to manipulate a robot by transoceanic fiberoptic cables and watched the procedure on a video monitor (Fig. 1–3). During the procedure, a local surgeon who was in attendance and could intervene if necessary closely monitored the patient. The surgery was completed in less than 1 hour, and the patient was discharged from the hospital 2 days later.

The fields of engineering, optics, biomaterials, artificial vision, and miniaturization will contribute to the conceptualization and realization of flexible robots capable of driving themselves through delicate structures. These robotic devices will be focused on overcoming the limitations of human dexterity during surgery.

Advances in molecular biology of the brain allow the understanding of various physiological and pathological processes. Using this new knowledge, neurosurgeons can combine the technological aspects of image guidance with prevention or early intervention of degenerative diseases such as Parkinson's disease, or pathologies such as ischemia and brain tumors.

REFERENCES

1. Zernov DN. Encephalometer: a device for determination of the location of brain parts of living humans. In proceedings of the Society of Physicomedicine: Moscow. 1889;2:70–86.
2. Dittmar C. Ueber die Lange des sogennanten Gefaesszentrums in der Medulla oblongata. *Ber Saechs Ges Wiss Leipzig (math Phys)* Moscow: Society of Psychomedicine 1889;25:449–469.
3. Spiegel EA, Wycis HT. *Stereoencephalotomy, Part I: Methods and Stereotactic Atlas of the Human Brain*. New York: Grune & Stratton; 1952.
4. Kelly PJ. Computer-assisted stereotaxis: new approaches for the management of intracranial intra-axial tumors. *Neurology* 1986;36:535–541.
5. Berger MS. Ultrasound-guided stereotactic biopsy using a new apparatus. *J Neurosurg* 1986;65:550–554.
6. Zamorano L, Nolte L, Kadi M, Jiang Z. Modification of stereotactic frame guidance arcs using optical encoder verniers. In: Maciunas RJ, ed. *Interactive Image-Guided Neurosurgery*. Park Ridge, IL: American Association of Neurological Surgeons; 1993:97–103.
7. Spiegel EA, Wycis HT, Marks M, et al. Stereotaxic apparatus for operations on the human brain. *Science* 1947;106:349–359.
8. Horsley V, Clarke RH. The structure and function of the cerebellum examined by a new method. *Brain* 1908;31:45–124.
9. Picard C, Olivier A, Bertrand G. The first human stereotactic apparatus: the contribution of Aubrey Mussen to the field of stereotaxis. *J Neurosurg* 1983;59:673–676.
10. Talairach J, David M, Toumoux P. *Atlas d'Anatomie Sterotaxique*. Paris: Masson; 1957.
11. Leksell LA. Stereotactic apparatus for intracerebral surgery. *Acta Chir Scand* 1949;99:229–233.
12. Todd EM. Sterotactic surgery of the basal ganglia. In: Codman, Shurtleff, eds. *Todd–Wells Manual of Stereotaxic Procedures*. Randolph, MA; 1967.
13. Brown RA. A computerized tomography-computer graphics approach to stereotactic localization. *J Neurosurg* 1979;50:715–720.
14. Friedman WA, Coffey RJ. Stereotactic surgical instrumentation. In: Heilbrun P, ed. *Stereotactic Neurosurgery*. Baltimore, MD: Williams and Wilkins; 1984:55–72.
15. Roberts DW, Strohbehn JW, Hatch JF, et al. A frameless stereotactic integration of computerized tomographic imaging and the operating microscope. *J Neurosurg* 1986;65:545–549.
16. Kwoh YS, Hou J, Jonckheere EA, et al. A robot with improved absolute positioning accuracy for CT guided stereotactic brain surgery. *IEEE Trans Biomed Eng* 1988;35:153–160.
17. Drake JM, Joy M, Goldenberg A, et al. Computer- and robot-assisted resection of thalamic astrocytomas in children. *Neurosurgery* 1991;29:27–33.
18. Heilbrun MP, McDonald P, Wiker C, et al. Stereotactic localization and guidance using a mashine vision technique. *Stereotact Funct Neurosurg* 1992;58:94–98.
19. Young RJ. Application of robotic stereotactic neurosurgery. *Neurol Res* 1987;9:123–128.
20. Watanabe E, Watanabe T, Manaka S, et al. Three-dimensional digitizer (neuronavigator): new equipment for CT-guided stereotaxic surgery. *Surg Neurol* 1987;27:543–547.
21. Olivier A, Germano IM, Cukiert A, Peters T. Frameless stereotaxy for surgery of the epilepsies: preliminary experience. *J Neurosurg* 1994;81:629–633.

22. Golfinos JG, Fitzpatrick BC, Smith LR, Spetzler RF. Clinical use of a frameless arm: results of 325 cases. *J Neurosurg* 1995;83:197–205.
23. Maciunas RJ, Galloway RL, Fitzpatrick JM, et al. A universal system for interactive image-guided neurosurgery. *Stereotact Funct Neurosurg* 1992;58:108–113.
24. Guthrie BL, Adler JR Jr. Computer-assisted pre-operative planning, interactive surgery, and frameless sterotaxy. *Clin Neurosurg* 1992;38:112–131.
25. Kato A, Yoshimine T, Hayakawa T, et al. A frameless, armless navigational system for computer assisted tomography. *J Neurosurg* 1991;74:845–849.
26. Mascott CR. The Compass Cygnus-PFS image-guided system. *Neurosurgery* 2000;46:235–238.
27. Barnett GH, Kormos DW, Steiner CP, et al. Frameless stereotaxy using a sonic digitizing wand: development and adaptation to the Picker Vistar medical imaging system. In: Maciunas RJ, ed. *Interactive Image-Guided Neurosurgery*. Park Ridge, IL: American Association of Neurological Surgeons; 1993:715–720.
28. Bucholz RD, Smith KR. A comparison of sonic digitizers versus light emitting diode-based localization. In: Maciunas RJ, ed. *Interactive Image-Guided Neurosurgery*. Park Ridge, IL: American Association of Neurological Surgeons; 1993:715–720.
29. Smith KR, Frank KJ, Bucholz RD. The Neurostation: a highly accurate, minimally invasive solution to frameless stereotactic neurosurgery. *Computerized Medical Imaging and Graphics* 1994;18:247–256.
30. Germano IM. The NeuroStation System for image-guided, frameless stereotaxy. *Neurosurg* 1995;37:348–349.
31. Germano IM, Villalobos H, Silvers A, Post KP. Clinical use of the optical digitizer. *Neurosurgery* 1999;45:261–270.

2

Sources of Error in Image Registration for Cranial Image-Guided Neurosurgery

CALVIN R. MAURER JR., TORSTEN ROHLFING, DAVID DEAN,
JAY B. WEST, DANIEL RUECKERT, KENSAKU MORI, RAMIN SHAHIDI,
DAVID P. MARTIN, M. PETER HEILBRUN, AND ROBERT J. MACIUNAS

Registration is the process of computing a mapping between coordinates in one space and those in another, such that points in the two spaces that correspond to the same anatomical point are mapped to each other. Registration of multimodal images makes it possible to combine different types of structural information [e.g., x-ray computed tomography (CT) and magnetic resonance (MR) images] and functional information [e.g., positron emission tomography (PET) and single photon emission tomography (SPECT) images] for diagnosis and surgical planning. Registration of images acquired with the same modality at different times allows quantitative comparison of serial data for longitudinal monitoring of disease progression/regression and postoperative follow-up. Registration of preoperative images with the physical space occupied by the patient during surgery is a fundamental step in interactive, image-guided surgery (IGS) techniques. Surgical navigation systems use the image-to-physical registration (IPR) transformation to track in real time the changing position of a surgical probe on a display of the preoperative images. Stereotactic procedures use the transformation to direct a needle (stereotactic biopsy) or energy (stereotactic radiosurgery) to a surgical target (e.g., tumor) visible in the images.

Many methods have been used to register medical images. Image-guided stereotactic surgical procedures have been performed since the early 1970s using stereotactic frame systems. Such systems generally include a reference frame that provides rigid skull fixation using pins or screws and establishes a stereotactic coordinate system in physical space, a method for stereotactic image acquisition, and a system for mechanical direction of a probe or other surgical instrument to a defined intracranial point. Most current systems relate image space to the physical coordinate space established by the reference frame by attaching a localizing system consisting of N-shaped fiducials during image acquisition. Frames permit neurosurgeons to perform biopsies and to resect deep-seated and previously inaccessible lesions. Frame-based techniques, however, have several limitations. The frames are bulky and may interfere with the surgical exposure. Patients complain about the weight of the frame and the pain associated with its application. The surgeon is typically limited to target points on a linear trajectory. And, perhaps most importantly, frame-based stereotactic systems do not provide real-time feedback to the surgeon about anatomical structures encountered in the surgical field. To address these limitations, a number of frameless IGS systems have been developed over the last decade.

For most types of monomodality and multimodality image-to-image registration (IIR), research has demonstrated that the most effective and accurate algorithms are those based on intensities. Point-based and surface-based methods can also be used for these applications, but they require a greater degree of user interaction and typically exhibit lower accuracy than intensity-based methods. Techniques based on points and surfaces do, however, play an important role in IPR, which is important in IGS and radiosurgery because the internal information necessary for intensity-based registration is typically unavailable in physical space intraoperatively.

In this chapter, we make a few general comments about image registration, note how it is related to image fusion, and present several applications of IIR and IPR transformations. Then we discuss three sources of error in image registration—geometrical distortion in preoperative images, error inherent in the registration process, and intraoperative brain deformation. We limit our discussion to frameless image registration (i.e., point-based, surface-based, and intensity-based registration).

■ Registration, Fusion, and Surgical Navigation

As already described, registration is the determination of a one-to-one mapping or transformation between the coordinates in one space and those in another, such that points in the two spaces that correspond to the same anatomical point are mapped to each other. This concept is illustrated in Figure 2–1. The left picture shows the patient's head during surgery; the middle and right pictures show CT and MR image slices of the patient's head, respectively. The arrows represent the one-to-one mapping between the same anatomical point—in this case a point on the cortical surface in the left hemisphere—in physical space, CT, and MR. The simplest mappings are rigid-body transformations, which are transformations in which the distances between all pairs of points are preserved. A rigid-body transformation can be decomposed into a rotation and a translation. Most methods used to register head images compute a rigid-body transformation, which assumes that the head is approximately a rigid body, or a rigid-body plus anisotropic scaling transformation, which is used to correct for scaling error (image voxel dimension error).

To make the registration beneficial in terms of medical diagnosis or treatment, the transformation or mapping that the registration produces must be applied in a clinically meaningful way by a system that will typically include registration as a subsystem. For IIR, the larger system, which might be an IGS system, may combine the two registered images by producing a reformatted version of one image that can be combined or fused with the other. Image reformatting is the mapping of image intensities onto points in a space that has been rotated and/or translated relative to the space in which the image was originally acquired. A common example is the creation of sagittal and coronal image slices from an image volume that was acquired with transverse slices. Another example is the reformatting of an image after it has been registered to some target image such that each voxel in the reformatted image represents the same anatomical location as the corresponding voxel in the target image. Fusion of one image with another image to which it has been registered and reformatted may be accomplished, for example, by simply summing intensity values in the two images voxel by voxel, by superimposing outlines from one image on the other image, or by encoding one image in hue and the other in brightness in a color image. Regardless of the method employed, image fusion should be distinguished from image registration, which is a necessary first step before fusion can be performed successfully. Nonetheless, several manufacturers of IGS systems refer to image registration as image fusion. Alternatively, the larger system may use the registration simply to provide a pair of movable cursors on two views linked via the registering transformation so that the cursors are displayed at corresponding points.

Image registration and fusion is useful for combining complementary structural information (e.g., soft tissue

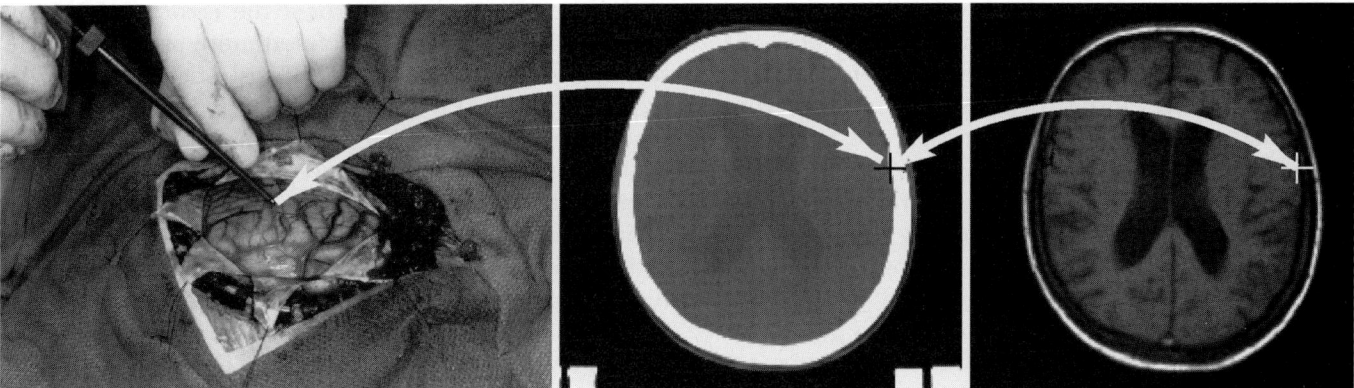

FIGURE 2–1. Concept of registration. Registration is the determination of a one-to-one mapping or transformation between the coordinates in one space and those in another, such that points in the two spaces that correspond to the same anatomical point are mapped to each other. The left picture shows the physical space occupied by the patient's head during surgery. The middle and right pictures show CT and MR image slices of the head, respectively. The arrows represent the one-to-one mapping between the same anatomical point—in this case a point on the cortical surface in the left hemisphere—in physical space, CT, and MR.

from MR with bone from CT). This is illustrated in Figure 2–2. Image fusion is also very useful for interpreting functional imaging and incorporating it into an IGS system for navigation.[1] When functional images such as PET, SPECT, functional MR (fMRI), and MR spectroscopy (MRS) are coupled with high-resolution anatomical images through image registration and fusion, the functional, metabolic, and biochemical properties can be linked to the anatomic structures in which they occur. Surgical navigation with an IGS system can then be employed to resect lesions on the basis not only of their structural abnormalities but also of their functional characteristics. Applications for structural–functional image fusion include the ability to differentiate between recurrent tumor and radiation necrosis, accurately identify a tumor's boundaries (particularly those surrounded by edema), and determine a particular pathology's relationship to eloquent cortex. The ability to identify eloquent cortex accurately is extremely beneficial, as these areas are often shifted greatly in the presence of a mass lesion. Registration of images acquired with the same modality at different times allows quantitative comparison of serial data for longitudinal monitoring of disease progression/regression and postoperative follow-up.

Surgical navigation systems use the IPR transformation to track in real time the changing position of a surgical probe on a display of the preoperative images, to direct a needle (biopsy) or energy (radiosurgery) to a surgical target located in the images, or to augment reality by superimposing information derived from the images (e.g., tumor contour) on the surgical scene viewed through a microscope[2] or head-mounted display.[3] Planning for a surgical procedure can be performed preoperatively with an IGS system. Intraoperatively, the surgeon can travel along the predetermined pathway to the desired target. Surgical navigation facilitates the use of smaller craniotomies for the complete resection of lesions. The location and size of the craniotomy can be determined exactly, and structures such as the frontal sinus, mastoid air cells, venous sinuses, and large draining veins can be avoided or at least anticipated. Once the bone flap is removed and the dura is opened, the IGS system can direct the surgeon to the area of the tumor, which may not be apparent from the overlying cortical surface. During cortical dissection to a tumor, vital vascular anatomy that is not necessarily grossly obvious can be identified and preserved. During gross total resection of a tumor, surgical navigation can demonstrate depth in relation to an instrument's position (i.e., anatomy deep to the area of dissection) so that vital vascular and neural structures can be avoided; display the actual extent of the tumor on the basis of its contrast enhancement or metabolic activity in three dimensions, which may not be appreciated when the tumor is infiltrating and grossly resembles normal brain parenchyma; and provide a frame of reference to help with intraoperative orientation during dissection. During resection of an arteriovenous malformation (AVM), surgical navigation using an MR angiography (MRA) image can help identify arterial feeding vessels.

Figure 2–3 illustrates two surgical navigation applications of the IPR transformation. The top row shows a sample screen from an IGS system in which the IPR transformation is used to display in real time the changing position and orientation of a tracked endoscope on triplanar reformatted preoperative CT image slices (bottom three panels), the endoscope video image (top right panel), and a synthetic (virtual) perspective rendering generated from the same viewpoint as the endoscope using the CT image (top left panel). By changing opacity values when generating the rendering, the physically visible surface can be made transparent and structures below the surface can be visualized. In this case, the synthetic rendering shows the optic nerve (arrows). The bottom row shows two images obtained at different orientations from an augmented reality (AR) system.[3] In the AR system, virtual objects, in this case a texture-mapped dot pattern representing the surface of a tumor segmented from an MR image and a cylinder representing an interactively manipulated biopsy needle, are overlaid on video images of the real-world scene viewed by the surgeon. Depth perception is provided by stereo disparity (each of these images is only one of a stereo pair seen by the surgeon in a head-mounted display), motion parallax, and perspective.

The application of a transformation produced by image registration for image fusion and surgical navigation is clinically useful only if coordinates in the two images or in the image and physical space that correspond to the same anatomical point are accurately mapped to each other. Registration error is the error of this mapping (registration error is defined more carefully in the section Error Inherent in the Registration Process). In Figure 2–3, the IPR transformation is used to correctly place internal anatomical objects onto the video images of the real-world scene. If there is error in the IPR transformation, the anatomical objects will appear in the wrong location. The rest of this chapter is concerned with three important sources of error in image registration: (1) geometrical distortion in preoperative images, (2) error inherent in the registration process, and (3) intraoperative brain deformation. There will always be some error. It is important for the surgeon to know the possible sources of registration error to minimize this error, to know the magnitude of registration errors typically obtained with different registration methods, and to better understand how IGS systems work and what some of their limitations are.

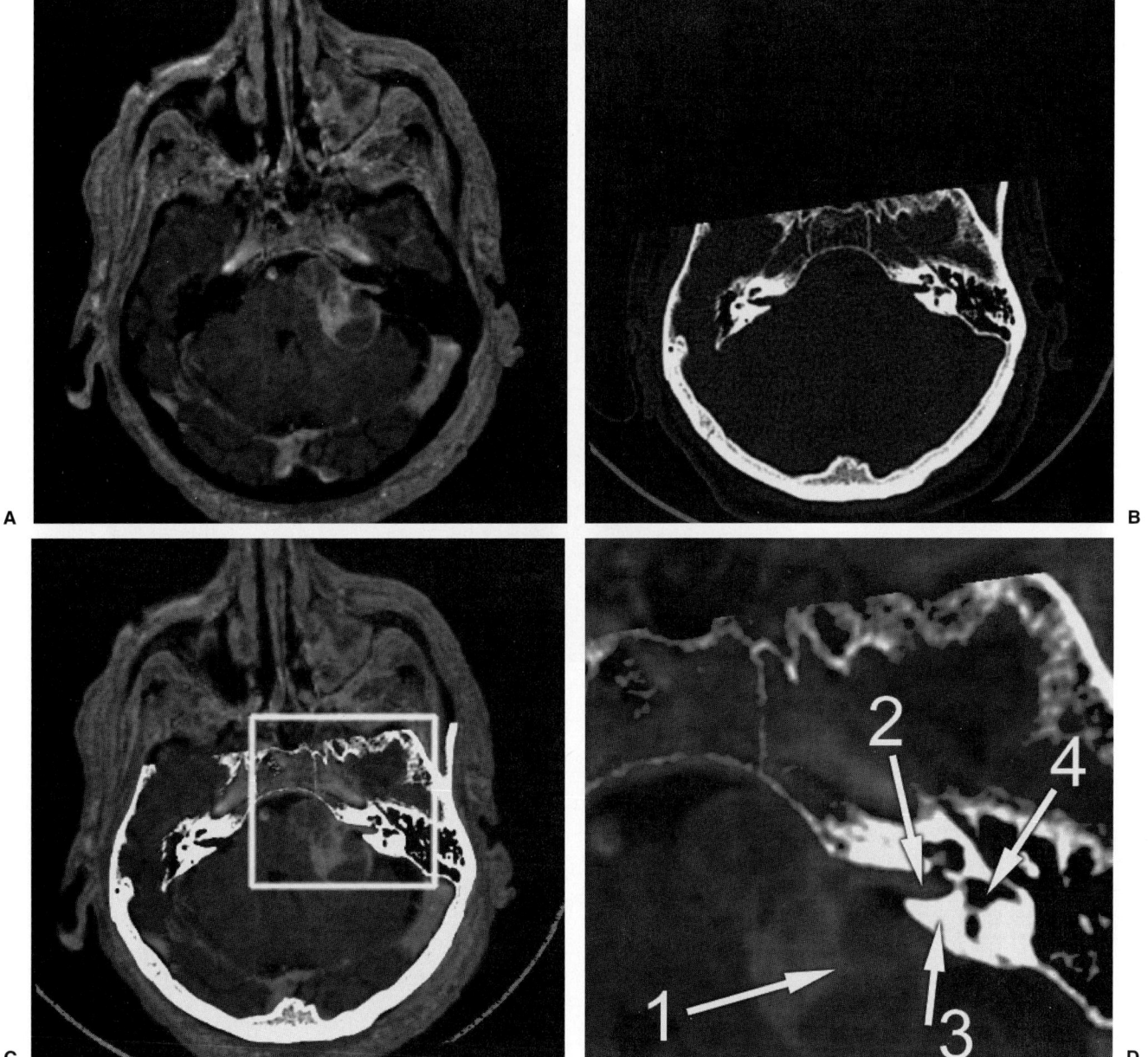

FIGURE 2–2. Example of image fusion. This is an application of the transformation determined by image-to-image registration (IIR). (A). A slice from an MR image (T_1-weighted gradient-echo sequence) of a patient with an acoustic neuroma. (B). A slice from a CT image from the same patient that has been registered (i.e., the transformation from CT to MR has been determined), and reformatted (i.e., a new slice has been interpolated from the original image such that each voxel in the reformatted CT slice represents the same anatomical location as the corresponding voxel in the MR slice). (C). A fusion of the MR and CT images. The bone was segmented from the reformatted CT image by thresholding and combined with (added to) the MR image. (D). A magnified image of the region inside the box highlighted in (C). Arrow 1 points to the tumor. Arrow 2 points to the acoustic nerve and tumor running through the auditory canal in the petrous bone. Arrow 3 points to the petrous bone. Arrow 4 points to one of the semicircular canals in the bone. The fused image is useful because it combines complementary image information—soft tissue from MR with bone from CT. (Adapted from Rohlfing T. *Multimodale Datenfusion fur die bildgesteurte Neurochirugie und Strahlentherapie* [Ph.D. thesis]. Berlin: Technical University Berlin; 2000.)

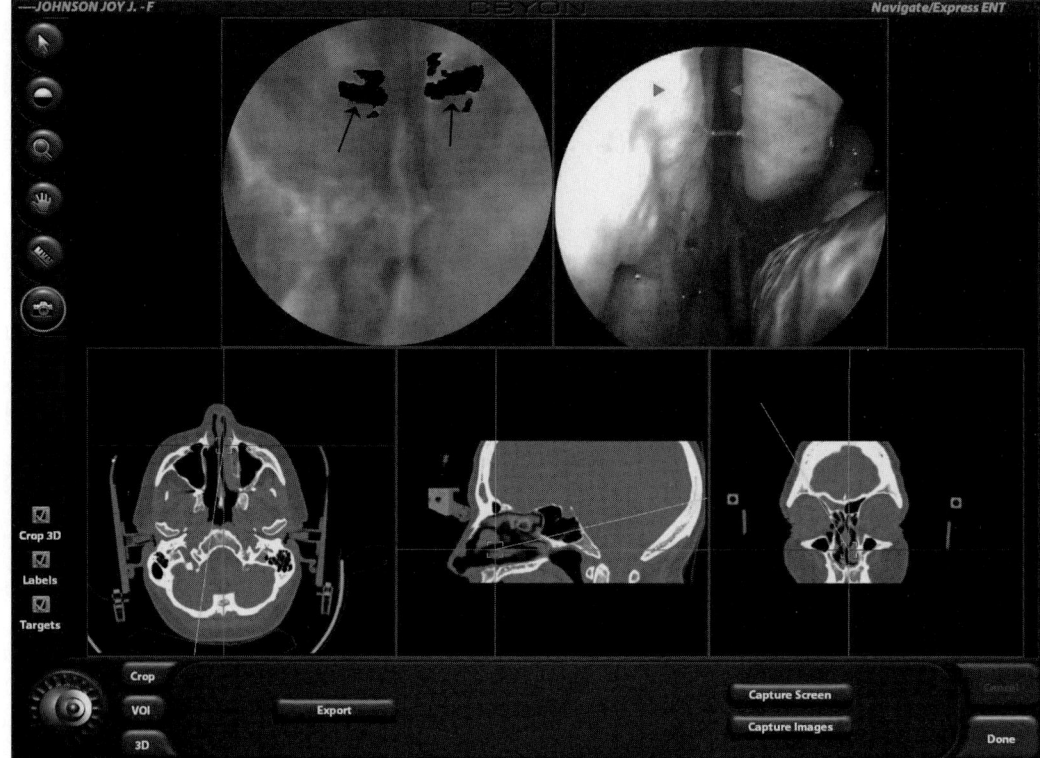
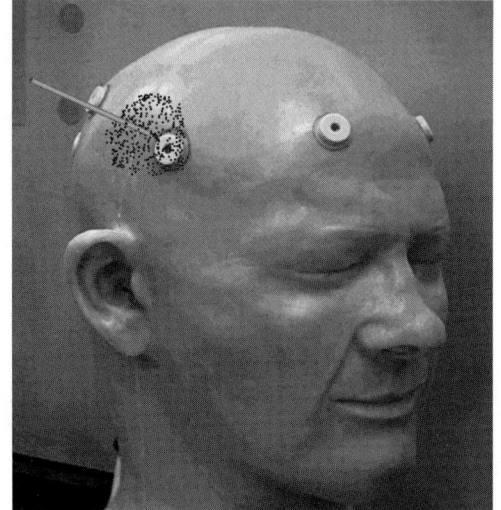
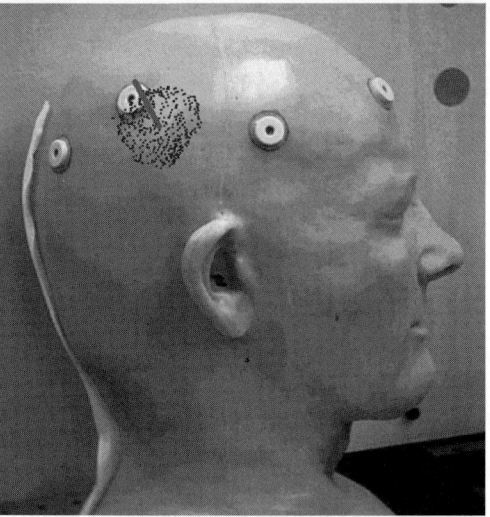

FIGURE 2–3. Applications of the transformation determined by image-to-physical registration (IPR). (A). A sample screen from a surgical navigation system in which the IPR transformation is used to display in real time the changing position and orientation of a tracked endoscope on triplanar reformatted preoperative CT image slices (bottom three panels), the endoscope video image (top right panel), and a synthetic (virtual) perspective rendering generated from the same viewpoint as the endoscope using the CT image (top left panel). By changing opacity values when generating the rendering, the physically visible surface can be made transparent and structures below the surface can be visualized. In this case, the synthetic rendering shows the optic nerve (arrows). (B,C). Two images obtained at different orientations from an augmented reality (AR) system.[3] In this AR system, virtual objects, in this case a texture-mapped dot pattern representing the surface of a tumor segmented from an MR image and a cylinder representing an interactively manipulated biopsy needle, are overlaid on video images of the real-world scene viewed by the surgeon. Depth perception is provided by stereo disparity (each of these images is only one of a stereo pair seen by the surgeon in a head-mounted display), motion parallax, and perspective. The IPR transformation is used to correctly place internal anatomical objects on the video images of the real-world scene.

Geometrical Distortion in Preoperative Images

The medical images we are interested in are three-dimensional (3-D) arrays of elements called voxels. Each voxel has an intensity value associated with it that represents the average value of some quantity. In CT, for example, the intensity represents the average x-ray attenuation coefficient over the region covered by the voxel. Spatial sampling (discretization) of the underlying continuous image constitutes a loss of information by partial volume averaging; structural information on the scale of the voxel dimension and smaller is lost. Point-based registration error is proportional to fiducial marker localization error, which decreases as the ratio of the fiducial marker size to voxel dimension increases. The effective total system accuracy, sometimes referred to as application accuracy, cannot be better than the voxel resolution.[a] Thus it is helpful to acquire images for IGS that have small voxel dimensions. Fortunately, current CT and MR scanners can easily produce images with voxel dimensions on the order of 1 mm or better in each direction.

Geometrical distortion in CT images

There are two common types of intensity artifacts in CT images. The first is streak artifacts, which are caused by the presence of electron-dense materials with such high x-ray absorption that the attenuation is outside of the dynamic range of the scanner. Thick bone such as the skull base, dental fillings, and the pins of some stereotactic frame systems often cause such artifacts. The other is beam hardening artifacts, which are a consequence of the fact that the x-ray beam is composed of a spectrum of photon energies. As the polychromatic x-ray beam transits through the patient and is increasingly attenuated, the lower energies are preferentially removed, causing an increase in the effective or average energy of the beam, thereby decreasing the calculated attenuation coefficient. These artifacts do not affect the geometrical fidelity of the image, but they can interfere with fiducial marker localization or surgical target identification.

The spatial fidelity of CT image slices is determined largely by the number, position, and operating characteristics of detecting sensors, and is, therefore, relatively constant between studies and independent of the specific patient imaged. Slice thickness is determined from the table positions corresponding to the image slices. Table position is accurately measured and recorded in current CT scanners. In our experience at several major university hospitals, quality assurance testing of CT scanners is very good and geometrical distortion in routinely acquired clinical CT image slices is very low. Nonetheless, we have on rare occasions observed problems with linear scale distortion (image voxel dimension error) or tilt angle error.[b]

A CT image volume is a stack of two-dimensional (2-D) image slices. If a CT image is acquired with the gantry tilted, and the image slices are simply stacked without accounting for the nonzero tilt angle, then the image volume will have a type of geometrical distortion called shear. If the tilt angle is known, it is straightforward to generate an image volume that is free of shear distortion. Most, if not all, current CT scanners produce image file formats that contain the gantry tilt angle in the image header. Unfortunately, many current IGS systems cannot account for a nonzero tilt angle in their software, and for such systems it is important to acquire a CT image without gantry tilt.

Because CT image volumes are stacks of sequentially acquired slices, any patient movement between slices distorts the image. In addition to the normal difficulties of keeping a person still, head movement can be caused by inertial jerking during each table advance in conventional CT image acquisition. Helical CT image acquisition involves continuous patient translation during x-ray source rotation and produces a complete image volume in a relatively short period of time. Some current CT scanners feature multiple detector arrays; multislice helical CT image acquisition is extremely fast. These scanner improvements reduce the risk of significant head movement during scanning and thus are quite useful for cranial IGS scan acquisition.

Geometrical distortion in magnetic resonance images

A detailed description of MR imaging is beyond the scope of this chapter; however, some fundamental understanding of spatial encoding is required to understand the source of geometrical distortion in MR images. Many excellent books and review articles exist for the interested reader (e.g., Haacke et al[5]).

The resonance of hydrogen protons placed in a magnetic field produces radio waves. The frequency of the

---

[a]It is possible with an image processing algorithm to determine the centroid of a fiducial marker in an image with subvoxel accuracy (e.g., Wang et al[4]). Such an algorithm can exploit knowledge about the marker (e.g., its shape and size). But it is generally not possible to manually identify a surgical target with accuracy better than the voxel dimension.

[b]The N-shaped fiducial localization systems typically used in stereotactic frame systems are immune to image voxel dimension error and tilt angle error. The development and success of point-based and surface-based frameless IGS systems is due in large part to substantial improvement in the geometrical fidelity of images produced by current scanners.

radio wave signal is proportional to the strength of the local magnetic field. The amplitude of the signal is proportional to the density of hydrogen protons. A large sample placed in a static and spatially homogeneous magnetic field produces a signal with only a single frequency. Images are created by encoding the spatial positions of the precessing hydrogen protons. This is accomplished by applying linear, orthogonal gradients on a static magnetic field. Because the resonant frequency is proportional to the strength of the local magnetic field, impressing a linear gradient on a static magnetic field will result in a proportional gradient of resonant frequencies.

Three different spatial encoding methods are used. The most important in terms of geometrical distortion is frequency encoding. A linear magnetic field gradient is applied while the MR signal is received. This gradient is commonly referred to as both the frequency-encoding gradient and the readout gradient. The spatial positions of precessing hydrogen protons are encoded by the frequencies of their emissions; the change in frequency is proportional to distance. The amplitudes (densities) and positions of the hydrogen protons in the object are decoded from the received signal using a Fourier transform.[5] Inhomogeneity in the static magnetic field causes an error in the frequency at that position and thus results in a spatial error in the frequency-encoding gradient direction. The magnitude of the geometrical distortion is proportional to the error in the static magnetic field: $\Delta x = \Delta B_0 / G_x$, where Δx is the spatial error in the frequency-encoding direction, ΔB_0 is the error in the static magnetic field, and G_x is the strength of the frequency-encoding gradient.

Phase encoding is another spatial encoding method. In this case, a linear magnetic field gradient is applied, but instead of being applied while the MR signal is received, it is applied momentarily just before the signal is received. MR signals are complex quantities (i.e., they possess both magnitude and phase). The briefly pulsed gradient alters the phase of the signal; the change in phase is proportional to distance. The densities and positions of the hydrogen protons in the object are determined by applying multiple pulses of gradually increasing amplitude and receiving a signal for each pulse.[5] Theoretically, there is no geometrical distortion due to static field inhomogeneity in the phase-encoding gradient direction. This is because the position of a hydrogen proton source depends on the difference in phase between pulsed phase-encoding gradients, which in turn depends on the difference in the strength of the magnetic field at that location. This change in the strength of the field is due only to the step increase in amplitude of the phase-encoding gradient and is independent of the strength of the static magnetic field at that location.

Spatial position in the third direction is achieved in two different ways. In the first way, a slice of interest is defined by applying a radio frequency (RF) excitation pulse while a slice-selection gradient is applied in the slice direction. The slice-selection linear magnetic field gradient defines a gradient in frequency that corresponds to a gradient in slice position. An RF pulse is applied with a range of frequencies that corresponds to the spatial range (position and thickness) of the image slice to be excited. An alternative method is to excite a thick slab (the size of the image volume) and encode position in the slice direction using phase encoding. In the first case, static field inhomogeneity causes a spatial error in the slice-selection gradient direction, and the magnitude of the geometrical distortion is: $\Delta z = \Delta B_0 / G_z$, where G_z is the strength of the slice-selection gradient. However, the strength of the slice-selection gradient is typically much higher than the strength of the frequency-encoding gradient, and geometrical distortion in the slice-selection gradient direction is generally less than 1 mm, unless there are very large static field inhomogeneities. Slice position phase encoding has the same absence of geometrical distortion due to static field inhomogeneity that in-plane phase encoding has.

Accurate spatial localization requires a static and spatially homogeneous magnetic field and linear, orthogonal gradients. Spatial inhomogeneity in the static field causes geometrical distortion in the frequency-encoding gradient direction. Current clinical MR scanners are designed and manufactured such that they have a very uniform static magnetic field when no object is present in the scanner. Static magnetic field inhomogeneities and gradient nonlinearities can be corrected, or at least minimized, by using shims and electronic compensation circuits.[6] The presence of an object in the scanner can cause static field inhomogeneity in several ways. Metal causes severe local warping of the static field, especially if the metal is ferromagnetic or has a ferrous component, as is the case with some types of stainless steel. Common sources of metal artifact in MR images of the head include dental fillings and appliances, implants (e.g., aneurysm clips), and shrapnel.[7] An area of zero or low signal is generally prominent near the metal, and is often surrounded by a region with visually obvious spatial distortion. The intensity distortion gradually returns to normal, and far from the metal the image may appear spatially accurate. Nonetheless, there can be subtle yet clinically significant geometrical distortion in areas of the image that appear normal. A stereotactic targeting error of approximately 20 mm has been reported in a patient with dental braces.[8] Severe geometrical distortion caused by a needle accidentally left in the scalp has been observed.[9] Spatial distortion due to static magnetic field inhomogeneity caused by a metal hairpin located in the magnet has been noted.[10]

Objects consisting of media with different magnetic susceptibilities induce perturbations in the static magnetic field. The object-induced static field inhomogeneity causes geometrical distortion in the frequency-encoding gradient direction.[11–12] Air and tissue have different magnetic susceptibilities, and the object-induced effect is strongest in regions near air–tissue interfaces. This includes the scalp and areas near air-filled cavities (e.g., the frontal sinus, ethmoidal air cells, sphenoid sinus, mastoid air cells, and nasopharynx). Object-induced static field inhomogeneity at the scalp surface can distort the image position of skin-affixed and bone-implanted[c] fiducial markers and the skin surface, and thus increase the error of point-based and surface-based registration methods that use this information. Figure 2–4 shows an example where the basilar artery is misregistered by approximately 3 mm because of geometrical distortion in the MR image. The cause of the registration error is probably object-induced geometrical distortion of both the fiducial points used to register the images and the position of the basilar artery. Since the magnitude of the distortion is inversely proportional to the frequency-encoding gradient strength, increasing the strength of the gradient will reduce the spatial error. The frequency-encoding gradient magnitude for this example was 1.5 mT/m. Many current MR image pulse sequences use a substantially higher gradient strength than that used for the image in Figure 2–4. Gradient-echo MR images are often acquired with frequency-encoding gradient magnitudes of approximately 5 mT/m; the object-induced geometrical distortion for such images would be approximately one-third of the distortion observed for the image in this figure. Spatial distortion due to magnetic susceptibility differences can also occur in the region surrounding a cavernous hemangioma because of hemosiderin deposits.[15]

Hydrogen protons in fat have slightly lower MR frequencies than protons in water molecules because of the influence of neighboring carbon atoms. Such differences in resonance frequencies are the basis for MRS, but in standard clinical MR images these differences cause spatial error in the frequency-encoding gradient direction that is analogous to the error caused by static field inhomogeneity. The spatial error of fat relative to water is often referred to as chemical shift. Because the distribution of fat is relatively homogeneous throughout the brain, chemical shift is generally not important in MR images of the brain (the chemical shift of subcutaneous fat is visually obvious, but is rarely, if ever, important for cranial neurosurgery). However, it is important not to use fiducial markers containing fat (e.g., vitamin E capsules) because the position of such markers will be shifted relative to the brain. When chemical shift is important, selective saturation or selective excitation MR imaging methods can be used to produce water-only (fat-suppressed) or fat-only images.

To minimize the problem of spatial distortion in the frequency-encoding direction due to static magnetic field inhomogeneity and chemical shift, there are several simple guidelines to follow when acquiring MR images for IGS:

1. *Use the highest frequency-encoding (readout) gradient strength possible.* Since the magnitude of geometrical distortion due to static field inhomogeneity is inversely proportional to the frequency-encoding gradient strength, increasing the strength of the gradient will reduce the spatial error. Using the smallest field of view and highest matrix dimension possible will help maximize the gradient strength. There is a trade-off between gradient strength and signal-to-noise ratio (SNR) (i.e., increasing the strength of the gradient will increase the image noise). Though the SNR in an MR image is generally a more important factor than spatial fidelity in diagnostic imaging, the opposite is true for therapeutic imaging, and it is sometimes acceptable to sacrifice some SNR to improve spatial fidelity.
2. *Consider using a volume gradient-echo pulse sequence.* Theoretically, no geometrical distortion due to static field inhomogeneity is expected in the phase-encoding gradient direction. Such sequences apply phase encoding in two directions.
3. *Use a global shim before each patient is scanned.* Global shimming will reduce static field inhomogeneity and thus geometrical distortion. Current MR scanners provide automatic global shim procedures that are fast and reliable.
4. *Avoid using fiducial markers containing fat or oil.*

Several methods for correcting geometrical distortion in the frequency-encoding gradient direction due to static field inhomogeneity are available. One general approach involves creating a map of the static field inhomogeneity. This can be accomplished by acquiring two gradient-echo images with slightly different echo times (TE) and calculating the phase difference between the two images.[16] The inhomogeneity map is used to compute the spatial error at each voxel and thereby undistort the image. This approach, which has been implemented at several institutions,[17–19] requires an additional image and special software that is not commercially available and thus is not widely used. A different approach requires two spin-echo images that are acquired with the identical imaging parameters, except that the frequency-encoding gradient is reversed.[14] A practical alternative to these correction methods is to acquire an MR image such as SPAMM (spatial modulation of magnetization).[20] This imaging method uses special pulse sequences to superimpose a grid on the image. Static field inhomogeneity distorts the grid lines, which, without distortion, are parallel and perpendicular to

---

[c]A bone-implanted marker typically has a base or post that is screwed into the outer table of the skull of the patient (see Fig. 2–5). An image marker, which is attached to the base during image acquisition, is located at or near the air–skin interface.

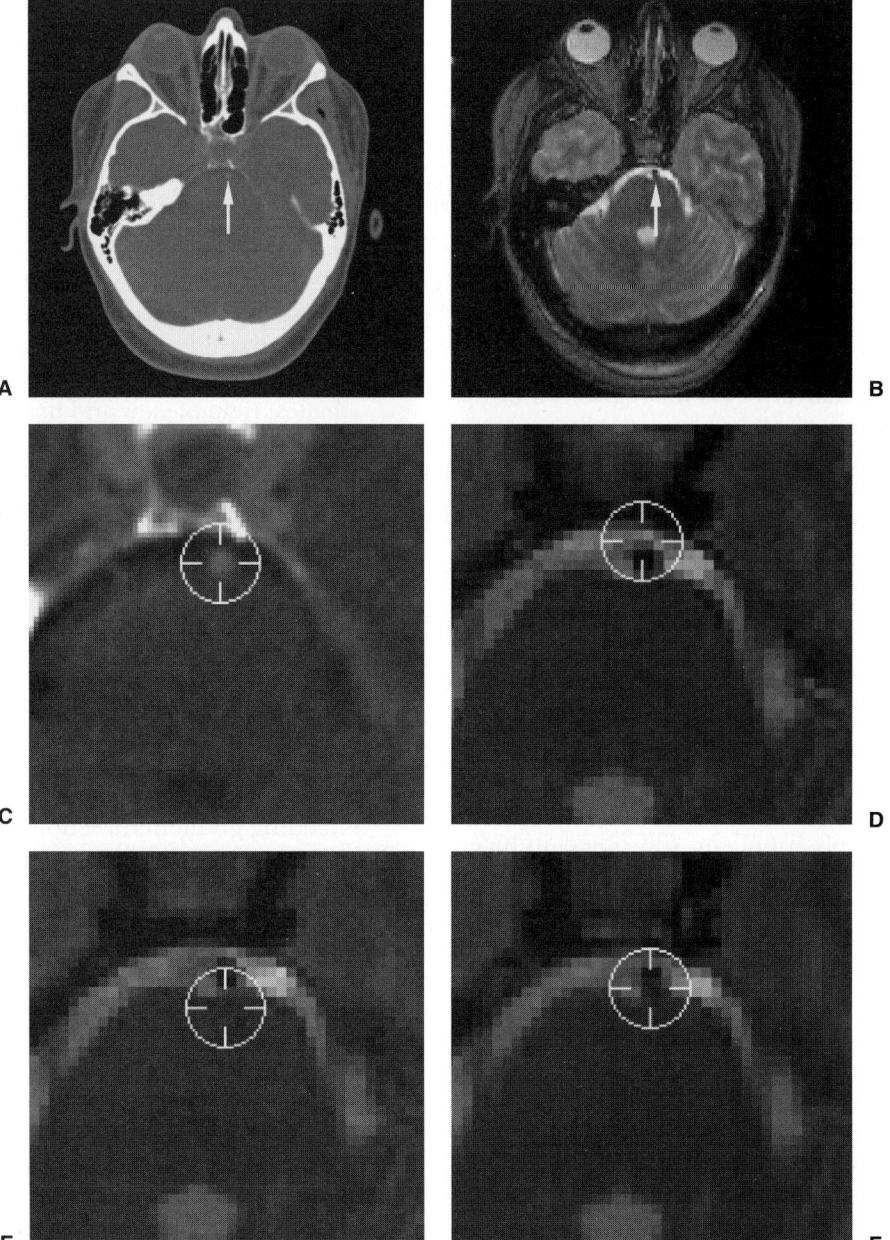

FIGURE 2–4. Example of the effect of geometrical distortion in MR on registration error. (A). Transverse CT and (B) MR image slices. The images were registered using five bone-implanted markers.[13] The arrows point at the basilar artery. (C–F). Enlargements of the region about the artery, which lies ventral to the pons. The position of the artery was manually identified in CT, where the artery appears slightly brighter than its surroundings. Periscope cursors were drawn at the user-identified position in CT (C) and at the corresponding positions (computed using the IIR transformation) in MR (D–F), where the artery appears darker than its surroundings. (D,E). A distorted pair of normally acquired MR images that were acquired with identical imaging parameters except that the frequency-encoding gradient (oriented in the anterior–posterior direction) was reversed. (F). A rectified image generated from (D) and (E) using the method in Chang and Fitzpatrick.[14] The cursor center is clearly anterior (D) or posterior (E) to the artery in the original (unrectified) images. It appears to be closer to the artery in the corrected image (F). The magnitude of TRE at the basilar artery due to geometrical distortion in the original (unrectified) MR images is approximately 3 mm. Geometrical distortion is substantial in this T_2-weighted spin-echo MR image primarily because the frequency-encoding gradient magnitude is relatively low (1.5 mT/m). (Modified from Maurer CR Jr, Aboutanos GB, Dawant BM, et al. Effect of geometrical distortion correction in MR on image registration accuracy. *J Comput Assist Tomogr* 1996;20:666–679. With permission.)

each other. Although this type of image can be used for correcting geometrical distortion, it can also be used to quickly visually assess whether substantial static field inhomogeneity and the associated spatial distortion is present in the therapeutic image.

Another type of geometrical distortion is scaling error (i.e., error in the image voxel dimensions), which results from error in the magnitudes of the linear gradients used for spatial encoding (miscalibration). This type of error is not uncommon and is extremely important when it occurs. The voxel dimensions of diagnostic images do not need to be known very accurately, and this may be why clinical MR scanners are sometimes poorly calibrated. In our experience with a variety of MR scanners at several institutions, scaling errors of 1 to 2% are not uncommon, and errors of 2 to 3% are not rare.[d] A scaling error leads to errors in the distances between points in the image. For example, if there is a 2% scaling error in an image with a 200 mm field of view, there is very little error in the distance between adjacent points, but an error of 4 mm between points at either side of the image. Scaling error is generally anisotropic (i.e., the scaling errors in the three dimensions are different from each other).

There are two major approaches for correcting scaling error in MR images. One obvious idea is to image a phantom (test object) of known shape and size.[22–24] It is important to use the identical scanning parameters for the patient and phantom images. This method is straightforward to implement, but it requires custom software and an extra phantom scan for each patient, and thus is not widely performed. Another approach, which is possible when both CT and MR images are acquired, is to register the MR image to the CT image and calculate the scaling factors as part of the registration procedure.[22] Typically, image volumes of the head are assumed to differ only by the position and orientation of the head in the scanner when the images were acquired, and thus algorithms that register head images frequently determine a six degree-of-freedom (DOF) rigid-body transformation that consists of three rotation and three translation parameters. In this approach, the registration algorithm determines a nine DOF transformation that consists of the six rigid-body transformation parameters plus three scale factors, one for each of the MR image axes. Several commercial IGS and radiosurgery planning systems implement this approach and calculate MR image scale factors, or equivalently, calculate correct voxel dimensions, as part of the MR-to-CT image registration process (though the fact that the system is doing this is often invisible to the user).

It is clear that MR images are useful for IGS and can provide accurate target localization. However, as discussed above, there are many causes of geometrical distortion in MR images, and it is prudent to use caution when performing IGS using only an MR image. Hardy and Barnett[8] recently stated, "At present, it is probably unwise to use conventional MR stereotaxy alone for stereotactic guidance unless the lesion is large (i.e., 2 cm or more); MR localization is used as an adjunct to conventional visuotactile definition of brain anatomy; or a means for detecting and/or correcting MR spatial distortion is part of the imaging protocol." For a variety of logistical and economic reasons, cranial IGS procedures at many institutions are commonly performed using only an MR image, and few sites perform distortion correction procedures. This is probably adequate for planning skin flaps and craniotomies, especially if the treatment MR image is acquired with a pulse sequence that minimizes geometrical distortion due to static field inhomogeneity. But for procedures that require high accuracy (e.g., stereotactic biopsy of lesions that are small or near critical structures, functional procedures, and radiosurgery), it may be helpful to acquire a static field inhomogeneity map or a screening MR image such as SPAMM for visual assessment of spatial distortion due to static field inhomogeneity, and to detect, and if necessary correct, scaling distortion in the treatment MR image either by scanning an appropriate test object or by obtaining a CT image of the patient and correcting scaling distortion as part of the MR-to-CT registration process.[e] Although some groups report that the use of appropriate MR scans can keep geometrical distortion below 1 mm,[25] the potential for clinically unacceptable distortion is sufficiently high to justify the time and effort necessary to obtain extra scans to detect and/or correct for spatial distortion in MR images for certain IGS procedures.

■ Error Inherent in the Registration Process

Point-based registration

Points are simple geometrical features that can be, and frequently have been, used for medical image registra-

---

[d]Several examples of clinically relevant scaling error have been reported: 1.0% in-plane and 1.9% axial mean error, with a maximum error in one patient of 3.7%,[21] a range of 0.4 to 1.7% in-plane and 1.3 to 3.0% axial error,[22] a maximum error of approximately 1%.[23] For eight patients who underwent stereotactic radiosurgery at the University of Rochester, scaling error determined using a nine DOF MR-to-CT image registration ranged from 0.6 to 1.9% in-plane and 0.9 to 2.4% axial error (unpublished data).

[e]Because software for correcting geometrical distortion due to static field inhomogeneity is not widely available, a practical alternative is to use available pulse sequences for screening and visual assessment. In this case, if substantial geometrical distortion is detected, the user will not be able to correct the distortion but will at least know that the MR image data cannot be fully trusted and will have an approximate estimate of the magnitude of the distortion.

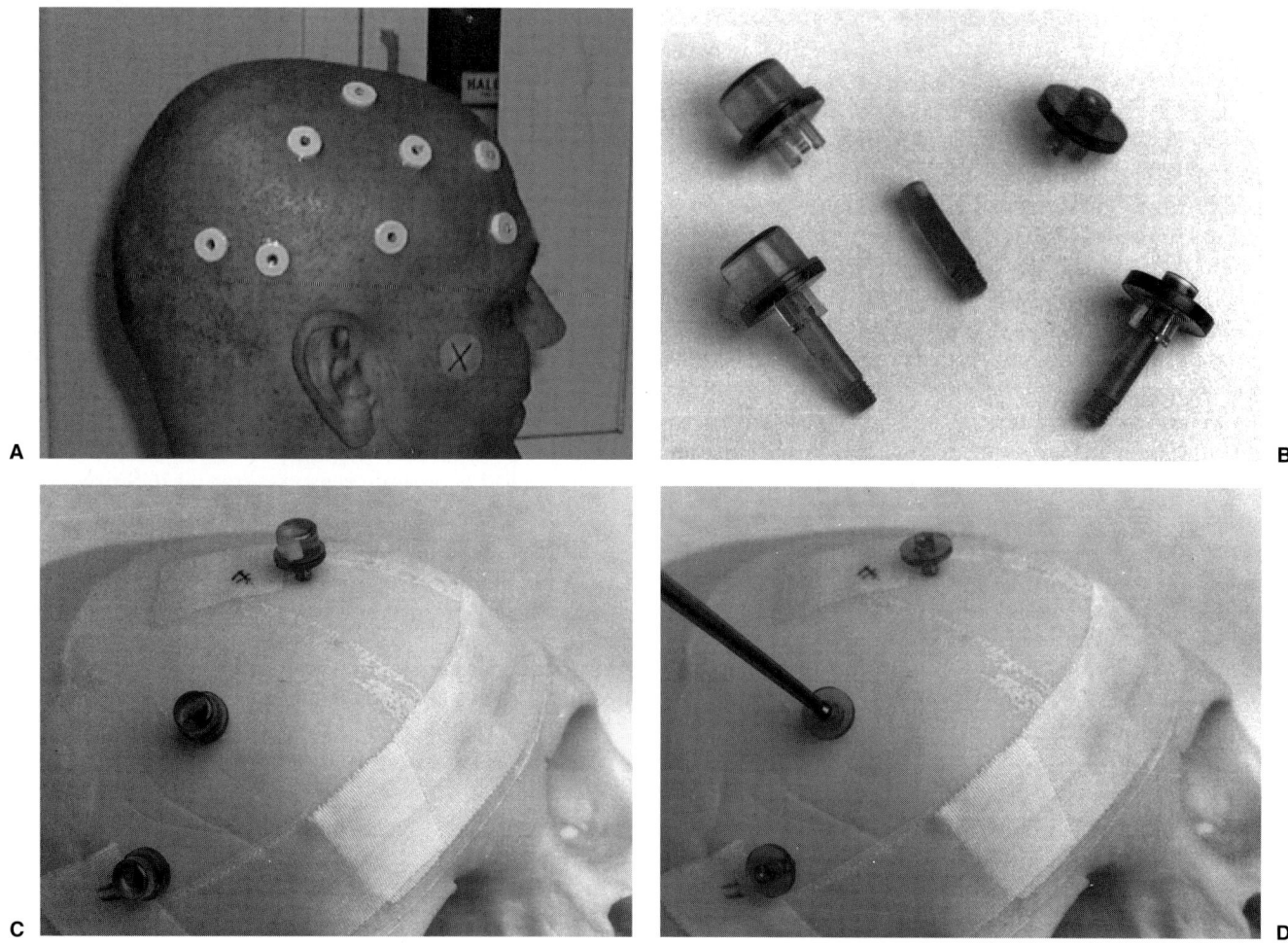

FIGURE 2–5. Fiducial markers. (A). Skin-affixed markers (multimodality radiographic markers, IZI Medical Products, Baltimore, MD) on a patient. (B–D). A bone-implanted marker system.[13] The image markers are constructed from hollow plastic cylinders that are filled with an aqueous solution of iothalamate meglumine and gadopentetate dimeglumine and sealed (B, left; C). The physical space markers (localization caps) are manufactured with a hemispherical divot whose position corresponds to the centroid of the image markers (B, right; D). The threaded ends of plastic marker bases or posts (B, center) are screwed into the outer table of the skull of the patient. (C). The image markers are attached to the bases during image acquisition. (D). The physical space markers are attached to the bases intraoperatively.

tion. Point-based registration involves determining the 3-D coordinates of corresponding points in two images (for IIR), or in an image and physical space (for IPR), and computing the transformation that best aligns these points. Because such points are taken to be reliable for the purpose of registration, they are often called fiducial points, or simply fiducials. A comprehensive introduction to point-based registration can be found in Fitzpatrick et al.[26]

Fiducials can be anatomical landmarks, skin-affixed markers, or bone-implanted markers (Fig. 2–5). Anatomical landmark localization is a manual, interactive process in which the fiducial points are defined in three dimensions. The landmarks must be visually identifiable in both spaces. For IIR, internal landmarks are generally used. Hill et al[27] suggest several possibilities, including a point anatomical structure (e.g., the apical turn of the cochlea); the intersection of two linear structures (e.g., a blood vessel bifurcation or confluence); a particular topographic feature on a surface structure (e.g., an identifiable part of a sulcus or gyrus); and the intersection of a linear structure with a surface structure (e.g., where a nerve passes through a foramen). For IPR, external landmarks are necessary (e.g., the nasion, the medial and lateral canthi, the tragus, and the tip of the nose). Alternatively, the fiducial may be a characteristic point within a fiducial marker that is attached to the patient (e.g., affixed to the skin or implanted in the cranium). For example, a common imaging fiducial marker is a hollow sphere or cylinder filled with contrast material, and the fiducial point for such a marker is generally defined as the centroid of the spherical or cylindrical cavity. Marker-based registration has two considerable advantages over landmark-based registration—the fiducial is independent of anatomy, and automatic algorithms for locating fiducial markers in images can take advantage of the marker's shape and size to accurately and robustly compute the fiducial point (e.g., Wang et al[4]). In our experience, manual localization of both anatomical landmarks and fiducial markers is easier and produces more accurate results when three orthogonal views, instead of one or two, are used simultaneously during the interactive visual identification process. A rendering is frequently provided for helping locate markers in the image, but manual localization is definitely more accurate when the position obtained using the rendering is refined using image slices. For localization of anatomical landmarks, intra-observer precision is always better than inter-observer precision.[28] An observer may have a clear idea of what to look for but is often not able to precisely communicate the localization procedure used (i.e., the cues that he or she is looking for) to another observer. Thus manual localization of anatomical landmarks typically produces more accurate registration results if the same person localizes the landmarks in both the image and the other image or physical space.

There are several error measures associated with point-based registration:

1. *Fiducial localization error* (FLE). This is the distance between the true position of a fiducial and its measured position (i.e., the error of localizing the fiducial point).
2. *Fiducial registration error* (FRE). This is the distance, after registration, between the measured position of the fiducial in one view and its measured position in the other view.
3. *Target registration error* (TRE). This is the distance, after registration, between the position of an anatomical location (e.g., a surgical target) in one view and the corresponding anatomical position in the other view.[13,29,30]

Figure 2–6 illustrates these errors. Of these three error measures, TRE is the most clinically relevant. For IIR, TRE indicates how well corresponding anatomical locations are aligned in registered images (e.g., in the fused image shown in Fig. 2–2). For IPR, TRE indicates how accurately the positions of tracked instruments are displayed on preoperative images (e.g., in the surgical navigation example shown in Fig. 2–3). Although FLE, FRE, and TRE are actually vector quantities, they are generally reported as scalar values that are the lengths of the vectors. The quantity FLE is almost always used to mean the statistical root-mean-square (rms) average of the localization error, which is the square root of its expected squared value (i.e., $\mathrm{rms}[\mathrm{FLE}] = \sqrt{\langle \mathrm{FLE}^2 \rangle}$, where the

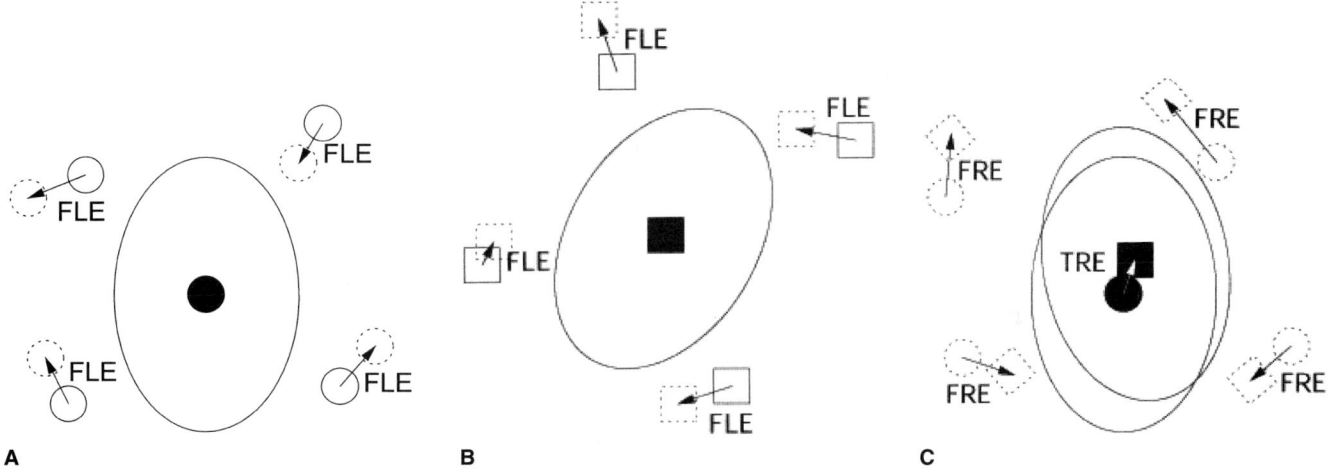

FIGURE 2–6. Illustration of point-based registration and the various types of errors. (A). One view (e.g., an image) of the head with four fiducial markers (solid circles) outside the head and one target (filled circle) inside the head. (B). A different view (e.g., another image or physical space) of the same head. For the second view, the fiducial markers are solid squares and the target is a filled square. The *fiducial localization error* (FLE) for each fiducial is the distance between the true position (center of solid circle or square) and the measured position (center of dashed circle or square) of the fiducial. Point-based registration is the determination of the transformation that best aligns the two sets of measured positions of the fiducials. (C). The *fiducial registration error* (FRE) for each fiducial is the distance, after registration, between the measured position of the fiducial in one view and its measured position in the other view. The *target registration error* (TRE) for the target is the distance, after registration, between the position of an anatomical location (e.g., a surgical target) in one view (center of filled circle) and the corresponding anatomical position in the other view (center of filled square).

brackets denote the expected value). The quantity FRE can refer to the registration error of an individual fiducial, in which case a subscript is often added. But FRE is almost always used to mean the rms average of the individual registration errors. The quantity TRE depends on the position of the target point. Generally TRE(**r**) is used to mean the registration error at a particular position **r**, and TRE is used to mean the registration error averaged over a set of target points or a volume of interest. Sometimes the subscript m is added (TRE$_m$) to denote that TRE was measured. The TRE using one registration method can be measured by using the transformation obtained using a different, and presumably more accurate, registration method as a reference gold standard.

Fiducial localization has error in both spaces. In physical space, the value of FLE depends on the tracking system and on the design of the fiducials. In an IGS system that uses optically tracked probes and instruments, the physical space FLE depends on several factors, including the type of optical position sensor and the number, configuration, and type [e.g., infrared light emitting diodes (IREDs), retroreflective spheres] of tracking fiducials.[31] In image space, factors that contribute to FLE include the shape and size of the fiducial marker, the voxel dimensions of the image (localization error decreases as the ratio of the fiducial size to voxel dimension increases[32,33]), the digital nature of the image (spatial and intensity quantization), the SNR of the image, the contrast of the fiducial relative to its background in the image, and geometrical distortion in the image. In theory, FLE adds in quadrature between the two spaces (i.e., the square of the "total FLE" of the system is approximately statistically equivalent to the sum of the squares of the FLE in each space).

There are statistical relationships among the expected values of FLE, FRE, TRE, the number of fiducials, and the shape of the fiducial configuration (see Appendix). The expected value of TRE is proportional to FLE. This means that the accuracy of the registration obtained when using fiducials (anatomical landmarks, skin-affixed markers, or bone-implanted markers) depends on the accuracy with which the fiducials are localized. It is thus very important to be careful when manually identifying fiducials in the image as well as when localizing the fiducials in physical space.

The statistically expected value of TRE depends on the shape of the fiducial configuration, but FRE does not. To illustrate some characteristics of the expected value of TRE, Figure 2–7 shows three different configurations of four fiducial markers, along with iso-TRE contours in midcoronal, midsagittal, and transverse image slices, for a patient with a lesion in the right orbitofrontal lobe. The iso-TRE contours were derived using Equation 2–2 in the Appendix by assuming rms[FLE] = 1.4 mm, for which rms[FRE] = 1.0 mm. This is representative of the situation when bone-implanted markers are used for cranial IGS.[f] The head image in this figure is a T_1-weighted gradient-echo MR image similar to those typically acquired for frameless cranial IGS. These images illustrate that TRE is smallest at the fiducial configuration centroid, that TRE increases as the distance of the target from the centroid increases, and that the iso-TRE contours are ellipsoidal.

Because TRE depends on the shape of the fiducial configuration, the configuration can affect the accuracy of navigation in IGS systems using fiducials to perform point-based IPR. The nature of the statistically expected value of TRE revealed by Equation 2–2 and illustrated in Figure 2–7 suggests several simple guidelines for fiducial marker placement:[30]

1. *Use as many markers as is feasible.* A minimum of three noncollinear fiducials is mathematically necessary to compute a 3-D image transformation. Additional markers improve the registration, which is clear given that TRE is inversely proportional to the square root of the number of fiducials. However, using more than 8 to 10 markers will provide little additional accuracy gain per extra marker.
2. *Place markers so that the centroid of their configuration is near the regions that are most critical during surgery.* TRE has its minimum value at the fiducial configuration centroid. Keeping the target close to the centroid minimizes d_k and thus minimizes the rotational component of TRE.
3. *Distribute the markers as far apart as is possible.* This helps maximize f_k and thus minimizes the rotational component of TRE. Markers placed in the field of the craniotomy itself will need to be removed during surgery, preventing re-registration in the event of a registration failure. Distributing the markers helps avoid placing them in the field of the craniotomy.
4. *Avoid linear, or almost linear, fiducial configurations.* If markers are placed in a near-collinear configuration, one of the principal axes will be oriented through the long axis of the configuration, the f_k value associated with that axis will be small, the ratio d_k/f_k will be large, and the rotational component of TRE will be large.
5. *Avoid placing markers on mobile areas of the scalp.* One of the assumptions in the TRE analysis is that localization error at each fiducial is identically distributed and uncorrelated. In the case of skin-affixed markers, deformation of the skin may cause correlated localization errors in the markers.

---

[f]When anatomical landmarks or skin-affixed markers are used for IPR in cranial IGS, FRE values between 1 and 3 mm are typical for 8 to 10 landmarks or markers. When bone-implanted markers are used, FRE values are generally 1 mm or less for three to five markers.

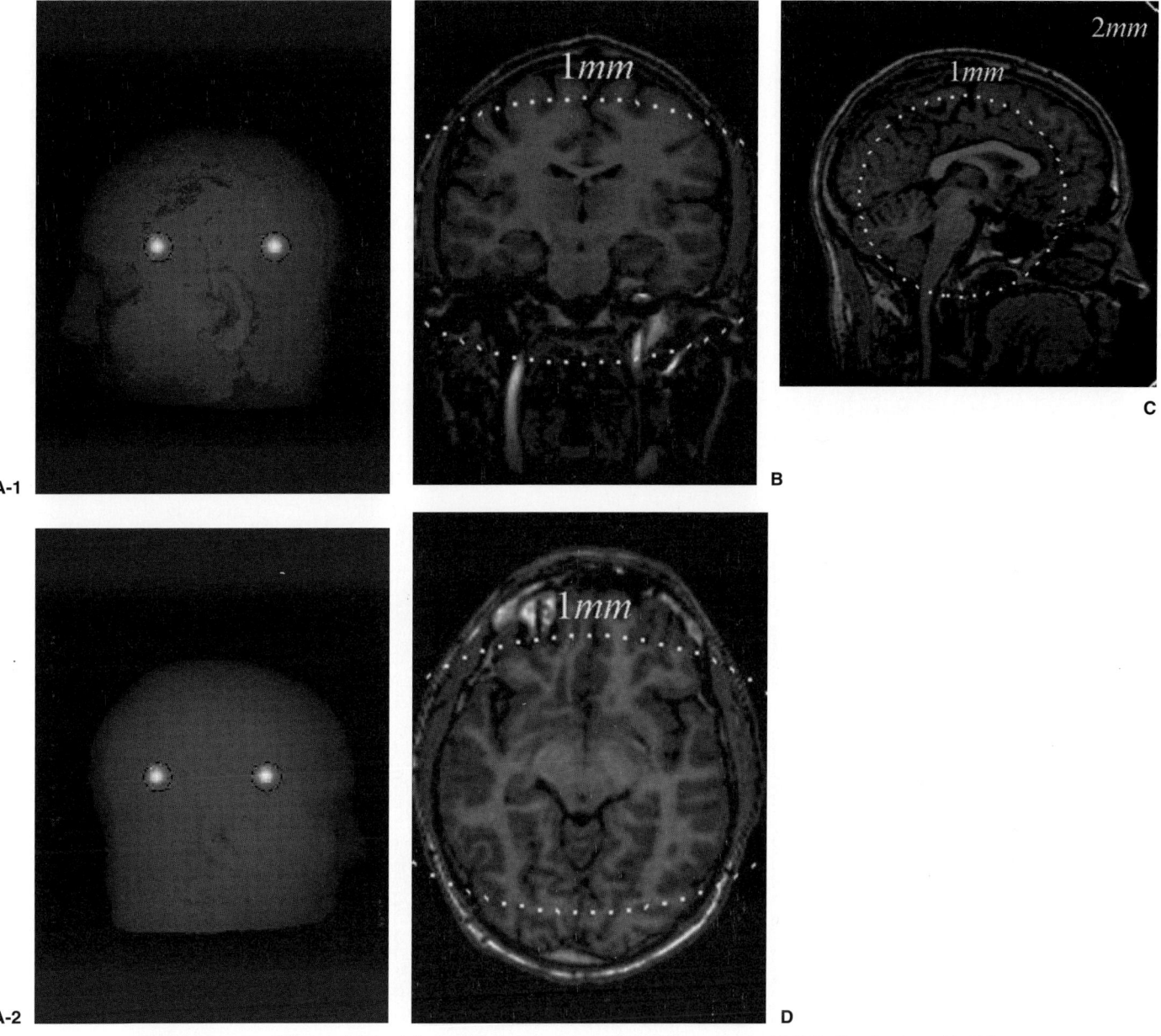

FIGURE 2–7. Effect of fiducial configuration on statistically expected TRE distribution. (A,E,I). Three different configurations of four fiducial markers. (B,F,J), (C,G,K), and (D,H,L). Iso-TRE contours (1, 2, 3, 4, 5, 10, and 20 mm) in midcoronal, midsagittal, and transverse image slices, respectively. These images illustrate that TRE is smallest at the fiducial configuration centroid, that TRE increases as the distance of the target from the centroid increases, and that the iso-TRE contours are ellipsoidal. The top row demonstrates that a widely separated fiducial configuration produces smaller TRE values than a clustered configuration. The middle row shows that a cluster of fiducials produces small TRE values only near the cluster. The bottom row illustrates the danger of using linear or near collinear fiducial configurations. The iso-TRE contours were generated for rms[FLE] = 1.4 mm, for which rms[FRE] = 1.0 mm. Missing contours indicate that TRE is above the value of the missing contour [e.g., in (G), contours for 1 and 2 mm are missing], which means that TRE values inside the 3 mm contour range between 2 and 3 mm. (Modified from West JB, Fitzpatrick JM, Toms SA, Maurer CR Jr, Maciunas RJ. Fiducial point placement and the accuracy of point-based, rigid-body registration. *Neurosurgery* 2001;48:810–817. With permission.) *(Continued on pages 24 and 25)*

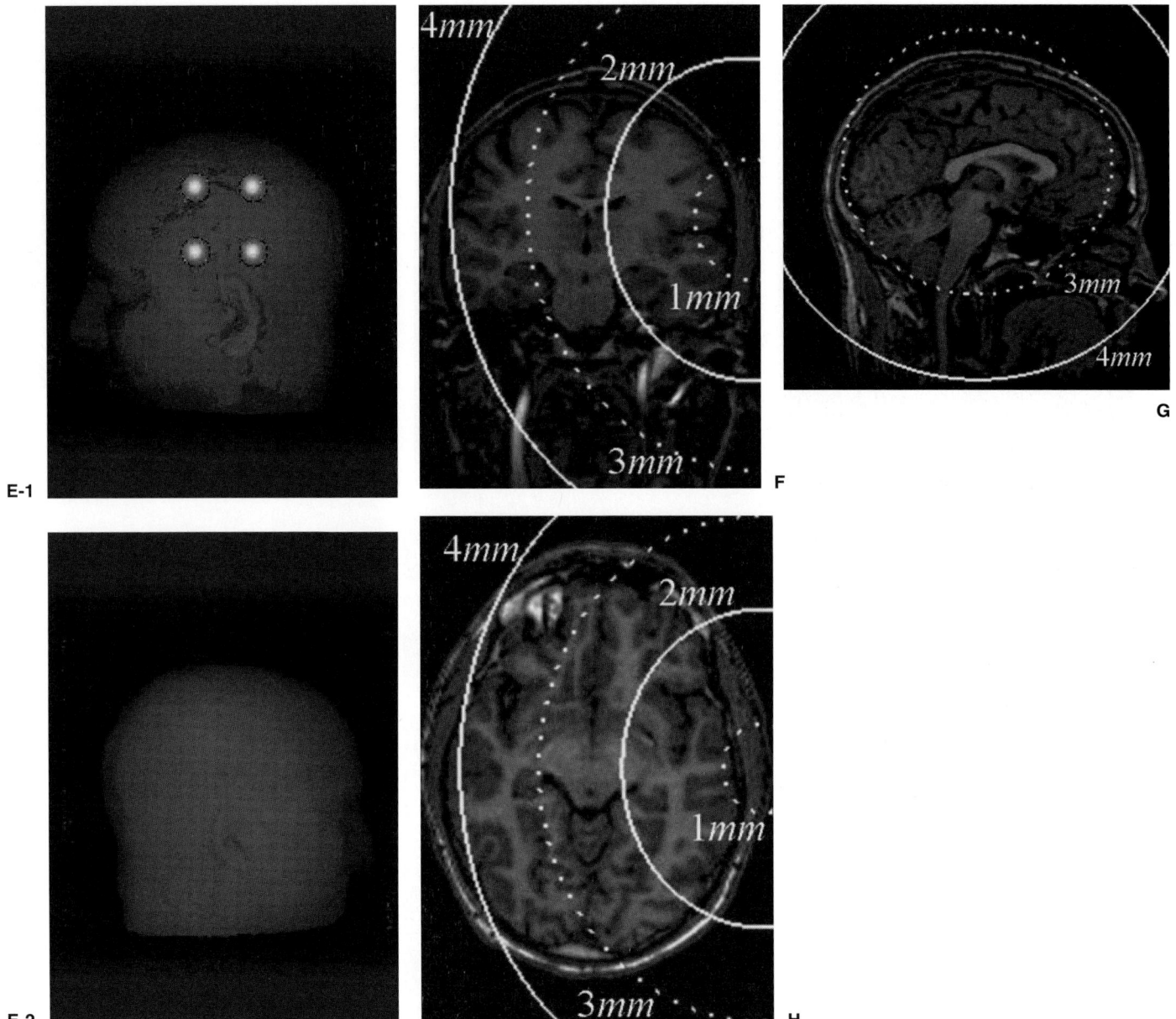

FIGURE 2–7. *Continued on page 25*

For cranial image-guided neurosurgery, Barnett[34] described a routine system of placing nine skin-affixed markers that adheres to these principles: "a pair just above the lateral aspect of the eyebrows, a pair on the lateral upper forehead, a pair on the asterions, one at the vertex, and a pair between the area just above the lateral aspect of the eyebrows and the vertex." This system produces a fiducial pattern for which the risk of marker displacement by head fixation devices and imaging headholders is minimized, and uses a sufficiently large number of markers so that there are still enough markers to obtain an accurate registration even if one or two of them cannot be used (e.g., if a marker falls off the skin because the adhesive does not stick, if a marker is not within the image field of view). An advantage of having a routine system of placement of a large number of markers (typically 8–10) widely distributed about the head is that a nurse or technician can easily apply the markers without regard to lesion location.

Of the three error measures discussed above, the most clinically relevant is TRE, but the only feedback currently available to the surgeon in most commercial IGS systems is FRE.[g] Because FRE is not dependent on the shape of the fiducial configuration, but TRE is, FRE is

---

[g]An even more serious problem is that some commercial IGS systems report an error measure, but the vendor does not explain what the measure is or how it is calculated.

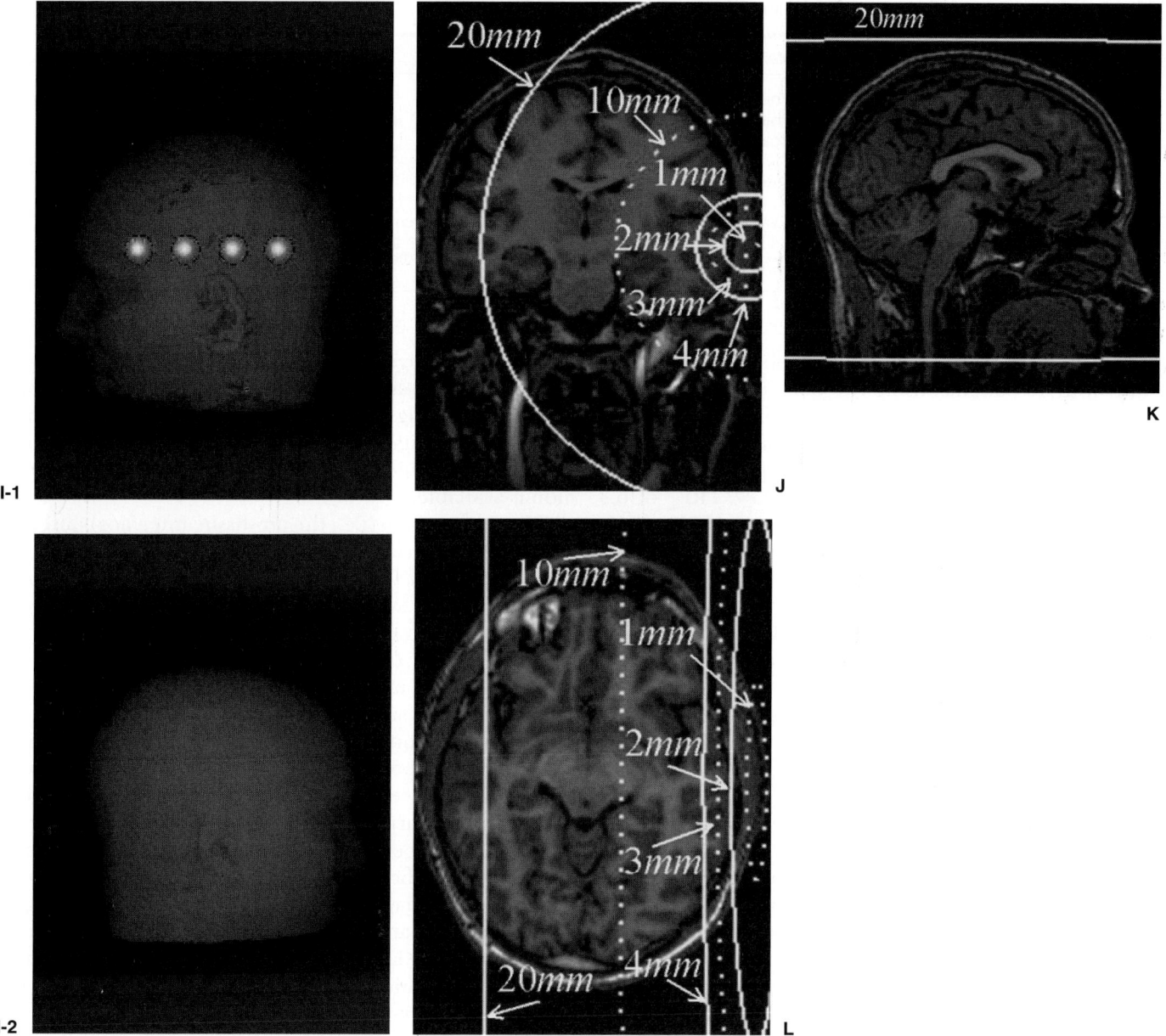

FIGURE 2-7. Continued from pages 23 and 24

often a poor indicator of TRE. This is clearly demonstrated in Figure 2–7 for three different fiducial configurations that have the identical value of FRE but produce very different values of TRE. Until commercial vendors incorporate statistical expected TRE distributions into their IGS systems, we believe that it is prudent to view the displayed FRE value with caution and to place fiducial markers according to the guidelines listed above. Also, at the risk of stating the obvious, one of the best measures of TRE is the surgeon's qualitative assessment of how accurately known external landmarks can be localized with the system after registration. We believe that it is extremely important that the surgeon identify and locate several external anatomical landmarks to visually assess and verify that the IGS system is working properly and that the registration is sufficiently accurate for the surgical procedure before using the system for surgical navigation.

The clinical accuracy of a bone-implanted marker system (see Fig. 2–5) was investigated using data acquired in a prospective clinical trial by six neurosurgeons at four medical centers from 63 patients undergoing craniotomies to resect cerebral lesions.[13] Using four bone-implanted markers as fiducials for registration and a fifth marker as a target for assessment of registration accuracy, the CT-to-physical TRE_m was found to be and 1.0 ± 0.5 mm (mean ± SD), with a 95% TRE_m of 1.8 mm. It is statistically expected that 1 out of every 20 pa-

TABLE 2–1. Target registration error

Type of Registration	Method	Mean ± SD	95%
CT-physical	Point-based, 10 anatomical landmarks	3.6 ± 1.6	6.3
CT-physical	Point-based, 10 skin-affixed markers	2.6 ± 1.2	4.5
CT-physical	Point-based, four bone-implanted markers	1.0 ± 0.5	1.8
CT-physical	Surface-based, skin surface	3.2 ± 1.4	5.6
CT-MR	Intensity-based, mutual information	0.8 ± 0.4	1.4

The bone-implanted marker-based TRE values were reported in Maurer et al[13] using data from 63 patients. The remaining values were calculated in an unpublished study with 40 patients, using five bone-implanted markers as a gold standard for assessment of registration accuracy. The 95% TRE values were calculated as mean + 1.645 SD by assuming that the TRE values are normally distributed. All values are in units of mm.

tients will have an error worse than the 95% value. In a study with 40 patients, using five bone-implanted markers as a gold standard for assessment of registration accuracy, we found that for the head, the CT-to-physical TRE_m for a registration performed using 10 anatomical landmarks was 3.6 ± 1.6 mm, with a 95% TRE_m of 6.3 mm (unpublished data). The CT-to-physical TRE_m for a registration performed using 10 skin-affixed markers (multimodality radiographic markers, IZI Medical Products, Baltimore, MD) was 2.6 ± 1.2 mm, with a 95% TRE_m of 4.5 mm (unpublished data). These error values are summarized in Table 2–1. The relatively poor accuracy and precision of registration performed using skin-affixed markers is probably due to deformation of the skin surface between the time of scanning and the time of treatment. The relatively poor accuracy of registration performed using anatomical landmarks is probably due to deformation of the skin surface, and also the difficulty in accurately determining the same anatomical landmark in the image and on the patient. Nonetheless, there are several neurosurgeons who routinely use anatomical landmarks for cranial IGS procedures and believe that they generally obtain registration errors of 2.0 mm or less. The relatively high accuracy of registration performed using bone-implanted markers (see Fig. 2–5) is due to the fact that the markers are anchored to the rigid cranium, and also to the fact that the markers can be localized accurately in both the image (by using a semiautomatic algorithm for finding the imaging marker centroid with subvoxel accuracy[4]) and physical space (by placing a ball-tipped probe in the hemispherical divot of the localization cap whose position corresponds to the centroid of the image markers).

Surface-based registration

The 3-D boundary or surface of an anatomical object or structure is an intuitive and easily characterized geometrical feature that can be used for medical image registration. Surface-based image registration methods involve determining corresponding surfaces in different images and/or physical space and computing the transformation that best aligns these surfaces. Whereas point-based registration involves aligning a generally small number of corresponding fiducial points, surface-based registration involves aligning a generally much larger number of points for which no point correspondence information is available.

The skin surface (i.e., the air–tissue interface) and the outer cranial surface are obvious choices that have been frequently used for both IIR and IPR of head images (Fig. 2–8). The surface representation can be simply a point set (i.e., a collection of points on the surface), a faceted surface (e.g., a set of triangles approximating the surface), an implicit surface, or a parametric surface (e.g., a B-spline surface). The skin surface is generally a high-contrast boundary in most image modalities, with the important exceptions of nuclear medicine scans with certain tracers and some echo planar MR images, and thus, not surprisingly, segmentation of the skin surface is relatively easy and fairly automatic for most types of images. The bone surface (e.g., the outer cranial surface in head images) is also an easily segmented high-contrast boundary in CT images. Extraction of many soft-tissue boundary surfaces is generally more difficult and less automatic. Segmentation algorithms can generate 2-D contours in contiguous image slices that are linked together to form a 3-D surface, or they can generate 3-D surfaces directly from the image (e.g., Gueziec and Hummel[37]). In physical space, skin surface points can be easily determined using laser range finders; stereo video systems; and articulated mechanical, magnetic, active and passive optical, and ultrasonic 3-D localizers. Bone surface points can be found using tracked A-mode[38] and B-mode[46] ultrasound probes. The computer vision sensors, 3-D localizers, and tracked A-mode probes produce surface point sets. Tracked B-mode probes produce a set of 2-D images (or a single compounded 3-D image) from which bone surface points need to be segmented.

There is a large body of literature in computer vision concerned with the surface-based registration problem. The approach normally used in the medical image processing community (and which is referred to in com-

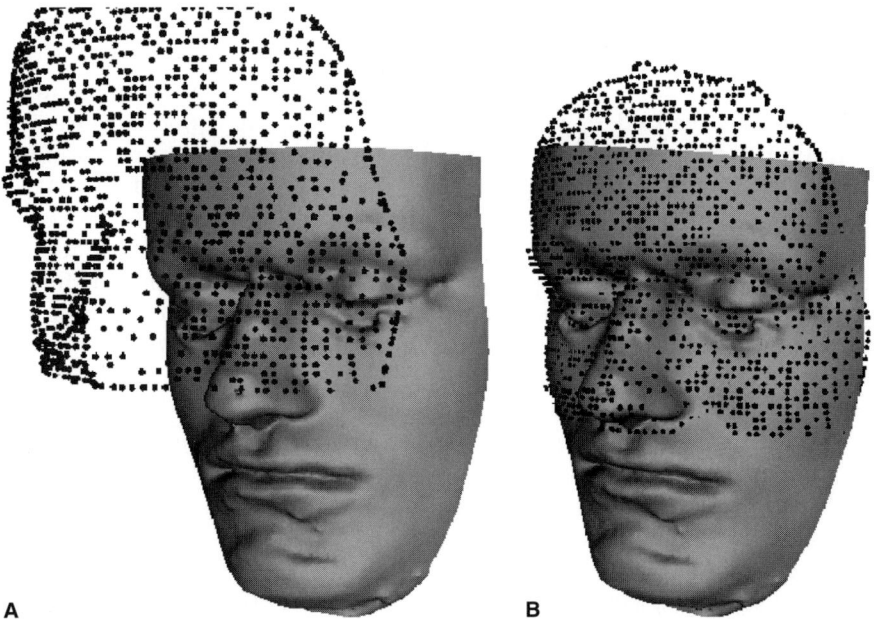

FIGURE 2–8. Illustration of surface-based registration of the head using the facial skin surface. The dots represent skin surface points acquired with a four-camera photogrammetry system. The surface rendering represents a triangle set model of the skin surface extracted from an MR image volume. (A). The initial position of the data sets. (B). The data sets after registration. The registration was performed using an independent implementation[35] of the iterative closest point algorithm.[36] The surfaces overlap only partially, which is a common situation in surface-based registration. The problem of partial overlap was dealt with by setting the weights of outliers to zero after the first search converged before running a second search.

puter vision as the "free-form" surface matching problem) is to search for the transformation that minimizes some disparity function or metric between the two surfaces. The disparity function typically used for surface-based image registration is the mean squared, and optionally weighted, distance[h] between points on one surface (the "data" point set) and corresponding points on the other surface (the "model" surface).[i] The principal difference between point-based registration, which minimizes the mean squared distance between two sets of corresponding points, and surface-based registration is the availability of point correspondence information. Whereas point-based registration can be solved using any of several algorithms with closed-form solutions, the lack of exact point correspondence information causes surface-based registration algorithms to be based on iterative search. Most algorithms calculate approximate point correspondence information for the current transformation at each iteration of the search. A detailed summary of surface-based registration algorithms can be found in in Fitzpatrick et al.[26]

Typically one surface contains more information than the other. The surface from the image that covers the larger volume of the patient or has the higher resolution is generally picked as the model shape. For example, when using the skin surface to perform CT-to-physical space registration, the triangle set representation of the CT skin surface typically contains $\sim 10^4$ to 10^6 vertices, whereas the number of physical space skin surface points typically is $\sim 10^2$ to 10^4. In this case, the CT triangle set is chosen as the model surface shape, and the physical space point set is chosen as the data point set.

All surface-based registration algorithms must search for the transformation that minimizes the disparity function or a variation thereof. This is a general nonlinear minimization problem that is typically solved using one of the common gradient descent techniques (e.g., see Press et al[39]). The search will typically converge to, or very close to, the correct minimum of the disparity function minimum if the initial transformation is within about 20 to 30 degree rotation and 20 to 30 mm translation of the correct solution. Thus it is very important that a good initial value of the transformation be provided to the algorithm (e.g., by using an interactive manual registration software interface or by manually identifying several anatomical landmarks and performing a point-based registration). To help minimize the possibility of the search getting stuck in a local minimum, many investigators perform the search in a hierarchical coarse-to-fine manner.

Point-based registration performed using skin-affixed or bone-implanted fiducial markers requires an additional scan for the image-guided surgical procedure. Surface-based registration, like point-based registration performed using anatomical landmarks, can potentially be used with historical (retrospectively acquired) images that typically were originally acquired for diagnosis. This

---

[h]Many variations of the cost (disparity) function are possible. For example, mean distance can be used rather than root-mean-square distance (i.e., L1 norm versus L2 norm).[21] Outliers can be handled using a thresholded distance, or by using a sigmoidal distance function (which is essentially a gradually tapered thresholded distance).

[i]The terms *data* and *model* arise from an industrial application: registration of digitized data from unfixtured rigid objects obtained using high-accuracy noncontact devices with an idealized geometrical (e.g., computer-aided design) model prior to shape inspection.[36]

aspect is frequently discussed as an advantage of these techniques, partly because it reduces the logistical difficulties of scheduling and acquiring an additional scan for treatment, but more importantly because of the economic benefit realized by not rescanning the patient. However, it is important to note that, although the economic consideration may be substantial, it does not alter the highly variable ways in which diagnostic images are acquired. Typically successful and accurate image registration is best obtained using prospectively acquired images following a protocol specifically designed for IGS. Examples of important image acquisition factors are field of view, voxel dimensions (especially slice thickness), and considerations that impact geometric fidelity. For CT this might include performing a spiral scan to minimize patient movement during image acquisition; for MR this might include using specific pulse sequences that minimize geometrical distortion due to static field inhomogeneity.

Surface-based registration techniques are currently used in several commercially available IGS systems for IPR. (The use of surface-based registration methods for IIR has recently been replaced in most systems by the use of intensity-based registration approaches.) For head applications, the skin surface is generally used for registration. The "model" skin surface is typically a triangle set that is relatively easily and fairly automatically generated for most types of images. The "data" surface points can be acquired by moving a tracked probe along the skin surface[40,41] or by using computer vision techniques (e.g., stereophotogrammetry using multiple calibrated cameras).[42,43] Several commercial vendors have recently demonstrated the use of lasers to acquire surface points. In one system, the optical tracking system, which is used for tracking surgical instruments by finding the positions of IREDs on the instruments, is also used to find skin surface points that are illuminated by shining a beam from what is essentially a laser pointer that emits both infrared as well as visible red light (the latter so that the user can see where the beam is being pointed). One of the commonly reported problems with surface-based IPR methods is that they take substantially more technical support and operator time to make them work, compared with fiducial point-based IPR methods. The new laser-based skin surface point acquisition methods may make data acquisition substantially easier and faster. Nonetheless, one of the main problems with skin surface-based IPR is accuracy and precision. In a study with 40 patients, using five bone-implanted fiducial markers as a gold standard, we found that for the head, the skin surface-based CT-to-physical TRE_m was 3.2 ± 1.4 mm (mean ± SD), with a 95% TRE_m of 5.6 mm (unpublished data). In a blinded evaluation of retrospective intermodality head image registration techniques, which also used bone-implanted fiducial markers as a gold standard, the mean skin surface-based CT-to-MR TRE_m was slightly greater than 5.0 mm, and more than 10% of the registrations had a TRE_m greater than 10.0 mm.[44,45] The probable reason for the relatively poor accuracy and precision of surface-based registration performed using the skin surface is deformation of the skin surface between the time of scanning and the time of treatment. The skin, especially in obese and older patients, is easily deformed, and skin thickness can change with the use of diuretics and steroids. The skin is often substantially deformed at the back of the head where it rests on the scanner table, on the sides of the head in MR images where ear pads are used for passive head restraint in the MR scanner head coil, and near the sites where Mayfield head clamp pins are implanted for head restraint in the operating room.

One possible approach to overcome this limitation is to perform surface-based IPR using a bone surface (e.g., the outer cranial surface). In pulse echo ultrasound, a short pulse of energy is transmitted into the body. Echoes in the received signal represent sound reflected at interfaces between regions of different acoustic impedance. The intensity reflection coefficient, which is the ratio of the pressure reflected to the pressure incident, is less than 0.1 for most soft-tissue interfaces, and is approximately 0.6 to 0.7 for bone–tissue interfaces. Thus echoes corresponding to bone–tissue interfaces have high signal amplitude and are easily identified. The distance from the transducer to the interface corresponding to an echo is easily calculated as $d = ut/2$, where d is the distance, u is the speed of sound, and t is the time interval between the initial sound pulse and the received echo. By tracking the position of an A-mode ultrasound transducer, it is possible to calculate the position of a bone surface point as the position of the ultrasound transducer face plus the distance to the bone–tissue interface along the ultrasound beam axis. Recent preliminary results on a phantom and several volunteers suggest that it is possible to achieve a bone surface-based CT-to-physical TRE ~ 1 to 2 mm using a tracked A-mode ultrasound-based system.[38] Bone surface points can also be found using tracked clinical B-mode ultrasound scanners.[46]

Intensity-based registration

Intensity-based registration involves computing a transformation between two images using image voxel values rather than geometrical features such as points or surfaces derived from the images. The term *intensity* refers to the scalar value of an image voxel. The physical meaning of the voxel intensity value depends on the image modality. The registration transformation is determined by iteratively optimizing some similarity measure computed from all voxel values. Because the images are generally 3-D images such as CT, MR, and PET, these measures are often referred to as voxel similarity measures.

A detailed description of intensity-based image registration is beyond the scope of this chapter; a good introduction can be found in Fitzpatrick et al.[26] But it is helpful to have some understanding of the most commonly used and successful algorithms, which are based on joint histograms and information theory. A joint histogram is a useful tool for visualizing the relationship between the intensities of corresponding voxels in two or more images. Such histograms are widely used with multispectral data (e.g., dual echo MR images). For two images A and B, the joint histogram is 2-D and is constructed by plotting the intensity a of each voxel in image A against the intensity b of each voxel in image B. Thus the axes of the histogram are the intensities in each image, and the value at each point in the histogram is the number of corresponding voxel pairs with that particular combination of intensities in the two images. Hill and Hawkes[47] observed that the appearance of joint histograms changes in a visually obvious way as correctly registered images are intentionally misaligned. Example joint histograms for MR and CT images and MR and PET images are shown in Figure 2–9. These joint histograms are functions of the two images and also of the registration transformation. The figure shows histograms for a correct registration and a translational misalignment of 5.0 mm. Although the appearance of the histograms for the two combinations of image modalities is quite different, there is an important similarity. Specifically, the intensity histograms are sharpest for the registered images, and they become noticeably blurred with misalignment. These plots provide insight into a concept of image registration that is based on entropy and information theory.

Information theory dates back to the pioneering work of Shannon in the 1940s.[48] Shannon, who was working at Bell Laboratories on the transmission of information along a noisy telephone line, devised a theory around a new measure of information. Its mathematical form is the same as the entropy defined in statistical thermodynamics, so he called this measure entropy.[j] Entropy is a measure of disorder. Its value can be computed from the joint histogram. Entropy increases with increasing misalignment as can be observed in the visual appearance of both a fused pair of images and the joint histogram (see Fig. 2–9). Minimizing the joint entropy, computed from a joint histogram, has been used as the basis for image registration.[50,51] However, joint entropy by itself does not provide a robust measure of image alignment. The use of this measure involves the implicit assumption that large regions in the two images being registered increase their degree of overlap as the images approach the correct alignment. If the overlap between large regions of the images is not maximal when the images are correctly aligned, then generally the joint entropy will not be minimal at this point. Intermodality image registration frequently involves registering images with very different fields of view, and usually the correct alignment will involve only part of each image. A solution to the overlap problem from which joint entropy suffers is to consider the information contributed to the overlapping volume by each image individually (the marginal entropies) as well as the combined information (joint entropy). Communication theory provides a technique for measuring the joint entropy with respect to the marginal entropies. This measure, introduced by Shannon,[48] is known as mutual information. Mutual information can qualitatively be thought of as a measure of how well one image explains the other, is generally relatively insensitive to the overlap problem, and is maximal at, or very close to, the correct alignment.

Intensity-based registration methods in general do not require that geometrical features such as points or surfaces be segmented from the images. The great attraction of mutual information in particular as a voxel similarity measure for image registration is that it makes no assumption about the relationship between the intensity of a particular anatomical structure in the modalities being aligned. As a result, it can be used for both intramodality registration and intermodality registration and is far more generally applicable than any other automatic IIR algorithm yet proposed. There is a considerable literature showing that mutual information is robust and accurate.[44,45,52–56]

As is the case for surface-based registration algorithms as discussed in the previous section, intensity-based algorithms require an iterative search for the transformation that minimizes the similarity measure (e.g., mutual information). Parameter spaces for intensity-based algorithms frequently have multiple local optima, and registration can fail if the optimization algorithm converges to the wrong optimum. Thus it is very important that a good initial value of the transformation be provided to the algorithm (e.g., by using an interactive manual registration software interface or by manually identifying several anatomical landmarks and performing a point-based registration).

In a comparative study of retrospective intermodality brain image registration techniques, intensity-based algorithms frequently registered CT and MR images with an accuracy of better than 2 mm, but such algorithms sometimes failed, leading to errors of 6 mm or more.[44,45] Thus a quality assurance method must be used to distinguish

---

[j]There is a humorous anecdote regarding the origin of the term entropy.[49] Apparently Shannon asked von Neumann what name he should give to his measure of uncertainty. Von Neumann answered, "You should call it 'entropy,' and for two reasons: first, the function is already in use in thermodynamics under that name; second, and more importantly, most people don't know what entropy really is, and if you use the word 'entropy' in an argument, you will win every time!"

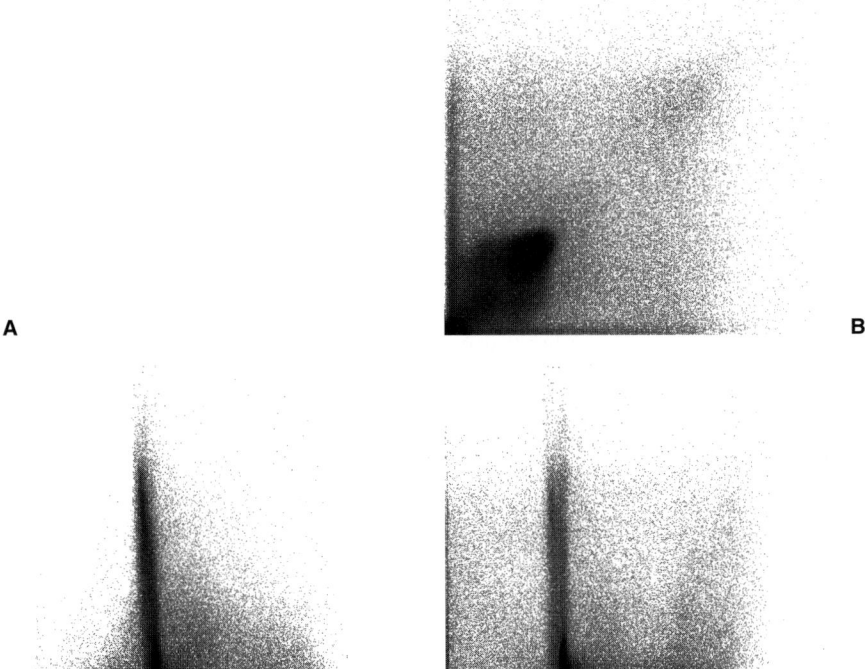

FIGURE 2–9. Examples of joint probability distribution functions (histograms) of image intensity. (A,B). Histograms for identical MR images of the head. (C,D). Histograms for MR (vertical axis) and CT (horizontal axis). (A,C). Histograms for registered images. (B,D). Histograms for images misregistered by a translation of 5 mm. The intensity histograms are sharpest for the registered images. The histograms are obviously blurred by the misregistrations.

between registration transformations that are clinically satisfactory and those that are not. As a result of efforts to quantify the accuracy of visual inspection as a means of failure detection in intermodality registration, it appears that when suitable interactive image viewing software is available, visual inspection can reliably detect a TRE greater than 2 mm for MR–CT registration[57] and 4 mm for MR–PET registration.[58,59] Figure 2–10 illustrates several methods of visual assessment for MR–CT registration.

Mutual information has been used successfully to register CT; many types of MR, including T_1-weighted, T_2-weighted, and proton density spin-echo and gradient-echo; and PET images. But there are situations where mutual information does not work very well. One example is the case where one of the images has a small number of slices (i.e., the image field of view is a thin slab). In this case the joint histogram is quite sparse and there can be too few voxels to compute mutual information accurately. Another example is the case where one of the images (e.g., MR) has severe intensity inhomogeneity (shading artifact). Mutual information is fairly robust to mild intensity inhomogeneity, but in severe cases, the relationship between the intensity values of anatomical structures in the two images is not spatially invariant. Although good results have been obtained for PET images acquired using [18F]-fluorodeoxyglucose (FDG) as a tracer, it is not clear whether similarly good results will be obtained for nuclear medicine scans acquired using receptor-specific tracers.

■ Intraoperative Brain Deformation

All IGS systems that use preoperative images assume that the head and its contents behave as a rigid body—that the intraoperative positions of anatomical structures of surgical interest are related to the positions of these structures in the preoperative image by a rigid-body transformation (sometimes scaling is also used to account for incorrect image voxel dimensions). Brain deformation between imaging and surgery or during surgery invalidates this assumption and consequently introduces an important source of error that is not detected by standard measures of registration error.

It is likely that brain deformation depends on many factors, including anesthetic practice, steroid use, osmotically active drug use, tumor size, tumor location, craniotomy size, extent of resection, and amount of cerebral atrophy. Debulking of tumors and aspiration of cysts often cause the wall of the resulting cavity to collapse. It is standard surgical practice to reduce intracranial pressure (ICP) prior to performing neurosurgical procedures. Steroids are often administered preoperatively to reduce inflammation. Intraoperatively, cerebral blood volume can be controlled by manipulating ventilation to alter carbon dioxide concentration in the blood and by tilting the bed to increase or reduce venous drainage. The water content of the brain can be reduced by administering an osmotically active drug (e.g., the sugar alcohol mannitol). Cerebrospinal fluid (CSF)

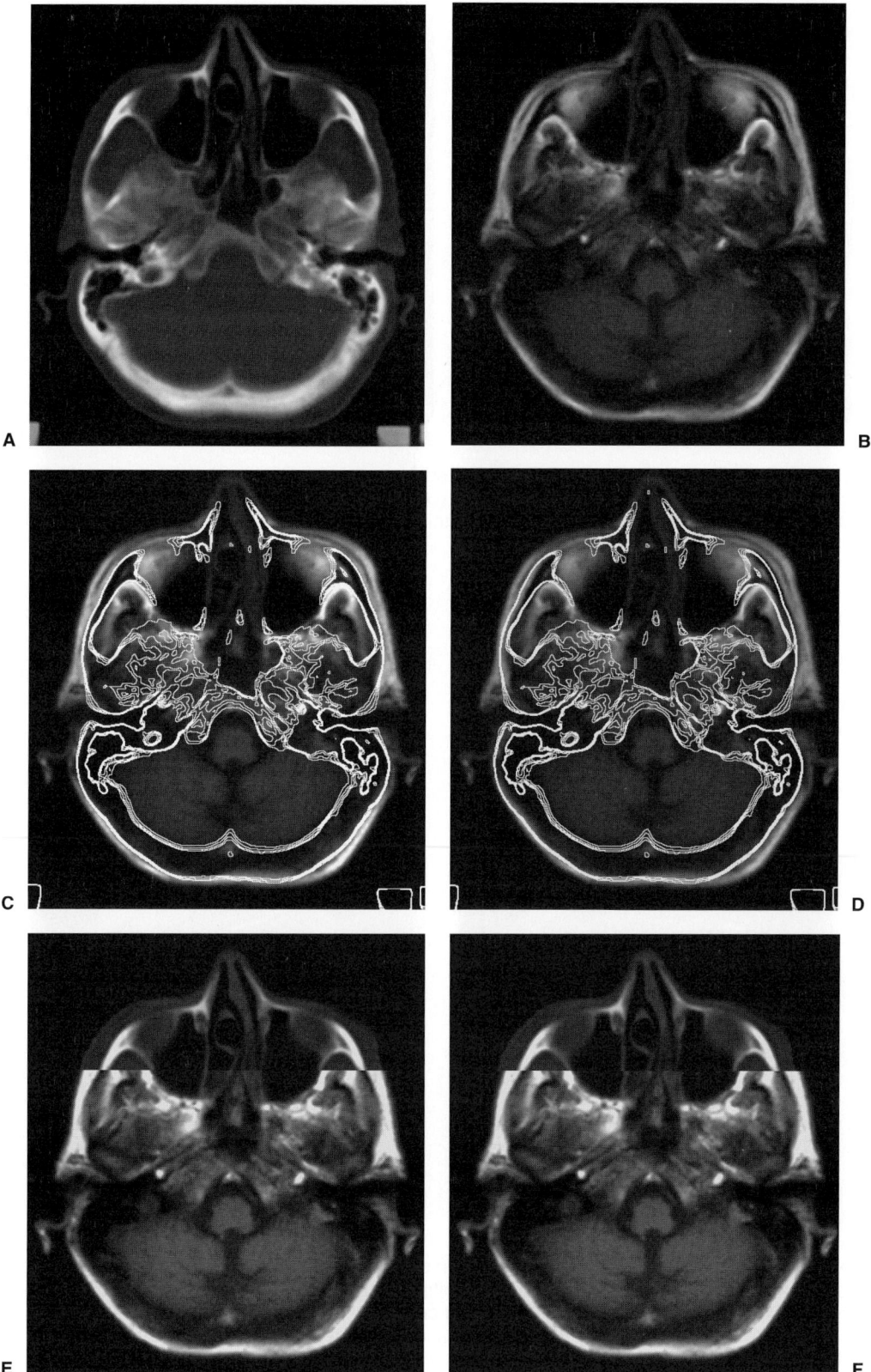

FIGURE 2–10. Visual assessment of registration accuracy. (A,B). Transverse slices from a CT (left) and MR (right) image of the same patient. (C–H). Several image fusion methods for visually assessing the accuracy of the CT-MR registration transformation. The left column shows images that are correctly aligned; the right column shows images that are intentionally misregistered by a lateral translation of 2 mm. (C,D). Bone edges extracted from CT and overlaid on MR. (E,F). *(Continued on page 32)*

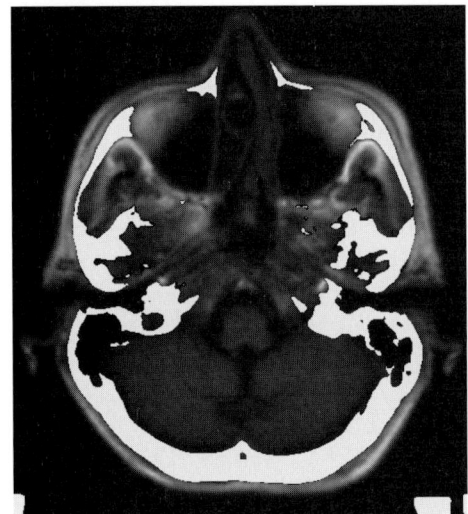 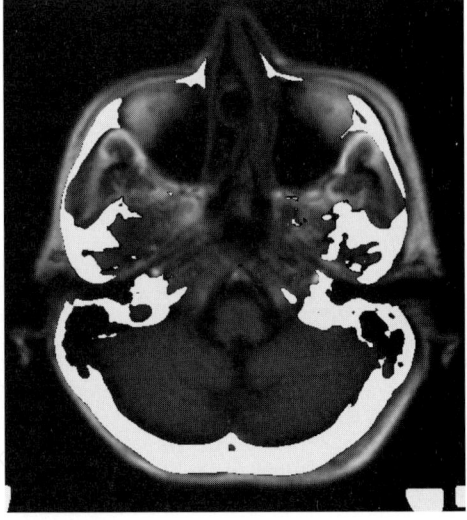

FIGURE 2–10. (*Continued from page 31*) Fused images with CT visible above an adjustable horizontal line and MR visible below the line. (G,H). Bone segmented from the CT image by thresholding and overlaid on the MR image. It is relatively easy to detect the 2 mm misregistration in all of these examples.

volume can be altered by reducing CSF production or by draining CSF (e.g., lumbar puncture). The effect these parameters have on ICP is well documented (e.g., Doczi[60]), but little is known about the resulting volume changes and brain deformation they cause in humans. Several groups have recently reported quantitative measurements of intraoperative brain deformation.[61–65] For craniotomies, deformation on the order of 10 mm has been observed at the cortical surface and on the order of 5 mm at subsurface structures such as the deep tumor margin. There is considerable variability in deformation among patients. However, in one study, regardless of the procedure, there was very little deformation of the midline, the tentorium, the hemisphere

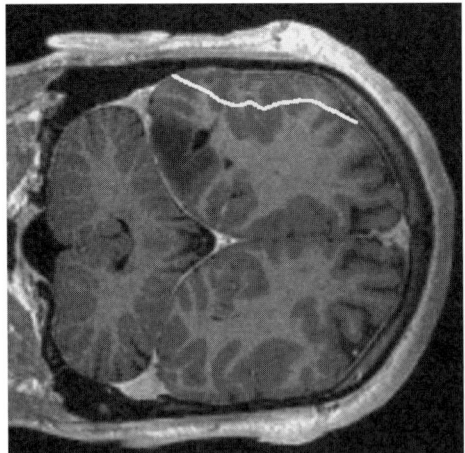 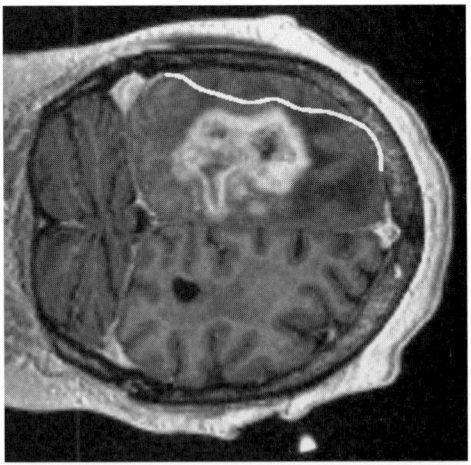

FIGURE 2–11. Examples of intraoperative brain surface deformation. These panels show coronal slices from MR image volumes of two patients that underwent intraoperative functional mapping of sensory, motor, or language areas using cortical stimulation. The brain surface was measured approximately 90 minutes after opening the dura but before performing resection of a tumor (white line). The images have been rotated to indicate the intraoperative orientation of the patient, with the direction of gravity vertical on the page. The patient's left side is at the top in each image. The inclination of the craniotomy for the patients was 6 degrees on the left and was 34 degrees on the right. The ends of the white lines represent the edges of the craniotomies. In both patients, the brain was sinking under much of the craniotomy, but in the patient shown on the right, there was a slight protruding region at the lowest edge of the craniotomy. (From Hill DLG, Maurer CR Jr, Maciunas RJ, Barwise JA, Fitzpatrick JM, Wang MY. Measurement of intraoperative brain surface deformation under a craniotomy. *Neurosurg* 1998;43:514–526. With permission.)

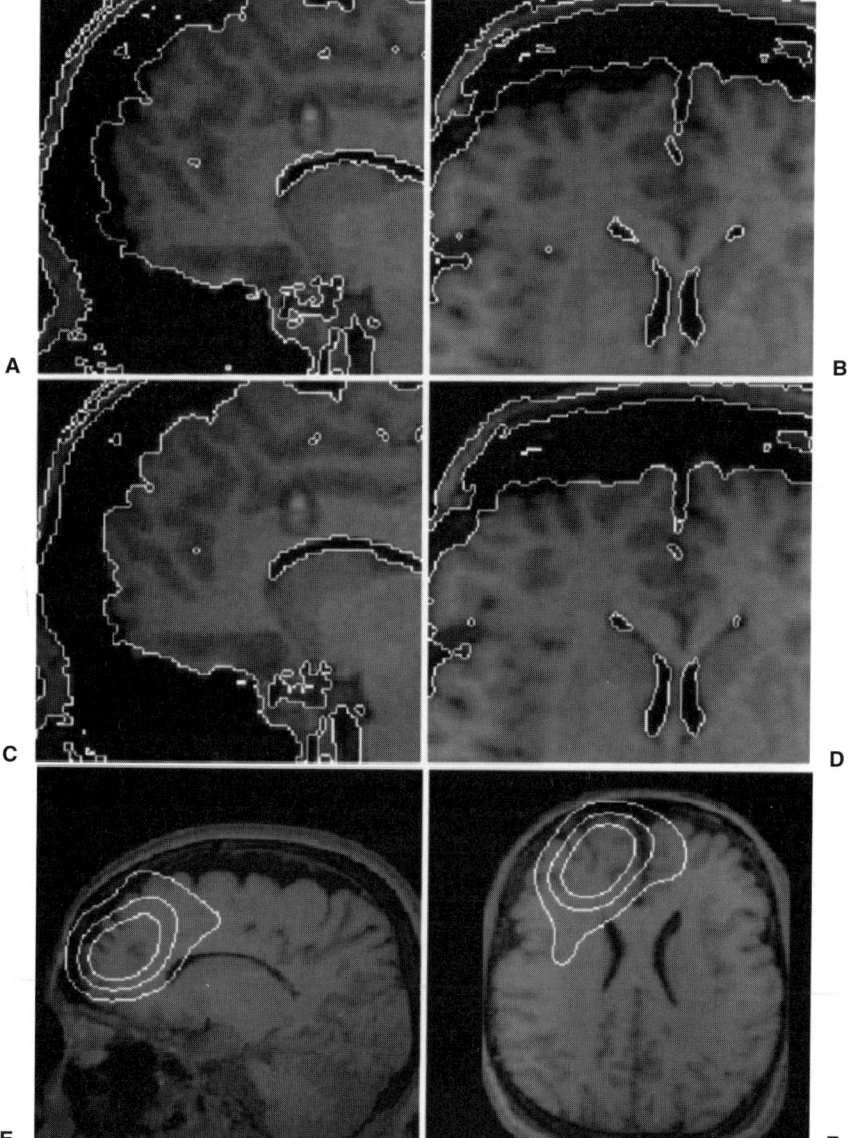

FIGURE 2–12. Intraoperative brain deformation. The top two rows show sagittal (A,C) and transverse (B,D) slices through an MR image volume acquired intraoperatively. The boundary of the brain obtained by thresholding a preoperative image is shown transformed and overlaid on the intraoperative image using a rigid-body registration transformation (A,B) and a 3-D B-spline deformation transformation (C,D). The results of the deformation algorithm provide substantially better alignment of the brain surface in the right frontal lobe. E and F show contours of constant deformation magnitude computed from the 3-D B-spline transformation superimposed on the sagittal and transverse slices from the preoperative image volume. The inner, middle, and outer contours represent deformation magnitudes of 4.5, 3.0, and 1.5 mm, respectively. (Modified from Maurer CR Jr, Hill DLG, Martin AJ, et al. Investigation of intraoperative brain deformation using a 1.5 Tesla interventional MR system: preliminary results. *IEEE Trans Med Imaging* 1998;17:817–825. © 1998 IEEE. With permission.)

contralateral to the procedure, and ipsilateral structures except those that are within 10 mm of the lesion or are gravitationally above the surgical site.[64] The absence of deformation across the midline may be due to mechanical support provided by the falx cerebri. Brain movement is unlikely to be a problem for stereotactic radiosurgery, procedures that involve twist drill openings (e.g., stereotactic biopsy, functional procedures), and procedures that involve nondeformable anatomy (e.g., skull base surgery). Little deformation was observed in one biopsy and one functional case.[64] Figures 2–11 and 2–12 show an example of brain deformation. Although in many patients the principal component of intraoperative brain deformation is oriented in the direction of gravity, in some patients the deformation is quite complicated.

The problem of brain deformation can be addressed by performing the IGS procedure using intraoperative imaging. Several intraoperative modalities have been used, including CT,[66] MR,[67–70] and ultrasound.[71–73] But brain deformation is also a concern for these systems if it is desirable to make intraoperative use of preoperative images (e.g., from other modalities) or information derived from preoperative images (e.g., a surgical plan). One approach to correct for intraoperative brain deformation is to acquire high-resolution images, in particular, MR, and compute a nonrigid deformation transformation between the preoperative image and the intraoperative image. Encouraging results have been reported using 3-D B-splines[64] and optical flow.[74] Figure 2–12 shows an example of non-rigid registrations performed using intraoperative MR image volumes. Another approach is to track an ultrasound probe and display the ultrasound image next to a reformatted image slice from a preoperative CT or MR image.[71] The two views can be fused or compared using a pair of movable linked cursors that are displayed at corresponding points. The surgeon can use this information to visually assess or quantitatively measure, and mentally compensate for, brain deformation. This is frequently helpful, although soft-tissue structures are often difficult to distinguish because of limited tissue contrast provided by ultrasound. A third approach is to build a patient-specific biomechanical model of brain tissue deformation based on segmentation of high-resolution preoperative images and deform it according to the governing equations of a mathematical description of tissue deformation using sparse intraoperative data (e.g., the cortical surface obtained using a laser rangefinder or stereo video cameras, limited anatomical landmarks or boundaries obtained using intraoperative ultrasound) to confine the deformation. Promising preliminary results have been obtained using multiphase consolidation theory, which considers the brain as a spongelike material where tissue motion is characterized by an instantaneous deformation at the area of contact followed by additional deformation resulting from exiting pore fluid driven by a pressure gradient.[75–77]

■ Appendix: Point-Based Registration Error Theory

Consider a set of N fiducial points that is registered to another set of points that differs from the first set by position, orientation, and noise that is added to each point (identical, independent, zero-mean, isotropic, normally distributed noise). Let σ^2 be the variance of the coordinate components of the random noise. In our case, the random noise represents the error of determining the positions of the fiducial markers. Thus $\sigma^2 = \langle FLE^2 \rangle/3$, and $rms[FLE] = \sqrt{3\sigma^2}$. Sibson[78] showed using perturbation theory that if the points are registered in a least-squares sense using a rigid-body transformation, then $FRE^2 \sim \sigma^2 \chi^2_{3N-6}$. This means that for a particular localization error (i.e., a particular value of $rms[FLE]$, or equivalently, a particular value of σ), there is a statistical distribution of FRE values for which the probabilities are given by the chi-square (χ^2) distribution with $3N$-6 degrees of freedom. It can be shown from this probability distribution that there is a statistical relationship among the expected value of FRE, FLE, and the number of fiducials N, which is described by

$$\langle FRE^2 \rangle = \frac{N-2}{N} \langle FLE^2 \rangle. \quad (2\text{–}1)$$

The expected value of FRE depends only on the expected value of FLE and the number of fiducials N, and is independent of the shape of the fiducial configuration.

Fitzpatrick et al[29] recently showed using perturbation theory that there is a statistical relationship among the expected value of TRE, FLE, the number of fiducials N, and the position of the target relative to the fiducials, which is described by

$$\langle TRE^2(\mathbf{r}) \rangle = \frac{\langle FLE^2 \rangle}{N} \left(1 + \frac{1}{3} \sum_{k=1}^{3} \frac{d_k^2}{f_k^2} \right), \quad (2\text{–}2)$$

where d_k is the distance of the target point $\mathbf{r}$ from the kth principal axis of the fiducial point set, and f_k is the rms distance of the fiducials from the kth axis (f_k is effectively the radius of gyration of the fiducial set about its kth principal axis). The constant inside the parentheses in Equation 2–2 represents the translational component of TRE; the summation term represents the rotational component. Several observations about the nature of the statistically expected value of TRE can be made based on inspection of Equation 2–2: (1) TRE (both its value at a particular position as well as its average over a region of interest) is proportional to rms [FLE]. (2) TRE is inversely proportional to $\sqrt{N}$, assuming that fiducials are added to the configuration such that their rms distance to the three principal axes (f_k) remains constant. (3) TRE depends on the position $\mathbf{r}$ of the target point. (4) TRE has its minimum value at the fiducial configuration centroid, and that value, which is $rms[FLE]/N$, is purely the translational component of registration error. (5) TRE increases as the distance of the target point from the principal axes increases. (6) The iso-error TRE contours are ellipsoidal. These observations are consistent with many published results.[13,27,79–80]

■ Acknowledgment

TR contributed to this chapter while supported by the National Science Foundation under Grant No. EIA-

0104114. DD and RJM acknowledge the support of the Research Foundation of the Department of Neurological Surgery and the Research Institute of University Hospitals of Cleveland.

REFERENCES

1. Maciunas RJ, Kessler RM, Maurer CR Jr, Mandava VR, Watt G, Smith G. Positron emission tomography imaging-directed stereotactic neurosurgery. *Stereotact Funct Neurosurg* 1992;58:134–140.
2. Edwards PJ, King AP, Maurer CR Jr, et al. Design and evaluation of a system for microscope-assisted guided interventions (MAGI). *IEEE Trans Med Imaging* 2000;19:1082–1093.
3. Maurer CR Jr, Sauer F, Bascle B, et al. Augmented reality visualization of brain structures with stereo and kinetic depth cues: system description and initial evaluation with head phantom. In: *Medical Imaging 2001: Visualization, Display, and Image-Guided Procedures*, vol. Proc. SPIE 4319, Bellingham, WA: The International Society of Optical Engineering 2001:445–456.
4. Wang MY, Maurer CR Jr, Fitzpatrick JM, Maciunas RJ. An automatic technique for finding and localizing externally attached markers in CT and MR volume images of the head. *IEEE Trans Biomed Eng* 1996;43:627–637.
5. Haacke EM, Brown RW, Thompson MR, Venkatesan R. *Magnetic Resonance Imaging: Physical Principles and Sequence Design*. New York: Wiley-Liss; 1999.
6. Webb PG, Macovski A. Rapid, fully automatic, arbitrary-volume in vivo shimming. *Magn Reson Med* 1991;20:113–122.
7. Shellock FG, Kanal E. *Magnetic Resonance: Bioeffects, Safety, and Patient Management*. 2nd ed. New York: Lippincott-Raven; 1996.
8. Hardy PA, Barnett GH. Spatial distortion in magnetic resonance imaging: impact on stereotactic localization. In: Gildenberg PL, Tasker RR, eds. *Textbook of Stereotactic and Functional Neurosurgery*. New York: McGraw-Hill; 1998:271–280.
9. Meuli RA, Verdun FR, Bochud FO, Emsley L, Fankhauser H. Assessment of MR image deformation for stereotactic neurosurgery using a tagging sequence. *Am J Neuroradiol* 1994;15:45–49.
10. Lunsford LD. Comment on "Evaluation of the spatial accuracy of magnetic resonance imaging-based stereotactic target localization for gamma knife radiosurgery of functional disorders." *Neurosurgery* 1999;45:1156–1163.
11. Ludeke KM, Roschmann P, Tischler R. Susceptibility artifacts in NMR imaging. *Magn Reson Imaging* 1985;3:329–343.
12. Posse S, Aue WP. Susceptibility artifacts in spin-echo and gradient-echo imaging. *J Magn Reson* 1990;88:473–492.
13. Maurer CR Jr, Fitzpatrick JM, Wang MY, Galloway RL Jr, Maciunas RJ, Allen GS. Registration of head volume images using implantable fiducial markers. *IEEE Trans Med Imaging* 1997;16:447–462.
14. Chang H, Fitzpatrick JM. A technique for accurate magnetic resonance imaging in the presence of field inhomogeneities. *IEEE Trans Med Imaging* 1992;11:319–329.
15. Kim JK, Kucharczyk W, Henkelman RM. Cavernous hemangiomas: dipolar susceptibility artifacts at MR imaging. *Radiology* 1993;187:735–741.
16. Schneider E, Glover GH. Rapid, in vivo proton shimming. *Magn Reson Med* 1991;18:335–347.
17. Dean D, Kamath J, Duerk JL, Ganz E. Validation of object-induced MR distortion correction for frameless stereotactic neurosurgery. *IEEE Trans Med Imaging* 1998;17:810–816.
18. Sumanaweera TS, Glover GH, Binford TO, Adler JR. MR susceptibility misregistration correction. *IEEE Trans Med Imaging* 1993;12:251–259.
19. Sumanaweera TS, Glover GH, Song SM, Adler JR, Napel S. Quantifying MRI geometric distortion in tissue. *Magn Reson Med* 1994;31:40–47.
20. Axel L, Dougherty L. MR imaging of motion with spatial modulation of magnetization. *Radiology* 1989;171:841–845.
21. Maurer CR Jr, Aboutanos GB, Dawant BM, et al. Effect of geometrical distortion correction in MR on image registration accuracy. *J Comput Assist Tomogr* 1996;20:666–679.
22. Hill DLG, Maurer R Jr, Studholme C, Fitzpatrick JM, Hawkes DJ. Correcting scaling errors in tomographic images using a nine degree of freedom registration algorithm. *J Comput Assist Tomogr* 1998;22:317–323.
23. Lemieux L, Barker GJ. Measurement of small inter-scan fluctuations in voxel dimensions in magnetic resonance images using registration. *Med Phys* 1998;25:1049–1054.
24. Schad LR, Lott S, Schmitt F, Sturm V, Lorenz WJ. Correction of spatial distortion in MR imaging: a prerequisite for accurate stereotaxy. *J Comput Assist Tomogr* 1987;11:499–505.
25. Bednarz G, Downes MB, Corn BW, Curran WJ, Goldman HW. Evaluation of the spatial accuracy of magnetic resonance imaging-based stereotactic target localization for gamma knife radiosurgery of functional disorders. *Neurosurgery* 1999;45:1156–1163.
26. Fitzpatrick JM, Hill DLG, Maurer CR Jr. Image registration. In: Sonka M, Fitzpatrick JM, eds. *Handbook of Medical Image Processing and Analysis*, vol 2. Bellingham, WA: SPIE Press; 2000:447–513.
27. Hill DLG, Hawkes DJ, Gleeson MJ, et al. Accurate frameless registration of MR and CT images of the head: applications in surgery and radiotherapy planning. *Radiology* 1994;191:447–454.
28. Dean D, Palomo M, Subramanyan K, et al. Accuracy and precision of 3D cephalometric landmarks from biorthogonal plain-film x-rays. In: Yongmin K, Seong MK, eds. *Medical Imaging 1998: Image Display*. Bellingham, WA: The International Society for Optical Engineering. Proc SPIE 3335;1998:50–58.
29. Fitzpatrick JM, West JB, Maurer CR Jr. Predicting error in rigid-body, point-based registration. *IEEE Trans Med Imaging* 1998;17:694–702.
30. West JB, Fitzpatrick JM, Toms SA, Maurer CR Jr, Maciunas RJ. Fiducial point placement and the accuracy of point-based, rigid-body registration. *Neurosurgery* 2001;48:810–817.
31. Khadem R, Yeh CC, Sadeghi-Tehrani M, et al. Comparative tracking error analysis of five different optical tracking systems. *Comput Aided Surg* 2000;5:98–107.
32. Bose CB, Amir I. Design of fiducials for accurate registration using machine vision. *IEEE Trans Pattern Anal Mach Intell* 1990;12:1196–1200.
33. Chiorboli G, Vecchi GP. Comments on "Design of fiducials for accurate registration using machine vision." *IEEE Trans Pattern Anal Mach Intell* 1993;15:1330–1332.
34. Barnett GH. Comment on "Fiducial point placement and the accuracy of point-based, rigid-body registration." *Neurosurgery* 2001;48:810–817.
35. Maurer CR Jr, Aboutanos GB, Dawant BM, Maciunas RJ, Fitzpatrick JM. Registration of 3-D images using weighted geometrical features. *IEEE Trans Med Imaging* 1996;15:836–849.
36. Besl PJ, McKay ND. A method for registration of 3-D shapes. *IEEE Trans Pattern Anal Mach Intell* 1992;14:239–256.
37. Gueziec A, Hummel R. Exploiting triangulated surface extraction using tetrahedral decomposition. *IEEE Trans Visualization Comput Graph* 1995;1:328–342.
38. Maurer CR Jr, Gaston RP, Hill DLG, et al. AcouStick: a tracked A-mode ultrasonography system for registration in image-guided surgery. In: Taylor CJ, Colchester ACF, eds. *Medical Imaging Computing and Computer-Assisted Intervention (MICCAI) 1999*, Berlin: Springer-Verlag; 1999:953–962.
39. Press WH, Teukolsky SA, Vetterling WT, Flannery BP. *Numerical Recipes in C: The Art of Scientific Computing*. 2nd ed. Cambridge: Cambridge University Press; 1992.
40. Maurer CR Jr, Maciunas RJ, Fitzpatrick JM. Registration of head CT images to physical space using a weighted combination of points and surfaces. *IEEE Trans Med Imaging* 1998;17:753–761.
41. Tan KK, Grzeszczuk R, Levin DN. A frameless stereotactic approach to neurosurgical planning based on retrospective patient-image registration. *J Neurosurg* 1993;79:296–303.

42. Colchester ACF, Zhao J, Holton-Tainter KS, et al. Development and preliminary evaluation of VISLAN, a surgical planning and guidance system using intra-operative video imaging. *Med Image Anal* 1996;1:73–90.
43. Grimson WEL, Ettinger GJ, White SJ, Lozano-Perez T, Wells WM III, Kikinis R. An automatic registration method for frameless stereotaxy, image guided surgery, and enhanced reality visualization. *IEEE Trans Med Imaging* 1996;15:129–140.
44. West JB, Fitzpatrick JM, Wang MY, et al. Retrospective intermodality registration techniques for images of the head: surface-based versus volume-based. *IEEE Trans Med Imaging* 1999;18:144–150.
45. West JB, Fitzpatrick JM, Wang MY, et al. Comparison and evaluation of retrospective intermodality image registration techniques. *J Comput Assist Tomogr* 1997;21:554–566.
46. Lavallee S, Troccaz J, Sautot P, et al. Computer-assisted spinal surgery using anatomy-based registration. In: Taylor RH, Lavallee S, Burdea G, Mosges R, eds. *Computer-Integrated Surgery: Technology and Clinical Applications.* Cambridge, MA: MIT Press; 1996:425–449.
47. Hill DLG, Hawkes DJ. Voxel similarity measures for automated image registration. *Visualization in Biomedical Computing (VBC) 1994.* Bellingham, WA: The International Society for Optical Engineering; 1994:205–216.
48. Shannon CE. The mathematical theory of communication (parts 1 and 2). *Bell Syst Tech J* 1948;27:379–423, 623–656. Reprint available at: http://www.lucent.com. Last accessed January 9, 2002.
49. Applebaum D. *Probability and Information: An Integrated Approach.* Cambridge, England: Cambridge University Press; 1996.
50. Collignon A, Maes F, Delaere D, Vandermeulen D, Suetens P, Marchal G. Automated multi-modality image registration based on information theory. In: Bizais Y, Barillot C, Di Paola R, eds. *Information Processing in Medical Imaging (IPMI) 1995.* Dordrecht, The Netherlands: Kluwer Academic; 1995:263–274.
51. Studholme C, Hill DLG, Hawkes DJ. Automated registration of truncated MR and CT datasets of the head. *Proc. Br. Mach. Vision Conf.* London: British Machine Vision Association; 1995:27–36.
52. Maes F, Collignon A, Vandermeulen D, Marchal G, Suetens P. Multimodality image registration by maximization of mutual information. *IEEE Trans Med Imaging* 1997;16:187–198.
53. Studholme C, Hill DLG, Hawkes DJ. Automated 3D registration of MR and CT images of the head. *Med Image Anal* 1996;1:163–175.
54. Studholme C, Hill DLG, Hawkes DJ. Automated 3D registration of MR and PET brain images by multi-resolution optimisation of voxel similarity measures. *Med Phys* 1997;24:25–35.
55. Studholme C, Hill DLG, Hawkes DJ. An overlap invariant entropy measure of 3D medical image alignment. *Pattern Recognit* 1999;33:71–86.
56. Wells WM III, Viola P, Atsumi H, Nakajima S, Kikinis R. Multimodal volume registration by maximization of mutual information. *Med Image Anal* 1996;1:35–51.
57. Fitzpatrick JM, Hill DLG, Shyr Y, West JB, Studholme C, Maurer CR Jr. Visual assessment of the accuracy of retrospective registration of MR and CT images of the brain. *IEEE Trans Med Imaging* 1998;17:571–585.
58. Pietrzyk U, Herholz K, Heiss WD. Three-dimensional alignment of functional and morphological tomograms. *J Comput Assist Tomogr* 1990;14:51–59.
59. Wong JCH, Studholme C, Hawkes DJ, Maisey MN. Evaluation of the limits of visual detection of image misregistration in a brain fluorine-18 fluorodeoxyglucose PET-MRI study. *Eur J Nucl Med* 1997;24:642–650.
60. Doczi T. Volume regulation of the brain tissue: a survey. *Acta Neurochir* 1993;121:1–8.
61. Dickhaus H, Ganser KA, Staubert A, et al. Quantification of brain shift effects by MR imaging. *Proc Annu Int Conf IEEE Eng Med Biol Soc* 1997;19:491–494.
62. Dorward NL, Alberti O, Velani B, et al. Postimaging brain distortion: magnitude, correlates, and impact on neuronavigation. *J Neurosurg* 1998;88:656–662.
63. Hill DLG, Maurer CR Jr, Maciunas RJ, Barwise JA, Fitzpatrick JM, Wang MY. Measurement of intraoperative brain surface deformation under a craniotomy. *Neurosurgery* 1998;43:514–526.
64. Maurer CR Jr, Hill DLG, Martin AJ, et al. Investigation of intraoperative brain deformation using a 1.5 Tesla interventional MR system. Preliminary results. *IEEE Trans Med Imaging* 1998;17:817–825.
65. Roberts DW, Hartov A, Kennedy FE Jr, Miga MI, Paulsen KD. Intraoperative brain shift and deformation: a quantitative analysis of cortical displacement in 28 cases. *Neurosurgery* 1998;43:749–758.
66. Butler WE, Piaggio CM, Constantino C, et al. A mobile computed tomographic scanner with intraoperative and intensive care unit applications. *Neurosurgery* 1998;42:1304–1311.
67. Black PM, Moriarty T, Alexander E III, et al. Development and implementation of intraoperative magnetic resonance imaging and its neurosurgical applications. *Neurosurgery* 1997;41:831–845.
68. Tronnier VM, Wirtz CR, Knauth M, et al. Intraoperative diagnostic and interventional magnetic resonance imaging in neurosurgery. *Neurosurgery* 1997;40:891–902.
69. van Vaals JJ. Interventional MR with a hybrid high-field system. In: Debatin JF, Adam G, eds. *Interventional Magnetic Resonance Imaging.* Berlin: Springer-Verlag; 1998:19–32.
70. Wirtz CR, Bonsanto MM, Knauth M, et al. Intraoperative magnetic resonance imaging to update interactive navigation in neurosurgery: method and preliminary experience. *Comput Aided Surg* 1997;2:172–179.
71. Bucholz RD, Yeh DD, Trobaugh J, et al. The correction of stereotactic inaccuracy caused by brain shift using an intraoperative ultrasound device. In: Troccaz J, Grimson E, Mosges R, eds. *CVRMed-MRCAS '97.* Berlin: Springer-Verlag; 1997:459–466.
72. Erbe H, Kriete A, Jodicke A, Deinsberger W, Boker DK. 3D-ultrasonography and image matching for detection of brain shift during intracranial surgery. In: Lemke HU, Vannier MW, Inamura K, Farman AG, eds. *Computer Assisted Radiology (CAR) 1996.* Amsterdam: Elsevier Science; 1996:225–230.
73. Koivukangas J, Louhisalmi Y, Alakuijala J, Oikarinen J. Ultrasound-controlled neuronavigator-guided brain surgery. *J Neurosurg* 1993;79:36–42.
74. Hata N, Nabavi A, Wells WM, et al. Three-dimensional optical flow method for measurement of volumetric brain deformation from intraoperative MR images. *J Comput Assist Tomogr* 2000;24:531–538.
75. Miga MI, Paulsen KD, Hoopes PJ, Kennedy, FE Jr., Hartov A, Roberts DW. In vivo quantification of a homogeneous brain deformation model for updating preoperative images during surgery. *IEEE Trans Biomed Eng* 2000;47:266–273.
76. Miga MI, Paulsen KD, Lemery JM, et al. Model-updated image guidance: initial clinical experiences with gravity-induced brain deformation. *IEEE Trans Med Imaging* 1999;18:866–874.
77. Paulsen KD, Miga MI, Kennedy FE Jr, Hoopes PJ, Hartov A, Roberts DW. A computational model for tracking subsurface tissue deformation during stereotactic neurosurgery. *IEEE Trans Biomed Eng* 1999;46:213–225.
78. Sibson R. Studies in the robustness of multidimensional scaling: perturbational analysis of classical scaling. *J R Statist Soc B* 1979;41:217–229.
79. Darabi K, Grunert P, Perneczky A. Analysing the relationship between fiducial position and the geometrical error of intraoperative navigation [abstract]. *Comput Aided Surg* 1997;2:224.
80. Evans AC, Marrett S, Collins DL, Peters TM. Anatomical-functional correlative analysis of the human brain using three dimensional imaging systems. *Medical Imaging III: Image Processing.* Bellingham, WA: The International Society for Optical Engineering; 1989:264–274.

3

Spinal Registration Accuracy and Error

IAIN H. KALFAS

Interactive frameless stereotactic technology has been successfully applied to spinal surgery. By linking digitized image data to spinal surface anatomy, image-guided spinal navigation facilitates the surgeon's orientation to unexposed spinal structures, thereby improving the precision and accuracy of the surgery. It is typically used to optimize the placement of spinal fixation screws and to monitor the extent of complex decompressive procedures. It can also be used as a preoperative planning tool.

The critical step in applying stereotactic technology to spinal surgery is the registration process. Both paired point registration and surface mapping techniques have been applied to image-guided spinal navigation. This chapter discusses the accuracy and errors of these registration techniques.

Over the last decade, the surgical options for managing complex spinal disorders have expanded through the continued evolution of spinal instrumentation devices as well as a variety of surgical approaches to the spine. However, intraoperative orientation to unexposed spinal anatomy provides difficulties to even the most experienced spinal surgeon. Regardless of the approach selected, much of the spinal anatomy in the surgical field is not directly visualized in the operative field. This is not problematic for routine decompressive procedures but can pose significant problems during the management of complex disorders such as fractures, neoplasms, and deformities.

Orientation to this unexposed spinal anatomy is critical to the success of complex spinal surgery. In particular, the variety of spinal fixation techniques that utilize the placement of bone screws into the pedicles of the thoracic, lumbar, and sacral spine; into the lateral masses and across joints of the cervical spine; and across the vertebrae of the thoracic and lumbar spine require a thorough understanding of the spatial relationships of the unexposed spinal anatomy to that portion of the spine seen in the surgical field. Although standard intraoperative imaging (i.e., fluoroscopy) can be helpful, it does not provide an axial plane image. For most spinal screw fixation procedures, the axial plane provides critical trajectory information that cannot be provided by either a sagittal or a coronal image.

The development of image-guided technology for spinal surgery was influenced by these difficulties of intraoperative spatial orientation during complex surgery as well as by the limitations of standard intraoperative imaging.[1,2] The initial application of stereotactic principles to spinal surgery was not intuitive. Unlike intracranial surgery, an external frame system was not practical for spinal surgery. Furthermore, the use of surface landmarks or fiducials could not be used because of skin movement with respect to bony landmarks.[3,4] This is less of a problem with intracranial applications because of the relatively fixed position of the overlying scalp to a set of attached fiducials.

The application of stereotactic technology to spinal surgery involves using the rigid spinal anatomy itself as a frame of reference for registration of the image data to the spinal anatomy. Two separate techniques of registration can be applied. Paired point registration involves matching selected points in the image data set to their corresponding points in the spinal anatomy.

Alternatively, the surface mapping technique involves selecting multiple nondiscrete points only on the exposed and debrided surface of the spine in the surgical field. This technique does not require the preselection of points in the image set, although several discrete points in both the image data set and the surgical field are frequently required to improve the accuracy of surface mapping. The positional information of these points is transferred to the workstation, and a topographic map of the selected anatomy is created and "matched" to the patient's image set.

Typically, paired point registration can be done more quickly than surface mapping. The average time needed for paired point registration is 10 to 15 seconds. The time needed for surface mapping is much longer, with difficult cases requiring as much as 10 to 15 minutes. This time difference can significantly impact the length of the navigational procedure and the surgery itself.[5]

Regardless of the technique used, the registration process represents the step during image-guided navigation that can have the greatest effect on navigational accuracy. Registration accuracy is dependent on the surgeon carefully selecting the correct reference points or performing the surface mapping process. If properly performed, registration will allow for the display of reformatted, multiplanar CT or MRI images to assist the surgeon with orientation to the unexposed spinal anatomy.

■ Navigational Technique

A variety of navigational systems have evolved over the past decade. The common components of most of these systems include an image-processing workstation interfaced with a two-camera optical localizer (Fig. 3–1). The optical localizer tracks infrared light emitted by a series of light-emitting diodes (LEDs) mounted on a customized handheld navigational probe or selected surgical instruments (Fig. 3–2). Alternatively, the optical localizer itself can be the source of infrared light, which is continuously reflected back to the camera system by passive reflectors attached to the probe or selected surgical instruments.

The computer workstation knows the dimensions of each navigational probe or customized trackable surgical instrument and also recognizes the spacing of the LEDs or passive reflectors. The infrared light that is transmitted from or reflected by these instruments is relayed to the computer workstation, which can then calculate the precise location of the instrument tip in the surgical field as well as the location of the anatomic point on which the instrument tip is resting.

When applying navigational technology to spinal surgery, the standard surgical exposure for a particular procedure is carried out. The registration process is performed immediately after surgical exposure and prior to any planned decompressive procedure. This preserves

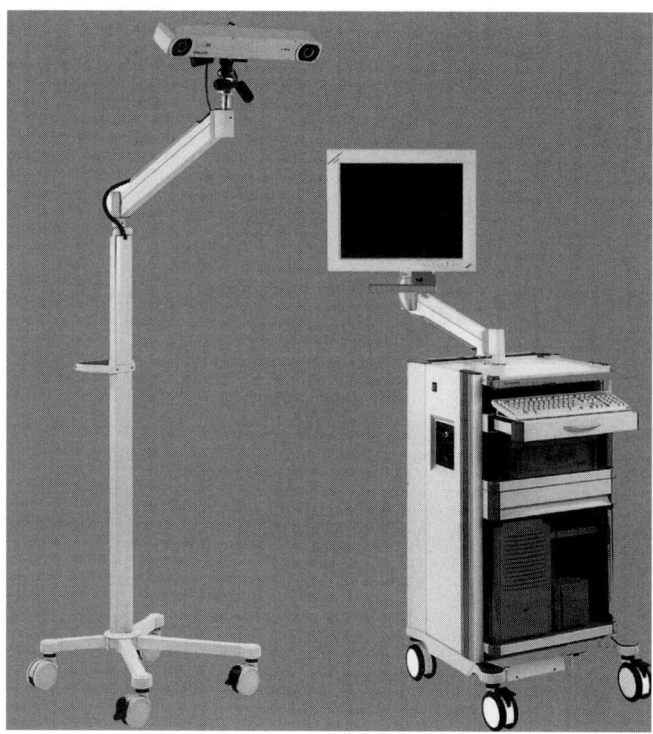

FIGURE 3–1. Image-guided navigational workstation with infrared camera localizer system.

the spinal anatomic landmarks that facilitate an easy and accurate registration process.

The registration process establishes a precise spatial relationship between the image space of the data and the physical space of the patient's corresponding surgical anatomy. If the patient is moved after registration, this spatial relationship is distorted, which creates navigational information that is inaccurate. This problem can be minimized by the optional use of a spinal tracking device consisting of a separate set of LEDs or passive reflectors mounted on an instrument that can be at-

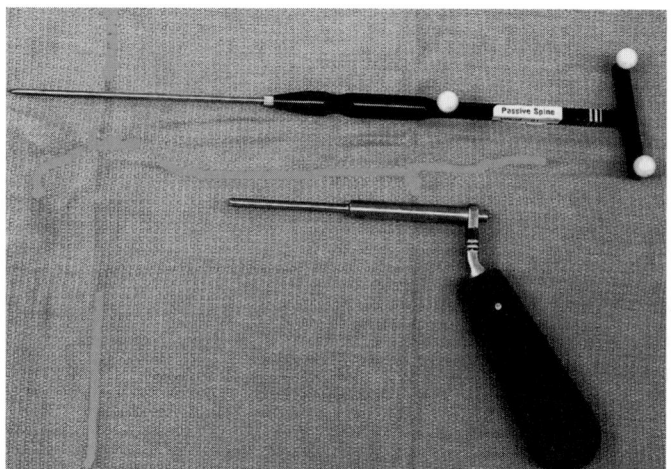

FIGURE 3–2. Navigation probe with drill guide for spinal surgery.

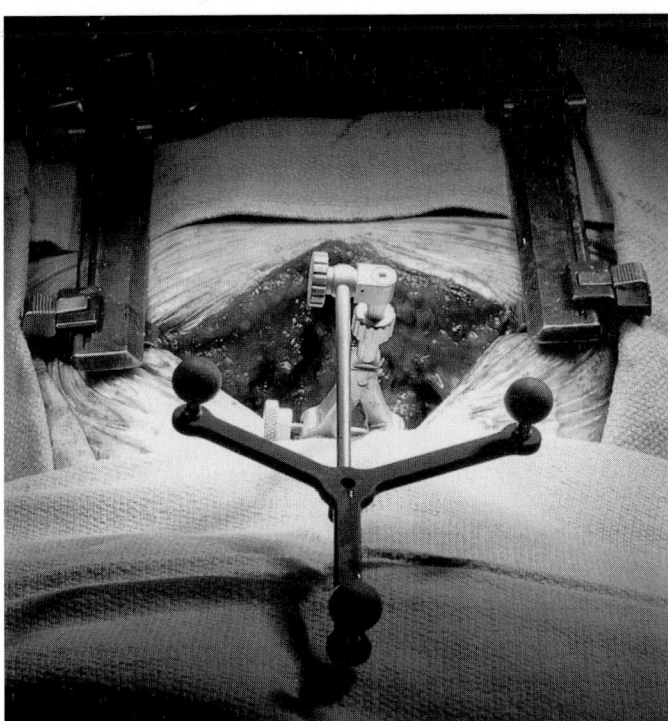

FIGURE 3–3. Reference frame attached to spinal anatomy. The reference frame monitors inadvertent movement of the spinal anatomy that may interfere with navigational accuracy.

tached to the exposed spinal anatomy (Fig. 3–3). The position of the reference frame can be tracked by the camera system. Movement of the frame alerts the navigational system to any inadvertent movement of the spine. The system can then make correctional steps to keep the registration process accurate and eliminate the need to repeat the registration process. The disadvantages of using a tracking device are the added time needed for its attachment to the spine, the need to maintain a line of sight between it and the camera, and the inconvenience of having to perform the procedure with the device placed in the surgical field.

Alternatively, image-guided spinal navigation can be performed without a tracking device.[1,2,5,6] This involves acknowledging the effect of patient movement on the accuracy of image-guided navigation and maintaining reasonable stable patient position during the relatively short amount of time needed (i.e., 10–20 seconds) for the selection of each appropriate screw trajectory. Patient movement can be caused by respiration, the surgical team leaning on the table, or a change of table position. Movement associated with patient respiration is negligible and does not require any tracking even in the thoracic spine. Although movement associated with leaning on the table or repositioning the table or the patient will affect registration accuracy, it can be easily avoided during the short navigational procedure. If inadvertent patient movement does occur, the registration process can be repeated.

Repeating the registration process is far more practical with the shorter paired point technique than it is with the more time-consuming surface mapping technique.

▪ Registration Accuracy

The ability to quantify and manipulate spatial information to relate one set of data to another is fundamental to surgical navigation. Accurately establishing the spatial relationships between image data and surgical anatomy is critical to the application of navigational technology to surgical procedures. Before the current, relatively inexpensive computing resources became available, stereotaxy relied on frame-based instrumentation and simple registration strategies. However, the advancement of computational power in the operating room has provided more efficient algebraic solutions to many of the registration tasks required for surgical navigation.

In the early seventeenth century, Pierre de Fermat and René Descartes independently recognized that two perpendicular lines could be used to identify any point within a plane.[7] The distance along each of these lines, termed x- and y-axes, from the origin (the intersection of the axes where each is typically assigned a value of 0) to a given point provides an ordered pair of numbers, or coordinates, unique to that point. This is referred to as the Cartesian coordinate system, in honor of Decartes, and may be extended to three dimensions, with x-, y-, and z-axes. This allows for each point in a given space to be uniquely and quantitatively defined.

Applying the coordinate system concept to image-guided spinal navigation involves recognizing the spinal anatomy as well as its corresponding image data set as two separate three-dimensional coordinate spaces. Each point in the two coordinate spaces can be assigned a specific x, y, and z coordinate value. There are six separate parameters relating these coordinates: the three angles of rotation by which the x, y, and z coordinate axes can be made parallel to one another and three distances along each of the axes by which the origins of the two coordinate systems can be superimposed. The spatial relationship between separate coordinate spaces can then be established by the registration process.

The most common method of registration in the spine involves determining a rigid-body transformation with the assumption that the morphology of each individual vertebra remains constant. The spatial relationship of one point at a single vertebral level to another point at that same vertebral level remains constant regardless of changes in patient position between image acquisition and operative alignment.

A series of complex mathematical calculations, termed transformation matrices, define the registration process.8,9 For each point existing in one coordinate space, the analogous point in a second coordinate space may be identified. Multiple matrices are required to account for each rotation and translation about the three axes as well as for scaling differences between separate coordinate spaces. Current computational power allows for these calculations to be done rapidly and accurately.

In the surgical setting, proper application of the registration process allows the surgeon to select a point in the exposed surgical field and view the corresponding point in the image data set on the computer workstation. Multiple planar images oriented either to the long axis of the spine or, more commonly, to the long axis of a selected trajectory are displayed in near real time as the surgeon moves the navigational probe through the field.

The accuracy of the registration process depends on several variables. The acquisition of preoperative spinal images can potentially affect accuracy, although standardization of image slice thickness, orientation, and spacing has minimized these problems. Potential problems associated with image transfer, improper tool specification, and software errors have also been significantly reduced.

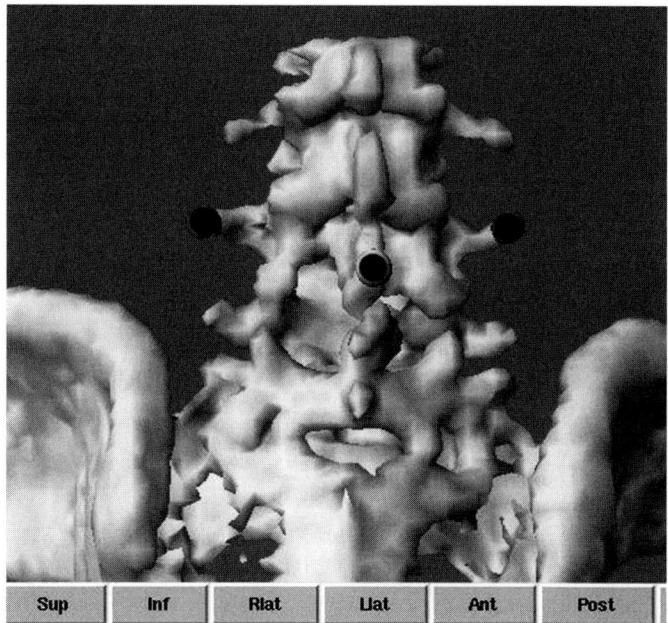

FIGURE 3–4. Navigational workstation screen demonstrating a paired point registration plan. Three discrete bony landmarks are selected at a single vertebral level. In this case the tips of the two transverse processes and the spinous process have been selected at the level to be instrumented. The paired point registration process is complete when the surgeon precisely places the probe on each of the three corresponding points in the surgical field.

■ Registration Techniques

Improper surgical technique is the primary source of registration error. Successful application of image-guided spinal navigation requires an understanding of the principles of registration, and failure to provide the necessary attention to detail assures less navigational accuracy.

The simplest and most commonly used method of achieving registration of separate coordinate spaces with surgical navigational systems is that of matching a set of ordered points visible to both the imaging study and the intraoperative digitizer.10–14 With this paired point technique, a minimum of three such noncolinear pairs of points is required for determination of the transformation, although many systems allow for the use of additional points. For image-guided spinal navigation, discrete bony landmarks that can be identified in the preoperative image set as well as the surgical field are used as registration points. These points typically can include the tip of a spinous or transverse process, a prominent facet or osteophyte, or any other reliably identified feature. Ideally, these registration points, or fiducials, should be confined to one vertebral level (Fig. 3–4). A separate registration is performed for each vertebral level undergoing navigation. This segmental registration process eliminates any potential distortion that can occur between the patient's preoperative scanned position (supine) and the intraoperative position (supine, prone, or lateral decubitus).

This paired point technique is limited in that it requires the surgeon to precisely identify points in the surgical field that correspond to those points selected in the image data set. A casual approach to this step may easily create significant registration errors. Points can be selected at the wrong level, on the wrong side, or at the wrong site on the correct landmark (i.e., 2–3 mm from the apex of a spinous process). Points that are too close together or are colinear or coplanar may also introduce significant registration error. Paired point registration may also be limited in its application to anterior spinal surgery or prior posterior spinal surgery. In both cases it may be difficult to identify the appropriate number of discrete landmarks to serve as fiducials.

With the surface-matching registration technique, an unordered set of points is used to match the surface of an anatomic structure to its corresponding surface in the image data set. A number of surface-matching techniques have been developed, the best known being the "hat and head" matching algorithm of Pelizzari and Chen.15,16 In this method, the navigational probe is sequentially placed on a series of arbitrarily selected points over the exposed anatomic surface (Fig. 3–5). The position of each point is subsequently relayed back to the workstation, which then

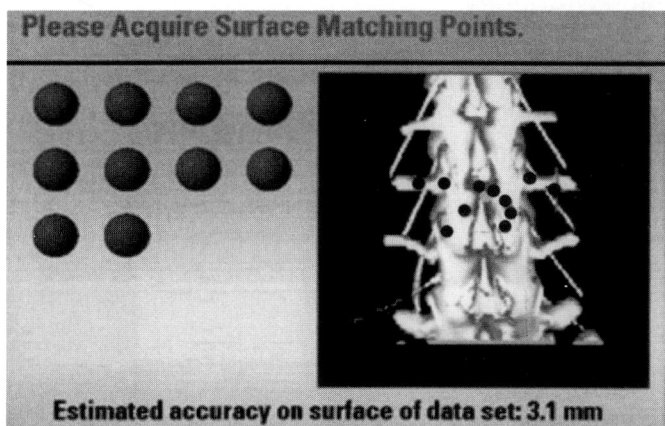

FIGURE 3–5. Navigational workstation screen demonstrating surface mapping registration. A series of points are selected over the exposed surface of the spinal anatomy. "Matching" of points with preselected data points in the image set is not necessary. The navigational workstation receives the series of selected points and creates a map of the registered spinal anatomy.

creates a "topographic map" of the selected anatomy and relates it to the stored image data.

This technique does not require the preselection of anatomic landmarks in the image data set, which makes surface mapping theoretically more easily applied than paired point registration to anterior spinal surgery and to the setting of previous posterior spinal surgery. Also, the surgeon is not required to match corresponding points in two separate coordinate spaces, which means there is less potential for user error.

However, surface mapping requires more time to complete than paired point registration, which necessitates the use of a reference frame during the registration and navigational steps. If a reference frame is not used and the patient is inadvertently moved after registration, the lengthy surface mapping technique must be repeated. This is not as much of a problem with the paired point registration because this technique can be more easily repeated than the surface mapping technique.

Another disadvantage of surface mapping is that it requires a thorough soft-tissue debridement of the exposed spinal surface. Without this debridement, false data points may be entered resulting in an inaccurate registration of the anatomy. This preparation of the spinal surface also contributes to the longer time needed for surface mapping as opposed to paired point registration.

When either registration process has been completed, most navigational workstations will calculate the error (expressed in millimeters). This is not a linear error but rather a volumetric calculation comparing the spacing of registration points in the surgical field with those corresponding points in the image data set. This figure is, at best, a relative indicator of accuracy.

Regardless of the registration technique used, a critical step of the navigational process in the spine is the verification of registration accuracy. This step is typically performed immediately after completing the registration process and is more of an absolute indicator of registration accuracy. The surgeon places the navigational probe on a discrete landmark in the surgical field. With the navigational system now tracking the movement and position of the probe, the trajectory line and cursor on the workstation screen will, if accurate registration has been achieved, move to the corresponding point in the image data set (Fig. 3–6A). If registration accuracy has not been achieved, the cursor and trajectory line may rest on something other than the point selected in the surgical field (Fig. 3–6B). If this occurs to a significant degree, the registration process must be repeated.

Glossop et al[17] assessed the in vitro accuracy of various registration techniques. The lumbar spine of a cadaver was implanted with four steel beads measuring one mm in diameter. A computed tomography (CT) scan of the spine was obtained and transferred to a navigational workstation. Registration was performed using either the implanted fiducial beads, a paired point technique (seven discrete anatomic landmarks), or a combination of the paired point technique and a surface mapping technique that involved the additional random selection of 30 to 35 points over the exposed spinal anatomy.

Following registration with each of the three techniques, guidewires were placed into the lumbar pedicles using navigational guidance. A second CT scan was obtained to determine the accuracy or wire placement using each individual registration technique. As predicted, registration using the implanted fiducials provided the smallest degree of insertion error followed by the combined paired point/surface mapping technique. The paired point technique had the highest error although the differences between the three techniques were small and within clinical tolerances.[17]

■ Clinical Application of Registration Principles

The practical clinical applications of strict registration principles to spinal surgery can be difficult and restrictive. Although intuitively it seems that every attempt to achieve greater navigational accuracy for spinal procedures should be made, there comes a point where additional accuracy is no longer needed. The concept of clinically relevant accuracy relates to the fact that only enough accuracy to achieve a specific clinical task (i.e., placing a 6 mm diameter pedicle screw into a pedicle that may measure 14–16 mm in diameter) is required. Once clinically relevant accuracy has been reached,

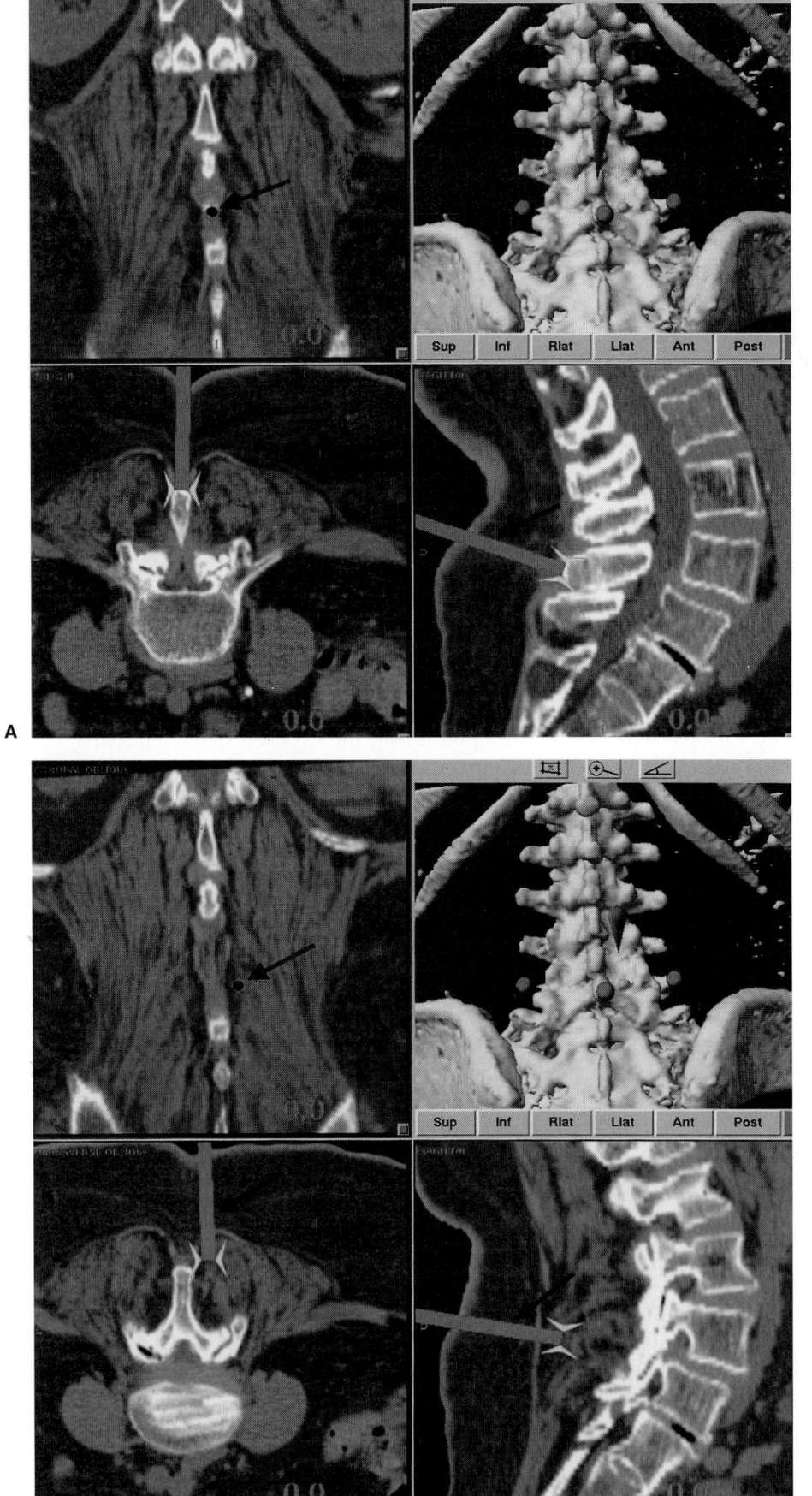

FIGURE 3–6. (A). Navigational workstation screen demonstrating satisfactory verification of registration accuracy. While the navigational probe is positioned on the L4 spinous process in the surgical field, the workstation screen should show the cursor and trajectory line in a correlative position in the CT image set. (B). Navigational workstation screen demonstrating an unsatisfactory verification of registration accuracy. If the navigational probe is positioned on the L4 spinous process in the surgical field but the workstation screen shows the cursor and trajectory line is a non-correlative position (i.e., not on the L4 spinous process), accurate registration has not been achieved and the registration process needs to be repeated before proceeding with spinal navigation.

more accuracy is not required. Attempting to achieve additional accuracy above the clinically relevant threshold requires more time and effort on the part of the surgeon in the operating room. This results in greater technical complexity of the navigational procedure, which in turn increases the overall length of the surgery. It defeats the purpose of bringing new technologies to the operating room, specifically to improve surgical precision, simplify the procedure, and reduce the operative time and morbidity.

The key to optimizing the design and use of image-guided navigational technology is to recognize realistic clinical expectations. The threshold of clinically relevant accuracy varies from one type of procedure to another. For example, the degree of accuracy required for placing C1–2 transarticular screws will be greater than that required for positioning lumbar pedicle screws. Clinical experience with navigational systems over the past several years has helped define realistic expectations in an effort to streamline the technology and make it as user-friendly as possible. Standardization and simplification of new technologies ultimately improve their rate of acceptance by surgeons. This is analogous to the evolution of various spinal fixation systems. In general, as each new generation of spinal fixation systems evolved they became easier to use and more versatile than the previous generations.

Registration is the critical step to image-guided spinal navigation. It is also the step that can take the most time to complete and introduce the most error to the process. There is a fine line between simplifying the registration process and sacrificing clinically relevant accuracy. However, simplifying the registration process simplifies the entire navigational procedure. This can realistically be done in most cases by using the paired point registration technique. This technique takes much less time than surface mapping and, if done correctly, provides the surgeon with enough accuracy for even C1–2 transarticular screw fixation. In addition, paired point registration gives the surgeon the option of using a reference frame. The minimal amount of time needed for the paired point technique also provides the surgeon the ability to repeat the registration procedure if the patient has been inadvertently moved after the initial registration. As already mentioned, re-registration using the surface mapping technique cannot be as easily and rapidly repeated, making spinal tracking a necessity in this case.

■ Conclusions

Image-guided spinal navigational technology has proven to be a versatile and effective adjunct for managing patients with complex spinal disorders. The registration process is the critical step for this technology to provide useful clinical information. However, it is also the greatest source of navigational error and time consumption. It is necessary for surgeons using spinal navigation systems to have a thorough understanding of the principles of spinal registration and to recognize the limitations of registration and navigational techniques. Image-guided spinal navigation is not a substitute for a surgeon's knowledge of the pertinent surgical anatomy or the correct surgical technique; it will not make an inexperienced surgeon capable. However, by providing clinically relevant accuracy for a variety of spinal procedures, it can make an experienced surgeon more effective and precise while minimizing or eliminating the need for intraoperative imaging, shortening the length of the procedure, and reducing the rate of patient morbidity.

REFERENCES

1. Kalfas IH, Kormos DW, Murphy MA, et al. Application of frameless stereotaxy to pedicle screw fixation of the spine. *J Neurosurg* 1995;83:641–647.
2. Murphy MA, McKenzie RL, Kormos DW, Kalfas IH. Frameless stereotaxis for the insertion of lumbar pedicle screws: a technical note. *J Clin Neuroscience* 1994;1(4):257–260.
3. Brodwater BK, Roberts DW, Nakajima T, Friets EM, Strohbehn JW. Extracranial application of the frameless stereotactic operating microscope: experience with lumbar spine. *Neurosurgery* 1993;32:209–213.
4. Bryant JT, Reid JG, Smith BL, Stevenson JM. A method for determining vertebral body positions in the sagittal plane using skin markers. *Spine* 1989;14:258–265.
5. Kalfas IH. Image-guided spinal navigation. *Clin Neurosurg* 1999;46:70–88.
6. Kalfas IH. Frameless stereotaxy assisted spinal surgery. In: Rengachary SS, ed. *Neurosurgery Operative Color Atlas*. Lebanon, PA: AANS Publications; 2000:123–134.
7. West BH, Griesbach EN, Taylor JD, Taylor LT. *The Prentice-Hall Encyclopedia of Mathematics*. Englewood Cliffs, NJ: Prentice-Hall; 1982:119–126.
8. Foley JD, Van Dam A. *Fundamentals of Interactive Computer Graphics*. Reading, MA: Addison-Wesley; 1984:245–266.
9. Lemieux L, Henri CJ, Wootton R, Collins DL, Peters TM. The mathematics of stereotactic localization. In: Thomas DGT, ed. *Stereotactic and Image Directed Surgery of Brain Tumors*. Edinburgh: Churchill Livingstone; 1993:193–216.
10. Day R, Heilbrun MP, Koehler S, McDonald P, Peters W, Siemionow V. Three-point transformation for integration of multiple coordinate systems: application to tumor, functional, and fractionated radiosurgery stereotactic planning. *Stereotact Funct Neurosurg* 1994;63:76–79.
11. Friets EM, Strohbehn JW, Hatch JF, Roberts DW. A frameless stereotaxic operating microscope for neurosurgery. *IEEE Trans Biomed Eng* 1989;36:608–617.
12. Heilbrun MP, Koehler S, MacDonald P, Siemionow V, Peters W. Preliminary experience using an optimized three-point transformation algorithm for spatial registration of coordinate systems: a method of noninvasive localization using frame-based stereotactic guidance systems. *J Neurosurg* 1994;81:676–682.

13. Maciunas RJ, Fitzpatrick JM, Galloway RL, Allen GS. Beyond stereotaxy: extreme levels of application accuracy are provided by implantable fiducial markers for interactive image-guided neurosurgery. In: Maciunas RJ, ed. *Interactive Image-Guided Neurosurgery*. Park Ridge, IL: American Association of Neurological Surgeons; 1993:259–270.
14. Roberts DW, Strohbehn JW, Hatch JF, Murray W, Kettenberger H. A frameless stereotaxic integration of computerized tomographic imaging and the operating microscope. *J Neurosurg* 1986;65:545–549.
15. Pellizzari CA, Chen GTY, Spelbring DR, Weichselbaum RR, Chen C. Accurate three-dimensional registration of CT, PET, and/or MR images of the brain. *J Comput Assist Tomogr* 1989;13:20–26.
16. Pellizzari CA, Levin DN, Chen GTY, Chen CT. Image registration based on anatomic surface matching. In: Maciunas RJ, ed. *Interactive Image-Guided Neurosurgery*. Park Ridge, IL: American Association of Neurological Surgeons: 1993:47–62.
17. Glossop ND, Hu RW, Randle JA. Computer-aided pedicle screw placement using frameless sterotaxis. *Spine* 1996;21:2026–2034.

4

The Optical Digitizer

ISABELLE M. GERMANO AND HAREL DEUTSCH

Image-guided neurosurgery stemmed from the need to maintain the advantages while overcoming the limitations of frame-based stereotaxy neurosurgery. Accuracy, the main benefit of a stereotactic system, is obtained by employing a rigid coordinate frame that provides a stable frame of reference and an aiming arc assembly that is mechanically stable as it holds the probe in position along a trajectory. Unfortunately, these components also produce the greatest limitations in the surgical space. Thus, several investigators have pursued novel technologies of interactive image-guided neurosurgery to provide accurate intraoperative cranial navigation without being constrained by the design limitations inherent to stereotactic frame systems.

Interactive image-guided neurosurgical systems include four fundamental components: a method for registration of image space to physical space, an interactive localization device, a computer and interface, and methods of real-time intraoperative feedback. Interactive localization devices include: mechanical arms, digitizers (sonic, optical, magnetic), machine-video devices, real-time ultrasonography, and intraoperative magnetic resonance and computed tomography (MR-CT).

Bucholz and colleagues first introduced the use of the optical digitizer for intracranial navigation in 1993.[1,2] Since its introduction, this interactive localization device has proved very helpful in image-guided neurosurgery. Consequently, it became an integral component of several currently marketed image-guided systems.[3-9] The senior author has been using the optical digitizer in her clinical practice since August 1993.[3,4] This chapter provides a brief technical overview of the optical digitizer and other components needed for neurosurgical navigation, and reviews the basic steps of the optical digitizer's clinical use for intracranial procedures.

■ Technical Overview

Navigation systems utilizing the optical digitizer include the following components: (1) the digitizer; (2) a light detector array or "cameras;" (3) a reference frame hosting "fixed" light-emitting diodes (LEDs), (4) surgical instruments with LEDs that can be tracked by the digitizer, and (5) a computer workstation and software to reformat and display preoperative images and to render intraoperative localization of the surgical instrument(s) overlapped to the preoperative images (Fig. 4–1). Additionally, some systems have a real-time intraoperative updating of the images using ultrasound or magnetic resonance imaging (MRI).[10]

Optical digitizer

The critical component of an image-guided system is the three-dimensional (3-D) digitizer, which determines position. The accuracy of the intraoperative localization will be limited by that of the digitizer used. Digitizers are computerized systems that provide coordinate addresses for any accessible point within their working volumes. They can be classified into two broad groups: linked and nonlinked. Linked digitizers require a mechanical link between the digitizer and the pointer used intraopera-

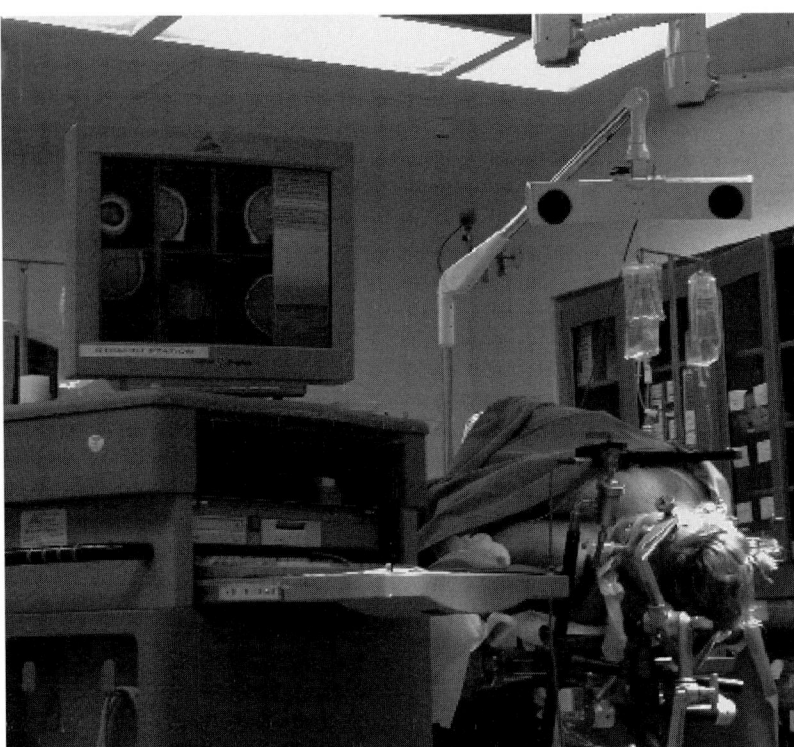

FIGURE 4–1. The computer workstation, optical digitizer, camera array, and reference arc demonstrating the intraoperative setup (StealthStation, Louisville, CO).

tively to confirm localization.[11] This type of digitizer is typically a mechanical arm and relies upon angle detectors located in joints within the arm to determine the position. By determining the angle of each joint, the position of the tip of the device can be determined with reference to its base. The base is connected with the patient's head, and the tip is registered to the preoperative images. Thus, by moving the tip of the arm one can determine its location relative to the preoperative images. The nonlinked digitizers, rather than relying on the link just described, rely upon the detection of signals generated by emitters or receptor arrays. A variety of digitizing technologies are currently available, including optical, sonic, and magnetic digitizers.[1,11–13] Most optical digitizers are based on multiple cameras fitted with linear-charged coupled devices and cylindrical lenses that detect LEDs or reflective devices within the surgical field.

Light detector array

The optical digitizer uses a camera array to detect the position of infrared light emitted by LEDs. These camera arrays are mounted on the reference frame and on the surgical instruments (see the section, Surgical instruments). Usually the detector array is placed 3 to 4 feet over the patient's lower extremities. There is a "sweet" location spot for the detection array, and this is displayed on the computer screen while the array is being positioned (see the section, Positioning and Registration).

Reference frame

The reference frame hosts a fixed set of LEDs, typically four or five, and is usually mounted to maintain a fixed relationship to the skull or spine throughout the surgery. This can be accomplished by mounting the reference frame to the head holder for cranial procedures, directly to the skull for skull base procedures, or to the spinous process for spinal cases.

Surgical instruments

Almost any instrument can be equipped with LEDs. Because the coagulation forceps are the most frequently used in microsurgery, the authors usually prefer to use this instrument for cranial navigation. For most instruments, a linear array of LEDs, typically three, is sufficient to obtain accurate localization of the instrument in space. For other instruments with a more complex 3-D shape, the LEDs, typically four, are mounted on a butterfly-shaped structure to provide for redundancy and allow for calibration of the instrument tip.

Computer workstation and software

Computer workstations use commercially available hardware. Examples include the StealthStation using a UNIX-based work station (Indigo graphics workstation, Silicon Graphics, Mountain View, CA) and the Cbyon suite (Cbyon, Palo Alto, CA) utilizing a dual processor PC running Windows 2000 software and its proprietary graphic engine.

Images can be displayed using a variety of reconstructed images. The three standard views, axial, sagittal, and coronal, with a 3-D reconstruction are often used for preliminary planning. Orthogonal views obtained in the trajectory of the probe are particularly helpful in planning a biopsy (Fig. 4–2).[14] The "probe view" is an interactive view that allows visualization of the planned path of microsurgical dissection. Additionally, neurophysiological atlases can be overlapped to standard views to facilitate surgical planning for movement disorders (Fig. 4–3).[15] Finally, image fusion using different modalities, such as functional MRI (fMRI), CT, positron emission tomography (PET), and others can be used to improve planning for functional cases. The position of the surgical instrument is represented by a crosshair on the above described images. The monitor displaying the images is usually kept to the surgeon's side. Some surgeons, however, prefer not to move the head from the operating field or microscope. Therefore, these views can be incorporated to a head-mounted display or to the optics of the operating microscope.[16,17]

■ Neuronavigation Procedure

Neuronavigation allows real-time feedback whereby the position of surgical instruments is projected over the preoperatively acquired images. Additionally, intraoperative update of the images can reflect the amount of resection performed. The option to have intraoperative, real-time feedback on the location of the surgical instruments adds the following steps to the neurosurgical procedure: preoperative imaging and data transfer according to established protocols, planning and virtual surgery, and registration (i.e., the process that allows "overlap" between the imaging and physical spaces). Although a learning curve is required to optimize the smoothness of such operations, they eventually become routine and do not interfere significantly with the overall surgical procedure.

Preoperative imaging and data transfer

As just described, image-guided neurosurgery allows the surgeon to obtain intraoperative real-time visualization

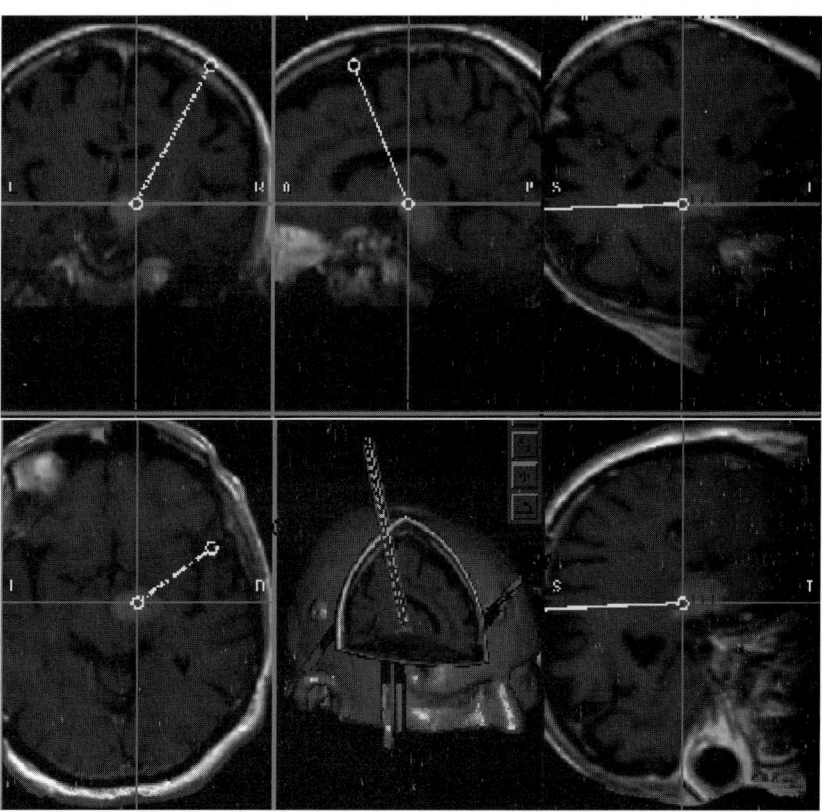

FIGURE 4–2. Intraoperative photo of the computer screen displaying magnetic resonance reformatted images used for surgical planning and intraoperative guidance. Clockwise from the upper left: coronal, sagittal, "trajectory" 1, axial, 3-D, and "trajectory" two. Trajectory views are images reformatted in planes orthogonal to the surgical instrument. These are particularly helpful when planning for a biopsy (StealthStation, Louisville, CO).

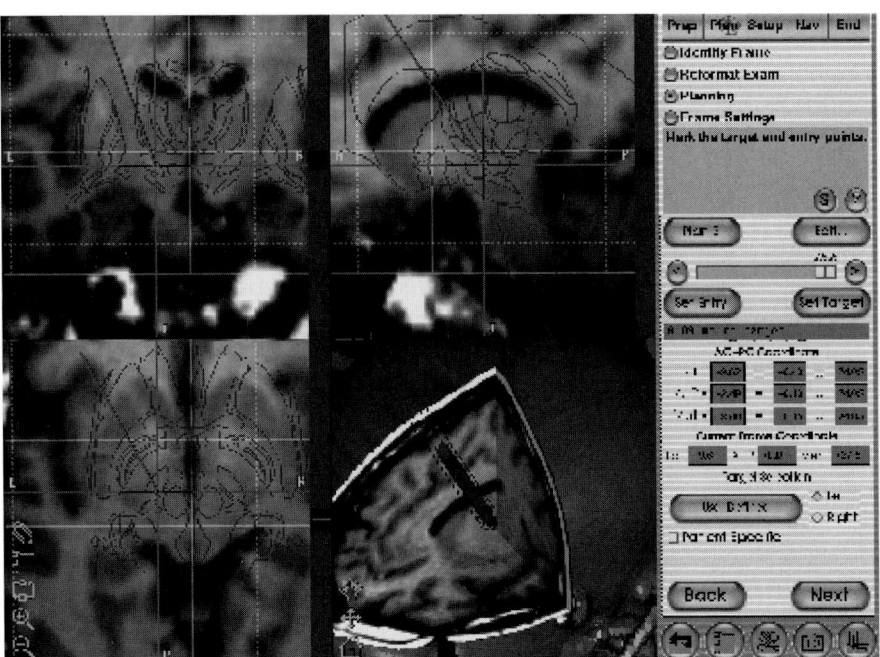

FIGURE 4–3. Intraoperative photo of the computer screen displaying magnetic resonance images. Clockwise from upper left: coronal, sagittal, axial, and 3-D. A patient-fitted Schaltenbrand neurophysiological atlas is displayed overlapped to the triplanar images to further assist the planning and intraoperative guidance of placement of a deep brain electrode in the subthalamic nucleus (StealthStation, Louisville, CO).

of the surgical instruments overlapped on the patient's preoperative images. To accomplish this, preoperative images need to be registered to the patient's anatomy and must be acquired using a specific protocol.[3,4] Two aspects must be taken into account prior to obtaining preoperative images for neuronavigation: protocol for image acquisition and use of fiducials.

Image acquisition

The protocol for image acquisition has a significant impact on the accuracy of the frameless system used. In particular the thickness and field of view of the preoperative images dictate the ultimate accuracy of the neuronavigation. In fact, the accuracy of the information obtained from the navigation system is equal to the thickness of the images plus the error inherent to each system used. Therefore, for a system that claims "one millimeter" accuracy, in the best circumstances this should be added to the 2, 3, or 4 mm thickness of the images used. Thus, when reading or hearing about the publicized "submillimetric accuracy" of frame-based or frameless systems the user should be aware that the claimed accuracy must be added to the thickness of the preoperative images. For this reason, it is advisable to use thin sections for preoperative images. Additionally, when planning the image acquisition scout, the surgeon should make sure that the region of interest is included. Thus, when planning for an entry point on the convexity, this must be part of the scanned field to allow accurate localization of the entry point intraoperatively.

Images are then transferred to the workstation over a local network using a conventional DICOM protocol or employing the archive media present on the scanners used, typically a digital archive tape (DAT) or CD-ROM.

Fiducials or markers

A variety of registration techniques offer alternative methods for mapping images to each other or to the physical space. Point-based registration methods define corresponding points in different images or physical space, determine their spatial coordinates, and calculate a geometric transformation between the volumes. These points, known as fiducials, may be extrinsic and must be applied to the patient prior to obtaining the preoperative images, or intrinsic and based on patient-specific anatomical landmarks. Registration using the patient's own anatomical landmarks is an appealing concept because it obviates the need to have trained personnel applying the fiducials. This method is currently used mostly for spine surgery. For cranial surgery, however, studies and clinical experience have shown that this process may be less accurate[18] than extrinsic markers and definitely more time consuming. Two types of markers have been used for extrinsic registration: adhesive markers that are affixed to the scalp, and implantable markers that are anchored to the skull. In both cases, these are applied before the acquisition of the images. We use adhesive markers because they are well tolerated by the patient and in our experience result in good accuracy.[3,4] We apply the markers the day of the scan (IZI Medical

Products, Baltimore, MD), and this is typically obtained the day of the surgical procedure. The markers are usually applied around the circumference of the head to achieve the highest accuracy. We apply 10 to 12 markers to allow us the greatest degree of freedom during the registration process (see discussion in the following text).

Planning and virtual surgery

As part of the conventional routine surgery, the surgeon displays x-ray films, CT and MRI slices, and even 3-D image reconstruction on light boxes along the wall of the operating room. These are used before and during the surgery, with the surgeon stepping away from the operating field as necessary to review where a particular structure lies before continuing safely with the surgery. After transferring and reformatting the preoperative images, the surgeon can use image-guided technology with commercially available software to create special "windowing" effects whereby layers of anatomy can be "cut out" through the use of a "transparent" window.

The rapid evolution of computer software allows ongoing improvement of the software used in neuronavigation. Surgical planning is performed using a multimodular software application for planning and interactive surgical assistance on intracranial or spinal procedures. Traditionally, the computation-intensive and time-consuming process necessary to create such images has hampered the 3-D display of medical data set. Recent advances in computer graphics have overcome most of these limitations. Interactivity in 3-D reconstruction is important in that it allows the surgeon and the physician in training to predict the desirable angle for viewing pathological abnormalities. We perform surgical planning for all procedures; however, this is particularly important for biopsies and functional cases where the precision of the entry point and the accuracy of the chosen trajectory determine the success of the surgery.[14,15]

New advances in computer technology allow "virtual surgery" before the operation by using sophisticated software that enables the surgeon to see the anatomy of interest and the structures beyond that anatomy. New algorithms in computation technology and 3-D imaging can generate a perspective volume rendering (PVR).[18-20] Using PVR, the user can "fly" through and around the data and generate virtual endoscopic views. This technique also allows viewing of tissues that would be inaccessible to conventional endoscopy. The main advantage of PVR, in comparison with surface rendering, is the accessibility of the whole volume at any stage of the "fly through" process. Figure 4–4 shows an example of virtual planning using virtual endoscopy.

Virtual reality simulation is becoming a standard part of the surgeon's training. Although virtual surgery will not replace current hands-on teaching about new surgical procedures, it will give surgeons a chance to learn complex anatomy inside-out and gain extra practice before the surgery is performed. The technology can also test surgical skills. Work in progress in different laboratories is exploring the possibility of developing reliable simulation models for evaluating whether the surgeon performs the steps of a procedure in the right order and in an appropriate length of time. Preoperative planning using virtual surgery is not only a powerful teaching tool, it allows the surgeon to optimize the approach and, thus, to perform minimally invasive and safer surgery.

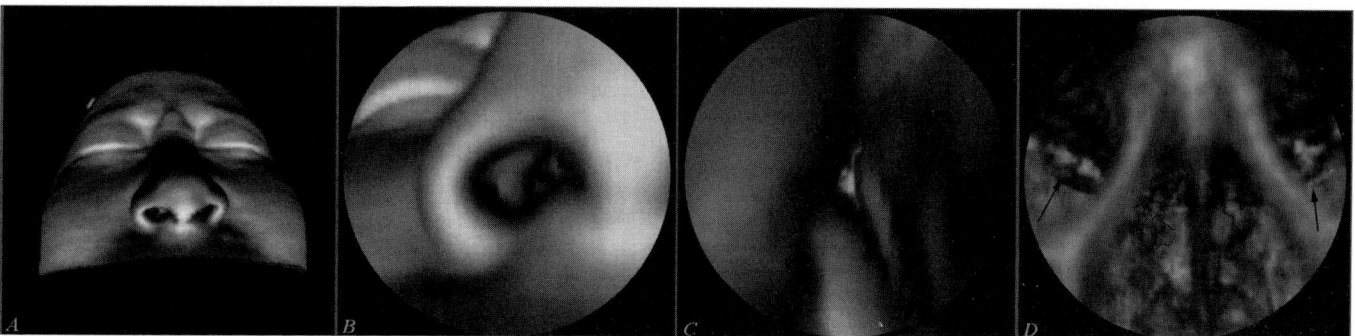

FIGURE 4–4. Photograph of the computer screen demonstrating virtual surgery using Volumetric Surgical Navigation software (Cbyon Inc, Palo Alto, CA). This navigation software allows for the "fly-through" approach through the patient's anatomy. Perspective volumetric images are updated at 15 frames/sec, turning any surgical tool into a virtual endoscope. (A). 3-D rendering of the patient's face. (B). Magnified view of the patient's nostril. (C). Virtual endoscopic view of the turbinate. (D). The surgeon can "see beyond" the tip of the instrument where carodit and optic nerves are located (arrows). (Courtesy of Ramin Shahidi, Ph.D.)

Positioning and registration

The registration of image space onto physical space requires a pointer with LEDs. By having three or more LEDs attached to a surgical instrument, the instrument's position in space can be tracked over time by triangulation techniques. These optical triangulation techniques are highly accurate and precise.

A variety of techniques offer alternative methods for achieving the mapping of images to the physical space. The two most used techniques are point-based and surface-based registration. The former is based on landmarks or fiducials as already described. The latter is based on fitting sets of points extracted from contours in one image set to surface models extracted from contours in other images or from physical coordinates of the patient's cranium. This technique, however, is less accurate than point-based registration.[21] Additional discussion on this topic can be found in Chapters 2 and 3 of this book.

The optical position sensor consisting of any array of three linear charge-coupled devices is positioned over the operating room table. In most units, the computer software will help the surgeon find the "best" location by determining the "sweet" spot of the camera alignment. The camera array will visualize and triangulate on all surgical instruments equipped with LEDs during the surgery. After proper positioning of the patient and before registration, the reference emitter is attached to the head holder (see Fig. 4–1). The reference emitter provides a fixed point in the physical space that covaries with the patient's head during any patient movement and is independent of movement at anytime. By registering image space through touching the fiducial markers with the pointer, the frame of reference established by the fiducial markers is calibrated and therefore continuously reestablished relative to this fixed point of the reference emitter. As a result, the patient may be moved in any surgically appropriate way throughout the course of surgery, making table tilting possible without needing re-registration.

After the patient is placed in the appropriate surgical position, registration of image space to physical space is carried out. Each marker has a central divot that corresponds to the geometric center of the imaging fiducial marker. The surgeon first recognizes and enters in the computer the location of all markers on the images. This is done by clicking with the computer mouse at the center of each marker. Then the center of each marker is touched by a nonsterile probe on the patient's head. By touching the markers with the pointer, the surgeon touches the point that corresponds to the fiducial point in the imaging fiducial marker. The registration is thus completed. At the end of the registration process, the surgeon must localize a few anatomical landmarks on the patient's head with the nonsterile probe and see in real time the projection of the probe on the preoperative images. This is necessary to visually confirm the accuracy of the registration process. A discrepancy between the location of the pointer on the patient's head and its projection on the preoperative images requires the registration process to be repeated until it is sufficiently accurate for the surgery to proceed.

Intraoperative real-time feedback and navigation

After the registration process is completed, the surgeon can visualize in real time the position of the surgical instruments overlapped on the computer-reconstructed images (Fig. 4–5). By having three or more LEDs attached to a surgical instrument, the instrument's position in space can be tracked over time by triangulation techniques. The LEDs on each instrument must be visible to the camera array at all times to receive the intraoperative feedback. We use mostly the bipolar cautery to guide our open craniotomies and a probe guide to guide the biopsies or functional cases. Various multiplanar display options are available to the surgeon. Whereas when planning the surgery we find it interesting to use multiple options, in most surgeries we deem it sufficient to have triplanar and 3-D images. Additionally, we use images displaying planes perpendicular to the axis or along the axis of the instrument to optimize the operative trajectory. Comprehension of such views, however, may sometimes be difficult and nonintuitive when the surgeon is new to this technology.

The digital scan information retains historical data and therefore is subject to becoming outdated during the course of surgical manipulation of tissue. Thus, the frameless equipment can be interfaced with image-guided technology capable of updating the images. Bucholz et al[9] first introduced the concept of such correction using ultrasound. This topic is reviewed in Chapter 15. Additionally, this information can be retrieved from intraoperative MR images, as described in Chapter 16.

■ Clinical Applications

Clinical experience with image-guided surgery using the optical digitizer has been growing over the past 10 years as the principles of "minimally invasive surgery" become general practice. The following is a brief overview of the uses of this technology in neurosurgery; details on each application can be found in Part II of this book.

Perhaps the most common application of frameless navigation is resection of subcortical and deep lesions,

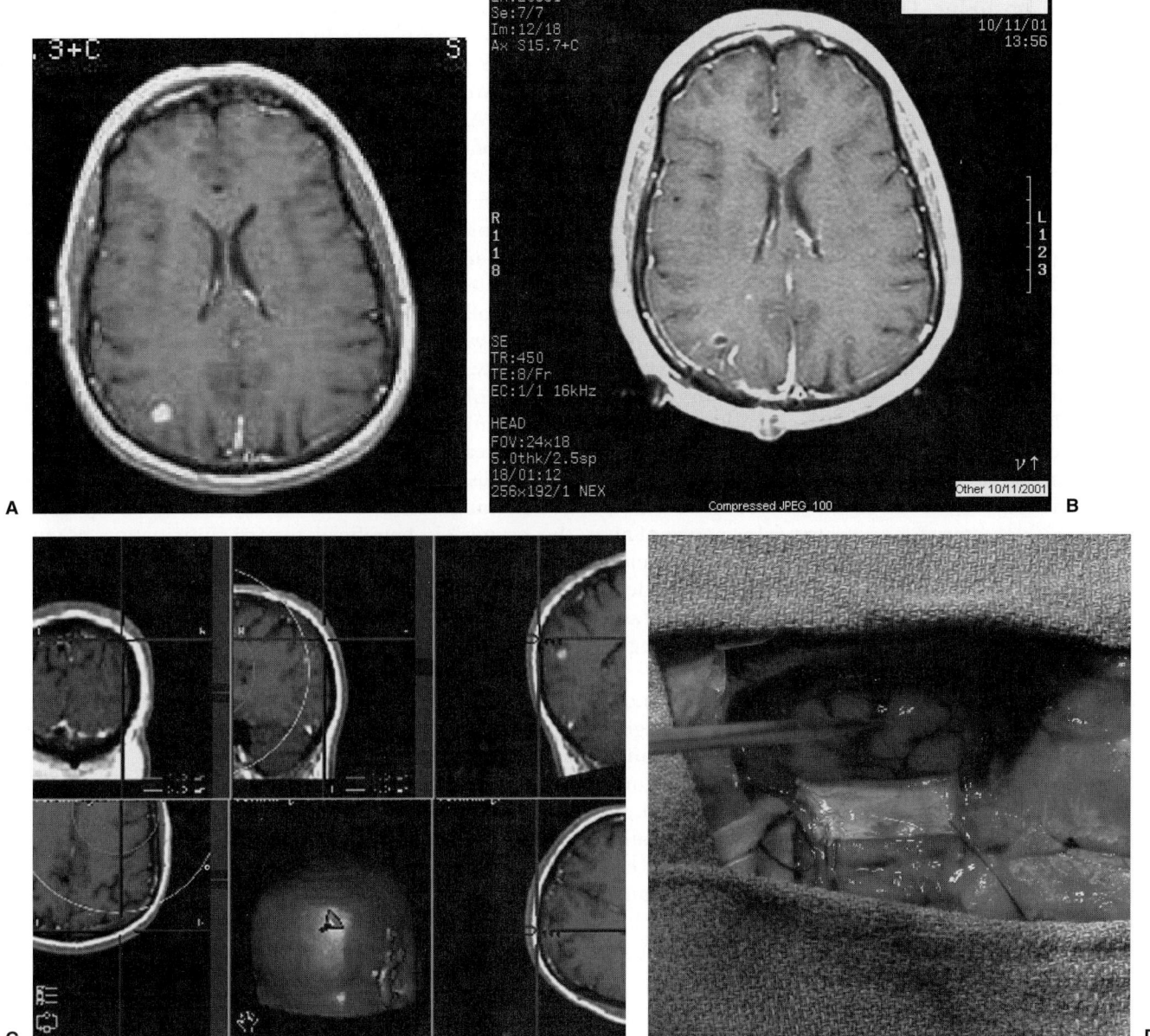

FIGURE 4–5. Magnetic resonance images of the brain after contrast in a patient with a right parietal cavernous angioma. (A). Before the surgery. (B). Twenty-four hours after image-guided resection showing gross total removal of the lesion. (C). Intraoperative photo of the computer screen displaying the views described in Figure 4–3. The crossing of the hairlines indicates the position in real time of the bipolar forceps on the brain seen in (D) (StealthStation, Louisville, CO). (D). Intraoperative photograph showing the pointer tip over the sulcus chosen to dissect to navigate to the lesion.

such as tumors and vascular malformations.[4,5,7,22] Image-guided technology allows the surgeon to perform preoperative planning and choose the least invasive pathway avoiding eloquent areas.[23–24] The location, shape, and size of the skin incision and bone flap can be tailored to minimize the overall bone exposure. The surface of the cortex can be predicted allowing exclusion of vascular structures from the opening. When the cortical exposure is completed, the real-time visualization of the surgical instrument on the preoperative images (see Fig. 4–5) allows the surgeon to choose the optimal cortical/sulcal location for the microsurgical dissection toward the lesion. Progress toward the lesion can be monitored dynamically on the computerized imaging studies (see Fig. 4–5). Upon arrival at the lesion, the resection can be guided by the same techniques enhancing the surgeon's assessment of complete resection and avoidance of normal tissue. Additionally, by fusing fMRI data and intraoperative mapping,[25] the surgeon can derive real-time guidance using electrophysiological information.

The use of frameless navigation for biopsies has increased over the past 10 years.[14,26] At the present time we routinely use frameless technology for diagnostic biopsies because it is a reliable technique and is well tolerated by patients.

Another neurosurgical field particularly well suited for image-guided neurosurgery is epilepsy surgery.[27,28] The identification of a seizure focus by depth electrode placement can be successfully performed using image guidance. When performing cortical resections, the identification of the seizure focus and preservation of normal function are facilitated by fusion and co-registration of multiple preoperative images, such as PET, ictal single photon emission computed tomography (SPECT), fMRI, and intraoperative recording.

Most functional neurosurgeons would agree that a rigid frame is necessary for accurate performance of ablative procedures and for implanting deep brain electrodes for surgical treatment of movement disorders. Nonetheless, image-guided surgery serves in many cases as an adjuvant for planning and intraoperative integration of neurophysiological recording.[15]

Neuronavigation has recently been used with more frequency for spinal instrumentation cases.[29,30] The goal of surgical orientation in the spine, as in intracranial work, is the localization and orientation of structures not visible in the surgical field. This process has traditionally been done with the guidance of intraoperative radiographs or fluoroscopy, but these technologies can be time-consuming and inaccurate.[31] Image guidance obviates some of these drawbacks and improves final location of the instrumentation.[32]

■ Clinical Benefits and Limitations

The number of neurosurgeons practicing image-guided stereotactic techniques is rapidly growing. Most of the commercially available systems employ the optical digitizer for navigation, implying that this is a user-friendly and helpful technology. In particular, the optical digitizer has been shown by different authors to offer several advantages compared with conventional techniques. Review of the literature shows that most articles describing the use of the optical digitizer for image-guided neurosurgery consistently report similar benefits such as increasing the efficiency of the craniotomy, minimizing the size of exposure and the invasiveness of the procedure, allowing an approach through the least eloquent path, defining resection boundaries that may not be apparent to the surgeon's eyes, and minimizing the manipulation of brain tissue outside the pathologic process.

Several reports have linked the subjective advantages of image guidance to more objective and quantifiable factors. We have described a decrease in length of hospital stay.[4] Additional described benefits include a greater degree of lesion resection with less collateral dissection, leading to improved clinical outcome and decreased morbidity.[33] The proper placement of the scalp incision and craniotomy flap prevents the need for extensive bone opening and thereby saves operative time. Directing and defining the approach to deep-seated subcortical tumors allow a minimal and precisely directed corticotomy, which might lessen perioperative neurological morbidity. Working around and within the lesion is greatly enhanced by spatial feedback reinforcing image-based knowledge of the tumor's relationship with eloquent areas and vascular structures. Even when the surgeon is dissecting along the surface of the capsular plane of a meningioma or metastasis the ability to "see around the corner" is beneficial toward anticipating potential hazardous structures or disorienting tumor lobules.

Line-of-sight problems have proven to be surprisingly minor during operative procedures with the optical digitizer. Naturally, a clear path must be maintained between the reference arc and the camera array during the procedure, which requires that the surgeon and nurses not cross this path. This is true for all types of digitizer, and several arrangements of the operating room table and equipment have been proposed to overcome this problem.[4] Electromagnetic digitizers are based on the detection of an electromagnetic field. Given that ferromagnetic material within the operating room environment can distort the electromagnetic field, a ferromagnetic-free environment must be maintained around the digitizer to ensure its proper functioning.[34] Similarly, the sonic digitizer needs an unobstructed acoustic path between the emitter and the detector array to ensure accuracy.[35]

Interference from surgical light sources has not proven to be a problem; the infrared wavelength of their emissions is not disruptive to surgery. The advantages of using infrared light over other types of light include its maximal accuracy, decreased sensitivity to ambient light, and small emitter size.

■ Conclusions

Image-guided neurosurgery using the optical digitizer is now widely applied for cranial and spinal procedures. This technology has been proven to be user-friendly and enables the surgeon to be minimally invasive. As the twenty-first century brings tremendous development of new technology, image-guided neurosurgery will be incorporated in additional technical advances.

REFERENCES

1. Bucholz RD, Smith KR. A comparison of sonic digitizers versus light emitting diode-based localization. In: Maciunas RJ, ed. *Interactive Image-Guided Neurosurgery*. Park Ridge, IL: American Association of Neurological Surgeons; 1993:715–720.
2. Smith KR, Frank KJ, Bucholz RD. The Neurostation: a highly accurate, minimally invasive solution to frameless stereotactic neurosurgery. *Computerized Medical Imaging and Graphics* 1994;18:247–256.
3. Germano IM. The NeuroStation System for image-guided, frameless stereotaxy. *Neurosurg* 1995;37:348–349.
4. Germano IM, Villalobos H, Silvers A, Post KP. Clinical use of the optical digitizer. *Neurosurgery* 1999;45:261–270.
5. Zamorano LJ, Nolte L, Kadi AM, Jiang Z. Interactive intraoperative localization using an infrared-based system. *Stereotact Funct Neurosurg* 1994;63:84–88.
6. Li Q, Zamorano L, Jiang Z, et al. Effect of optical digitizer selection on the application accuracy of a surgical localization system: a quantitative comparison between the Optotrak and flashpoint tracking systems. *Comp Aid Surg* 1999;4:314–321.
7. Gumprech HK, Widenka DC, Lumenta CB. BrainLab Vector vision neuronavigation system: technology and clinical experience in 131 cases. *Neurosurgery* 1999;44:97–104.
8. Lee JY, Lundsford LD, Sunbach BR, Jho HD, Bissonette DJ, Kondziolka D. Brain surgery with image guidance: current recommendations based on a 20-year assessment. *Sterotact Funct Neurosurg* 2000;75:35–48.
9. Bucholz RD, Yeh D, Trobsugh S, et al. Correction of stereotactic inaccuracy caused by brain shift using the intraoperative ultrasound device. In: Proc CVRMed-MRCA'97, Grenoble, France, 1997: 459–466.
10. Nimsky C, Ganslandt O, Kober H, Buchfelder M, Fahlbusch R. Intraoperative magnetic resonance imaging combined with neuronavigation: a new concept. *Neurosurgery* 2001;48:1082–1089.
11. Watanabe E, Watanabe T, Manaka S, et al. Three-dimensional digitizer (neuronavigator): new equipment for CT-guided stereotaxic surgery. *Surg Neurol* 1987;27:543–547.
12. Goerss SJ, Kelly PJ, Kall B, Stiving S. A stereotactic magnetic field digitizer. *Stereotact Funct Neurosurg* 1994;63:89–92.
13. Barnett GH, Kormos DW, Steiner CP, et al. Frameless stereotaxy using a sonic digitizing wand: development and adaptation to the Picker Vistar medical imaging system. In: Maciunas RJ, ed. *Interactive Image-Guided Neurosurgery*. Park Ridge, IL: American Association of Neurological Surgeons; 1993:715–720.
14. Germano IM, Queenan JV. Clinical experience with intracranial brain needle biopsy using frameless surgical navigation. *Comp Aid Surg* 1998;3:33–39.
15. Germano IM, Weisz DJ, Silvers A, Shrivastava R, Yang BY. Surgical techniques for stereotactic implant of deep brain stimulators. *Sem Neurosurg* 2001;12:213–223.
16. Barnett GH, Steiner CP, Weisenberg J. Adaptation of personal projection television to a head-mounted dysplay for intraoperative viewing of neuroimaging. *J Image Guid Surg* 1995;1:109–112.
17. Visarius H, Gong J, Scheer C, et al. Man-machine interfaces in computer-assisted surgery. *Comput Aided Surg* 1997;2:102–107.
18. Shahidi R, Tombropoulos R, Grzeszczuk R. Clinical applications of three-dimensional rendering of medical data sets. *Proceedings IEEE* 1998;86:555–568.
19. Shaidi R, Wang B, Epitaux M, Grzeszczuk R, Adler J. Volumetric image guidance via a stereotactic endoscope. In: Colshester A, Delp S, eds. *Medical Image Computing and Computer-Assisted Interventions*. First Intern Conference Proceedings, Boston, MA. 1998:241–252.
20. Shahidi R, Argiro V, Napel S, et al. Assessment of several virtual endoscopy techniques using computed tomography and perspective volume rendering. *Proceedings of Visualization in Biomedical Computing*, 4th International Conference Proceedings, Hamburg, Germany. 1996:521–528.
21. Villalobos H, Germano IM. Evaluation of multimodality registration in frameless stereotaxy. *Comp Aid Surgery* 1999;4:45–49.
22. Barnett GH, Steiner CP, Weisenberg J. Intracranial meningioma resection using frameless sterotaxy. *J Image Guid Surg* 1995;1:46–52.
23. Zamorano L, Matter A, Saenz A, et al. Interactive image-guided surgical resection of intracranial arteriovenous malformations. *Comp Aid Surg* 1998;3:57–63.
24. Matz P, McDermaott M, Gutin P, et al. Cavernous malformations: results of image-guided resection. *J Image Guid Surg* 1995;1:273–279.
25. Krombach GA, Spetzger U, Rhode V, Gilsbach JM. Intraoperative localization of functional regions of sensorimotor cortex by neuronavigation and cortical mapping. *Comp Aid Surg* 1998;3:64–73.
26. Barnett GH, Miller DW, Weisenberger J. Frameless stereotaxy with scalp-applied fiducial markers for brain biopsy procedures: experience in 218 cases. *J Neurosurg* 1999;7:313–319.
27. Olivier A, Germano IM, Cukiert A, Peters T. Frameless stereotaxy for surgery of the epilepsies: preliminary experience. *J Neurosurg* 1994;81:629–633.
28. Dealmeida AN, Wheatley BM, Olivier A. Advanced surgical approach for selective amygdalohippocampectomy through neuronavigation. *Neurosurgery* 2001;42:109–197.
29. Nolte LP, Visarius H, Arm E, et al. Computer-assisted spine surgery: a technique for accurate transpedicular screw fixation using CT data and 3D optical localizer. *J Image Guid Surg* 1995;1:88–93.
30. Lavalle S, Sautot P, Troccaz J, et al. Computer-assisted spine surgery: a technique for accurate transpedicular screw fixation using CT data and a 3D optical digitizer. *J Image Guid Surg* 1995;1:65–73.
31. Theodore N, Sonntag VKH. Spinal surgery: the past century and the next. *Neurosurgery* 2000;46:767–776.
32. Foley KT, Simon DA, Rampersaud YR. Virtual fluoroscopy: computer-assisted fluoroscopic navigation. *Spine* 2001;26:347–351.
33. Paleologos TS, Wadley JP, Kitchen ND, Thomas DG. Clinical utility and cost-effectiveness of interactive image-guided craniotomy: clinical comparison between conventional and image-guided meningioma surgery. *Neurosurgery* 2000;47:40–47.
34. Mascott CR. The Compass Cygnus-PFS image-guided system. *Neurosurgery* 2000;46:235–238.
35. Reinhardt HF, Horstmann GA, Gratzl O. Sonic stereometry in microsurgical procedures for deep-seated brain tumors and vascular malformations. *Neurosurgery* 1993;32:51–57.

5

The Mechanical Arm System

EIJU WATANABE

Orientation is one of the most important factors in successful intracranial surgery. Surgical plans are based mainly upon images generated by computed tomography (CT) or magnetic resonance imaging (MRI). They are sometimes based on functional images such as functional MRI (fMRI), magnetoencephalographs (MEGs), and near infrared spectroscopic topography (NIRS) that are obtained as part of preoperative examinations, especially when patients have lesions in the vicinity of eloquent areas. In such cases, the surgery is planned intimately upon those images in determining the resection line to protect eloquent areas such as the motor strip, language area, or visual cortex.

However, transferring the surgical plan to the real operating field presents a dilemma—one that the surgical navigation system was developed to resolve. The first navigation system was reported by Roberts in 1985.[1] He used an ultrasonic three-dimensional (3-D) localizing system to detect the visual field of a microscope.[2] In 1986, a navigating system using a mechanical arm and dubbed "neuronavigator" was reported by Watanabe et al.[3] Figure 5–1 shows a recent model of our neuronavigator linked to a laptop computer.

Prior to the appearance of navigation systems, the stereotactic surgical frame was used to guide the needle into the brain. In 1947 Spiegel and Wycis[4] developed the first stereotactic frame. The needle control was based upon a pneumogram that delineated only the shape of the ventricles. Everything was located in relation to the anterior commissure and posterior commissure that were identified by the pneumoventriculograph. After the development of CT and MRI, stereotaxy had been guided by digital images. By means of these tomographic images, the targeting method has become more direct and more accurate. However, the frame itself became a hindrance for surgical procedures in open-cranium surgery. Consequently, the need arose for a frameless navigation system.

■ Method

As already mentioned, in 1987 Watanabe et al described their "neuronavigator," an arm-based, frameless guiding system (so named for its similarity to a car-navigating system designed at that time).[3] Several mechanical arm systems based on similar concepts were subsequently developed.[5–7]

The system works in general as follows. A mechanical arm system samples 3-D coordinates of the operating point and transfers them to a personal computer. The arm has six joints that allow the tip to be introduced into the surgical field. Each joint has a potentiometer that conveys the angle of the joint to the computer. The computer, running on Windows 98, calculates the 3-D location of the arm tip using these angles and arm length with trigonometry.

Preoperative CT or MRI images were acquired with three markers placed on the nasion and bilateral ear tragi. Capsules (about 4 mm in diameter) containing oily materials such as vitamin D are used as markers for MRI, and metallic balls (3 mm in diameter) are used for CT. These images are transferred to the computer via Ethernet. After the patient's head is fixed to the skull clamp, the arm tip points to the three fiducial points to register the 3-D location of these points on the com-

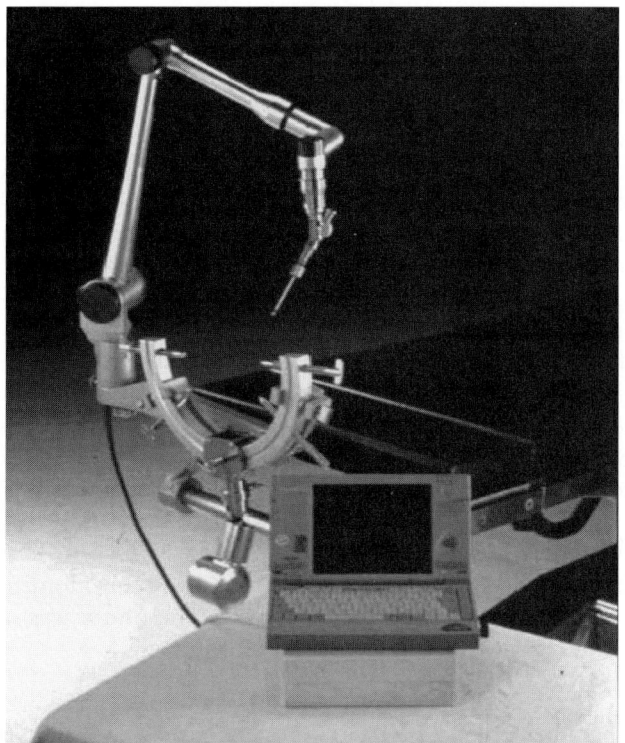

FIGURE 5–1. Basic construction of the neuronavigator, using a laptop PC running Microsoft Windows.

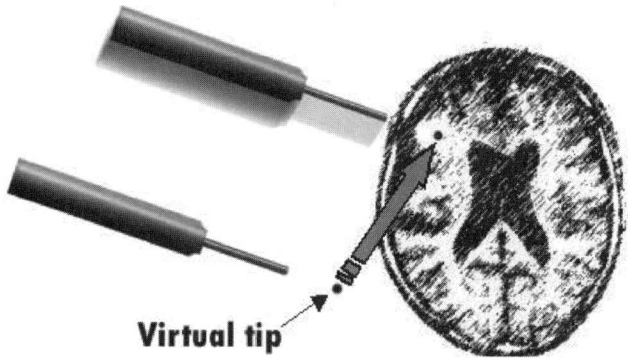

FIGURE 5–2. Designing of a craniotomy by the neuronavigator using a virtual tip. The craniotomy is easily designed in terms of proper size and placement using this method.

puter. The computer then creates a conversion matrix with which points in the surgical field are transferred onto the CT/MRI coordinates.

We usually use series of two-dimensional (2-D) slice images in three coordinates (axial, coronal, and sagittal). These triplanar images may be displayed in paging mode or fixed mode. Crosshair cursors are displayed on the corresponding images indicating the position of the arm tip.

■ Applications in Neurosurgery

The navigator is most often used to detect the localization of tumors. It is especially helpful when the tumor is located deep in the brain. To guide the surgeon to the target, the navigator tip is introduced from time to time into the operating field to check the orientation during the approach.

Virtual tip

Sometimes, it may be helpful when the system indicates the location of the point some distance ahead to the actual tip. For example, when we are dissecting the white matter toward the tumor, it is more informative when the navigator indicates the location of the point before we reach it, which allows us to know the existence of the cistern of large vessels before we encounter them. To achieve this function the navigator system is equipped with a virtual tip that indicates a point located at a desired distance ahead of the actual tip (Fig. 5–2). This is realized by simply retracting the arm tip by the desired length or by telling the computer to elongate the last segment in the software.[8–10]

The virtual tip is helpful in several situations. As just described, the virtual tip allows the surgeon to know the location of important structures such as large vessels before the surgeon actually encounters these structures. For this purpose the virtual tip is usually located 5 to 10 mm ahead of the actual tip. In cases where the tumor is located on the surface of the brain, as in convexity meningioma, the virtual tip helps to locate the tumor from the scalp surface before the skin incision is made. In this way, the craniotomy is easily designed in terms of desirable size and location. For this purpose, the virtual tip is usually placed at 20 to 30 mm ahead of the actual tip.

Combination with magnetoencephalographs

Daily more surgeons are using magnetoencephalography to measure the functional map of the brain such as motor cortex, sensory cortex, and language area. When we combine the functional mapping with the intraoperative navigation system, we can enhance our ability to protect functionally important areas during surgery. With the 37-channel squid system, the sensory evoked field is obtained, indicating the location of the sensory cortex. The median nerve is stimulated at the wrist, and the evoked magnetic field is averaged 200 times. The primary somatosensory cortex (Brodmann's area 3b) and then the central sulcus are determined by the sensory dipole. The sensory dipole is overlayed on the patient's MRI images, which are used as a guide for the navigator. When its location is transferred onto the patient's cortex with the navigator, the central sulcus and the motor cortex are easily recognized.

Combination with near infrared spectroscopic topography

NIRS is a relatively new noninvasive method of measuring the regional cerebral blood volume (rCBV) dynamics coupled with neuronal activities. Details of NIRS are described by Watanabe et al.[10] Near infrared light with wavelengths of 780 and 840 nm is used. The infrared light is guided to the scalp surface through an optical fiber bundle (2 mm in diameter). The reflection of infrared light is received by a probe placed on the scalp 30 mm away from the transmitting probe and is guided to a silicon photodiode by an optical fiber. Signal intensities of the near infrared light of the two wavelengths for each channel are separated and analyzed to obtain the relative change of total hemoglobin concentration in the brain tissue. Twenty-four channels of NIRS probes (12 on each side) are mounted on the scalp to cover the prospective focus region. The rationale of this method to detect the physiological activities of the brain is evaluated using motor activation[10] or language activation.[11]

We use this method to detect the epileptogenic focus for the resection surgery of intractable epilepsy.[12] In some cases, especially with neocortical foci, NIRS clearly delineates the location of the focus. In such cases, the navigator is used to locate the subdural grid electrode to place it correctly on the assumed seizure focus.

■ Clinical Experience

A recent type of an arm-based navigator (Neuronavigator, Mizuho Company, Tokyo, Japan) was installed at the Tokyo Metropolitan Police Hospital in 1990. Since then, more than 400 surgeries have been performed using navigator guidance. About 70% of these cases were glioma surgery, 10% were epilepsy surgery (electrode implantation or focus resection), and 10% were meningioma.

The CT or MRI images are transferred through an Ethernet connection by file transfer protocol (FTP). Homemade software is used to convert CT/MRI images into "bmp" image format. This procedure is usually done on a second PC workstation with similar specifications, and reformatted images are transferred to the navigator computer by optical disk.

The mechanical accuracy of the neuronavigator has been evaluated by phantom testing as about 1.5 mm (0.8 mm SD). The overall accuracy in the surgery including the errors in fiducial registration is about 2.5 mm. This is the result when we use surface markers placed in nasion and tragi. Several authors report that the accuracy becomes better when the bone pegs, which are fixed to the skull, are used for fiducial points.[12a]

Illustrative cases

Case 1

This 42-year-old male was operated for a tumor in the right parietal area (Fig. 5–3). Preoperative MEG showed the sensory dipole, which was back-traced and projected onto the MRI image (star in Fig. 5–3). The central sulcus was identified according to the sensory dipole, showing that the tumor was located in the primary sensory cortex.

Surgery was conducted under neuronavigator guidance to remove the tumor while saving the motor strip. The MEG-defined hand area and the MRI-defined tumor boundary were projected onto the cortex after the dura was opened. The cortical somatosensory evoked potential (SSEP) after median nerve stimulation was recorded from the cortical surface at several points around the central sulcus. The inversion of N20 and P20 was documented at the sulcus that was identified as the central sulcus by the navigator. The motor strip was easily identified and protected in the operating field. The tumor was successfully removed inducing no motor paresis.

Case 2

This patient showed monoparesis in his right hand. MRI revealed an enhanced mass lesion. MEG revealed the sensory dipole indicating that the mass was lying in the motor cortex (Fig. 5–4). During the operation, it was extremely difficult to detect the tumor with visual inspection or palpation. The tumor was partially excised preserving the motor cortex just outside of the lesion. The patient showed no worsening of preoperative hand paresis. The histological examination showed oligodendroglioma grade II.

Case 3

An 8-year-old girl with intractable epilepsy was referred to our clinic for surgical treatment. Her seizure started with a tingling sensation in the right arm sometimes followed by secondary generalization. Under electroencephalogram (EEG) and NIRS monitoring, a seizure monitoring was performed. A seizure began in the left parietal area. Ictal single photon emission computed tomography (SPECT) showed the hyperperfusion in the left postcentral area. NIRS showed rCBV increase in the same area as that in ictal SPECT immediately after the seizure onset lasting for about 25 seconds (Fig. 5–5). The rCBV began to increase 5 seconds after spike discharge in the left parietal area. The subdural electrodes were implanted using the navigator to cover the hyperperfusion area detected by NIRS. Subdural recording demonstrated the seizure spike onset in the left postcentral area, which confirmed the findings in NIRS and SPECT. The small corticectomy was done in the left postcentral area guided by a neuronavigator. Considerable seizure reduction was obtained after the surgery.

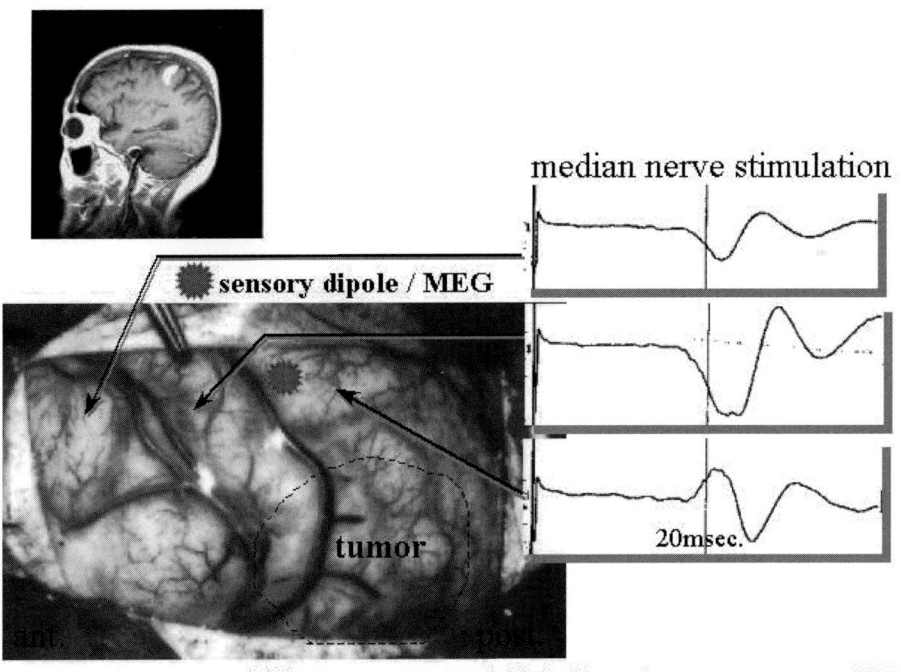

FIGURE 5–3. Case 1. The primary sensory cortex was defined by magnetoencephalograph (represented by the star). The tumor and the central sulcus were defined by the navigator and these locations were confirmed by cortical somatosensory evoked potential.

■ Discussion

There are several possible methods to choose for navigation, including the mechanical arm system,[5–7,13,14] electromagnetic system,[15] or light emission guiding system.[16]

The major advantage of the mechanical arm system is its simplicity. Lawton et al[17] demonstrated that in one institution neurosurgeons preferred the mechanical arm system to other types of navigating systems and that many neurosurgeons appreciate its simplicity.

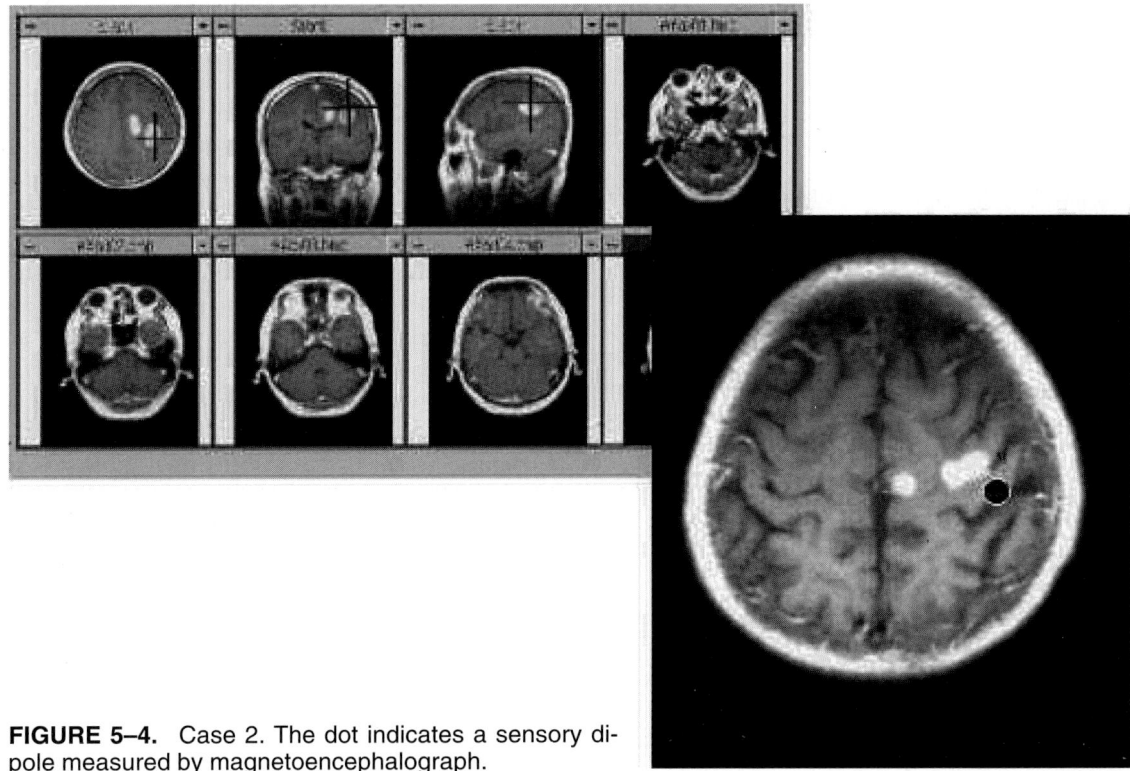

FIGURE 5–4. Case 2. The dot indicates a sensory dipole measured by magnetoencephalograph.

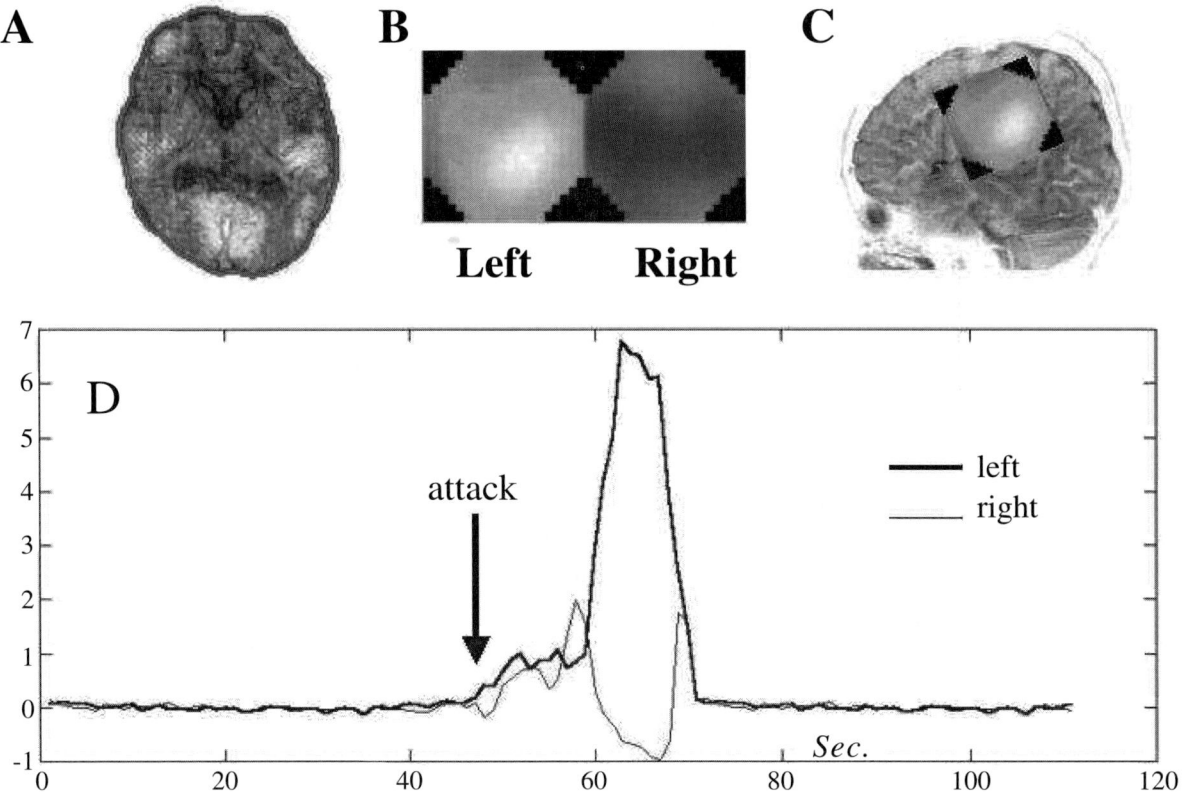

FIGURE 5–5. Navigation system applied in epilepsy surgery in case 3. Near infrared spectroscopic topography and cerebral blood volume (NIRS-rCBV) were monitored during epileptic seizure. (A). Ictal single photon emission computed tomography (SPECT) showed hyperperfusion area in the left parietal area. (B). A hyperperfusion area was also depicted by NIRS suggesting the location of the seizure focus. (C). NIRS map was overlaid on the magnetic resonance image. (D). NIRS-rCBV time course indicates the abrupt increase of rCBV in the left parietal region. These image data were transferred onto the cortical surface by a navigator during surgery, guiding the location of a subdural grid electrode.

Brain shift

We must be careful of the fact that the brain tissue deviates when considerable amounts of cerebrospinal fluid or tumor tissue are removed. In a practical sense, however, it is often recognized that merely opening the dura mater does not cause significant deviation of the intracranial tissue. As long as we use the preoperative CT/MRI images in navigation, this problem cannot be avoided. The easiest way to overcome this problem is to get orientation at the earlier phase of the surgery. A fundamental solution for this problem would be a real-time image-updating technique such as intraoperative CT or MRI.

■ Conclusions

The mechanical arm system was one of the first frameless stereotactic systems to demonstrate the usefulness of navigational surgery. It has future promise for use in translating the information of functional mapping into the surgical field. As has been shown here, MEG is one of the effective alternatives to localize the somatosensory cortex of the individual brain. Using this type of guidance, we could easily achieve lower postoperative morbidity in shorter operation time. Functional MRI is also a powerful candidate for preoperative functional mapping, which may be used in combination with navigation.

The neuronavigator has been proved helpful in routine neurosurgery. It is especially beneficial for tumor surgery near eloquent areas or in epilepsy surgery. It is expected that the mechanical arm system will continue to be utilized as a basic technology of frameless stereotactic surgery.

REFERENCES

1. Roberts DW, Strohbehn JW, Hatch JF, et al. A frameless stereotactic integration of computerized tomographic imaging and the operating microscope. *J Neurosurg* 1986;65:545–549.

2. Friets EM, Strohbehn W, Hatch JF, Roberts DW. A frameless stereotactic operating microscope for neurosurgery. *IEEE Trans BME* 1989;36:608–617.
3. Watanabe E, Watanabe T, Manaka S, Mayanagi Y, Takakura K. Three-dimensional digitizer (neuro-navigator): a new equipment for CT guided stereotaxic surgery. *Surg Neurol* 1987;27: 543–547.
4. Spiegel EA, Wycis HT, Marks M, et al. Stereotactic apparatus for operations on the human brain. *Science* 1947;106:349–350.
5. Moesges R, Schloendorff G. A new imaging method for intraoperative therapy control in skull base surgery. *Neurosurg Rev* 1988;11:245–247.
6. Reinhardt H, Meyer H, Amrein E. A computer-assisted device for the intraoperative CT-correlated localization of brain tumors. *Eur Surg Res* 1988;20:51–58.
7. Takizawa T. Isocentric stereotactic three-dimensional digitizer for neurosurgery. *Stereotact Funct Neurosurg* 1993;60:175–193.
8. Watanabe E, Kosugi Y. Intraoperative neuronavigator system in neurosurgery and computer surgery. In: Fujino T, ed. *Simulation and Computer-Aided Surgery*. Chichester: John Wiley & Sons; 1993:157–162.
9. Watanabe E. The neuronavigator: a potensiometer-based localization arm system. In: Maciunas RJ, ed. *Interactive Image-Guided Neurosurgery*. Park Ridge, IL: American Association of Neurological Surgeons; 1993:135–148.
10. Watanabe E, Yamashita Y, Maki A, Ito Y, Koizumi H. Noninvasive functional mapping with multichannel near infrared spectroscopic topography in humans. *Neurosci Lett* 1996;205:41–44.
11. Watanabe E, Maki A, Kawaguchi F, et al. Noninvasive assessment of language dominance with near infrared spectroscopic mapping. *Neurosci Lett* 1998;256:49–52.
12. Watanabe E, Maki A, Kawaguchi F, et al. Noninvasive cerebral blood volume measurement during seizures using multichannel near infrared spectroscopic topography. *J Epilepsy* 1998;11: 335–340.
12a. Alp MS, Dujovny M, Misra M, Charbel FT, Ausman JI. Head registration techniques for image-guided surgery. *Neurol Res* 1998;20: 31–37.
13. Guthrie BL, Kaplan R, Florek D. Stereotactic neurosurgical operating arm system. *Stereotact Funct Neurosurg* 1992;58:144–145.
14. Watanabe E, Mayanagi Y, Kosugi Y, Manaka S, Takakura K. Open surgery assisted by the neuronavigator: a stereotactic articulated, sensitive arm. *Neurosurgery* 1991;28:792–800.
15. Kato A, Yoshimine T, Hayakawa T, et al. A frameless, armless navigational system for computer-assisted neurosurgery. *J Neurosurg* 1991;74:845–849.
16. Zamorano LJ, Nolte L, Kadi AM, Jiang Z. Interactive intraoperative localization using an infrared-based system. *Neurol Res* 1993; 15:290–298.
17. Lawton MT, Golfinos JG, Geldmacher T, et al. A comparative clinical evaluation of current frameless stereotactic systems: accuracy, performance, and surgeon preference. *Perspect Neurol Surg* 1998; 9:47–62.

6

The Magnetic System

CHRISTOPHER R. MASCOTT

Image-guided neurosurgery has rapidly evolved in recent years, paralleling advances in computer technology and computerized imaging. Guidance depends on correlating an imaging data set with real space at the time of surgery. To accomplish this, surgical space needs to be defined with regard to a frame of reference. Traditionally, a stereotactic frame with rigid skull fixation has been used at the time of image acquisition to define space on the imaging data set as well as in real space at the time of surgery. Greater computer power and volumetric imaging have now made it possible to correlate volumetrically acquired images with surgical space by using surface landmarks on the patient's head, rather than frame placement, for imaging and surgery.[1] However, surface anatomical landmarks and skin markers do not have the same accuracy as a frame with skull fixation.

■ Frameless Image-Guided Surgery

In the absence of a frame, surgical space must be defined by rigid fixation of the head to the operating table at the time of surgery using a head holder. Subsequent surface registration of patient landmarks requires a probe that can be tracked within the defined space. A variety of methods have been employed to track probes in space. Some systems use a probe on a digitized articulated arm attached to the head holder.[2-3] Others use ultrasonic emission and triangulation.[4-6] Many systems use optical tracking and triangulation of a probe that is active (light emitting diodes)[7] or passive (reflective markers).[8] This requires an array of markers rigidly attached to the head holder that function as a frame of reference.

An alternative is to define space within a magnetic field by attaching a magnetic field generator to the head holder and then tracking a probe with an attached magnetic receiver.[9-10] This is the principle of the Cygnus-PFS system (Compass International, Rochester, MN) described in this chapter.

■ Magnetic Field Referencing of Stereotactic Space

A static magnetic field is used as a frame of reference once the patient's head is immobilized in three-point fixation. The magnet is attached to the head holder and remains immobile from the time of registration onward. When the patient is draped, the magnet remains concealed under the drapes. The receiver and probe are exchanged for an alternate sterile receiver and probe. Defining space with a magnetic field allows excellent continuous tracking of a probe during surgery because there is no interference with probe tracking such as that experienced with optical tracking systems where a line of sight must be maintained between the tracking cameras, reference markers, and probe markers. In theory, interference from metal objects within the surgical field may compromise tracking accuracy. In practice, this has not been an issue (see discussion of accuracy later in this chapter).

Applications and setup

Because stereotactic space is defined in relation to a magnet, the Cygnus-PFS system allows unprecedented

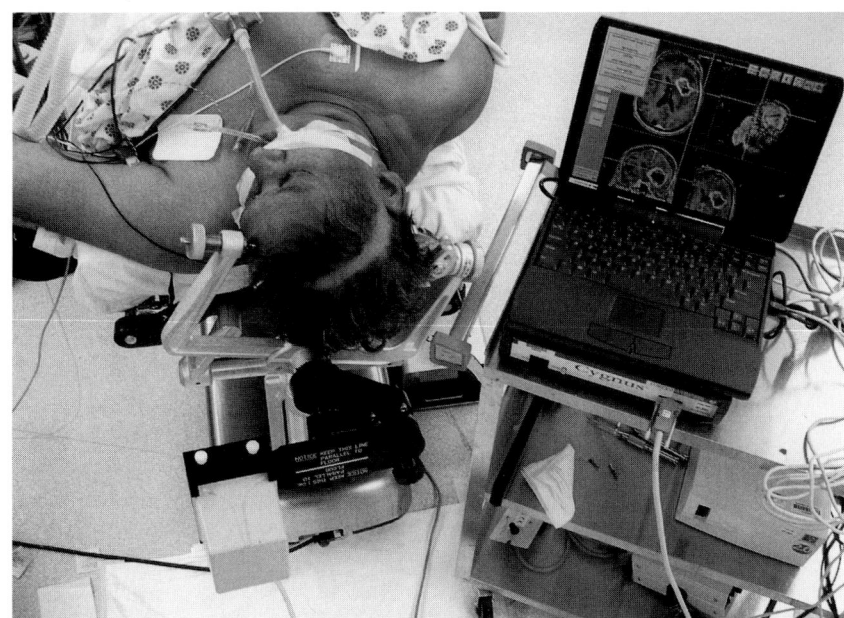

FIGURE 6–1. Cygnus-PFS setup for surgery illustrating magnet attached to head holder via L-shaped bracket, laptop computer, and magnetic control unit under computer (Compass International, Rochester, MN).

portability—neither tracking cameras nor cumbersome articulated arm systems are required. The core of the Cygnus-PFS system is the magnet with a control unit and a laptop computer (Fig. 6–1).[9] This allows for easy transport between hospitals. The magnet attaches to the outer starburst of a three-point head holder via an adjustable L-bracket. An optional stand with a touchscreen control panel/monitor is available for more sedentary use (Fig. 6–2).

Data acquisition is very efficient and requires less than 5 minutes. This is accomplished via an ethernet card or using an outboard digital archive tape (DAT) drive connected to the small computer system interface (SCSI) port of the laptop. The computer then builds three-dimensional models of the head for registration of landmarks in image space. A second data set can then be correlated to the primary data set, [i.e., computed tomography (CT) with magnetic resonance imaging (MRI)] thus allowing simultaneous use of two data sets during surgery (Fig. 6–3). Under "Image Registration," landmarks and fiducials are selected on the imaging data set for subsequent correlation with the homologous landmarks in real space on the patient at the time of surgery. This process of image and subsequent patient registration is similar in all commonly used image-guidance systems. The Cygnus-PFS laptop allows all the preoperative planning to be performed anywhere.

At the time of surgery, after the patient is positioned and in three-point fixation, the Cygnus-PFS magnet is attached to the head holder via an L-bracket. The laptop is connected to the electromagnetic control unit and the appropriate patient study is loaded. A nonsterile magnetic field receiver and probe are attached to the Cygnus control unit, and patient landmarks are registered on the patient by touching these with the probe. Following registration and draping, the receiver and probe are exchanged for a sterile receiver and probe and the system is ready for intraoperative use.

Features

The Cygnus-PFS has many of the same features as other image-guidance systems, including target volume planning, trajectory planning, and image correlation (image fusion). Image correlation can be used to correlate CT with MRI (see Fig. 6–3), different MRI sequences [i.e., spoiled gradient echo (SPGR) with fluid attenuated inversion recovery (FLAIR)], or functional imaging. Preoperative planning and image correlation with the Cygnus-PFS are particularly user-friendly and usually take less than 5 minutes.

Unique hardware features include not only a biopsy needle holder, but different-length probes that can be angled or straight and also used as suction probes. This is particularly useful during surgery because suction is the most commonly held tool during surgery. In this manner, image guidance can continuously demonstrate the position of the suction tip without the need to pick up a dedicated probe. We find this more practical than tracking bipolar cautery or any number of other surgical instruments. The Cygnus-PFS probes, including the suction probes, are all disposable, which is also a unique feature of increasing importance in contemporary practice.

The Cygnus-PFS has a number of extremely intelligent, useful, and instructive software features. Upon completion of patient registration at surgery, a registra-

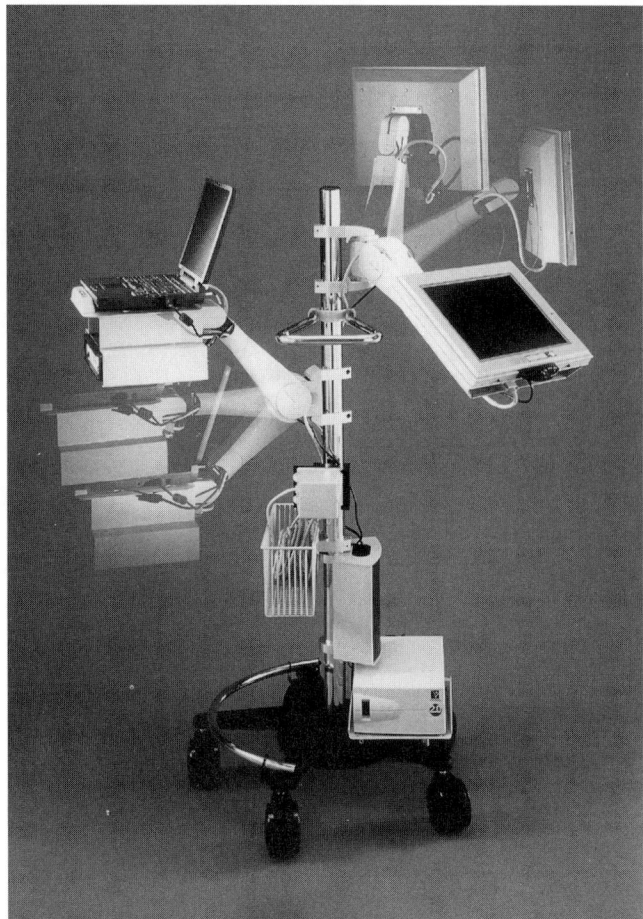

FIGURE 6–2. Optional Cygnus-PFS stand featuring movable touch-screen monitor (Compass International, Rochester, MN).

tion screen gives a calculated global accuracy (root mean square error), as do all image-guidance systems. In addition, a readout of the individual calculated error for each correlation point is given (Fig. 6–4). This is not readily available with many systems. Of particular interest, a feature called Show Registration on Images displays side-by-side images of landmarks in "image space" versus "real space" (Fig. 6–5). This feature has proven very instructive for understanding the source of inaccuracies at the time of patient registration, leading to higher true surgical accuracy.

During surgery there are a number of useful options. In addition to three orthogonal views (axial, coronal, and sagittal) a fourth "trajectory view" is available for simultaneous viewing (Fig. 6–6). Unlike trajectory views of some other systems, the orientation of the trajectory and the target can be altered by simply rotating the probe and receiver until a more anatomically and surgically intuitive picture is obtained. This obviates the need for multiple trajectory views. There is a simple one-step magnification feature that provides ideal enlargement of images (2× magnification) for smaller lesions. A single icon click switches between the primary imaging set and a second, correlated data set if this has been preplanned.

■ Lessons Regarding Accuracy in Image Guidance

Calculated accuracy

The relationship between image space and real space is basically a topological one, where each point in one needs to correspond to a point in the other. By selecting a finite number of points in image space and correlating these with equivalent points in real space, the image-guidance system finds an algorithm of the best match between the two sets. If a point moves (e.g., a skin marker near a head-holder pin site), the algorithm for the overall best match may or may not identify the true worst point. This is very well illustrated when performing a patient registration with the Cygnus. At any time, re-registering a point or eliminating a point will change the calculated accuracy values of all the other points because the algorithm tries to find the best match for the entire cohort of points and not points one at a time (see Fig. 6–4). We have found that having this information clearly presented leads to a better understanding of image guidance and does not really complicate the registration process. As expected, calculated accuracy is higher when using skull-implanted screw fiducial markers (Leibinger, Freiburg, Germany) than with adhesive skin markers or anatomical landmarks. The goal with most image-guidance systems is to obtain a calculated accuracy of less than 3 mm. Calculated accuracy usually improves to 1 mm or less when implanted skull fiducials are placed. Cygnus calculated accuracy on registration with implanted screw fiducials was 1.0 mm ± 0.4 mm ($n = 33$) as opposed to 2.0 mm ± 0.5 mm ($n = 56$) for skin markers.

True accuracy

It must be kept in mind that calculated accuracy does not represent true surgical accuracy, which depends on a number of factors. Stereotaxis with a frame and using CT imaging, which does not have the field distortions of MRI, can attain 1.0 mm accuracy at best.[11,12] All information regarding calculated accuracy must be compared with true surgical accuracy, preferably by verification of intraoperative anatomical landmarks. Visual verification of true accuracy should be obtained by selecting clearly recognizable anatomical landmarks during surgery. In Figure 6–6, the probe is placed so that it is almost touching the dome of an anterior communicating artery aneurysm seen on the images. This is an illustration of good true surgical accuracy.

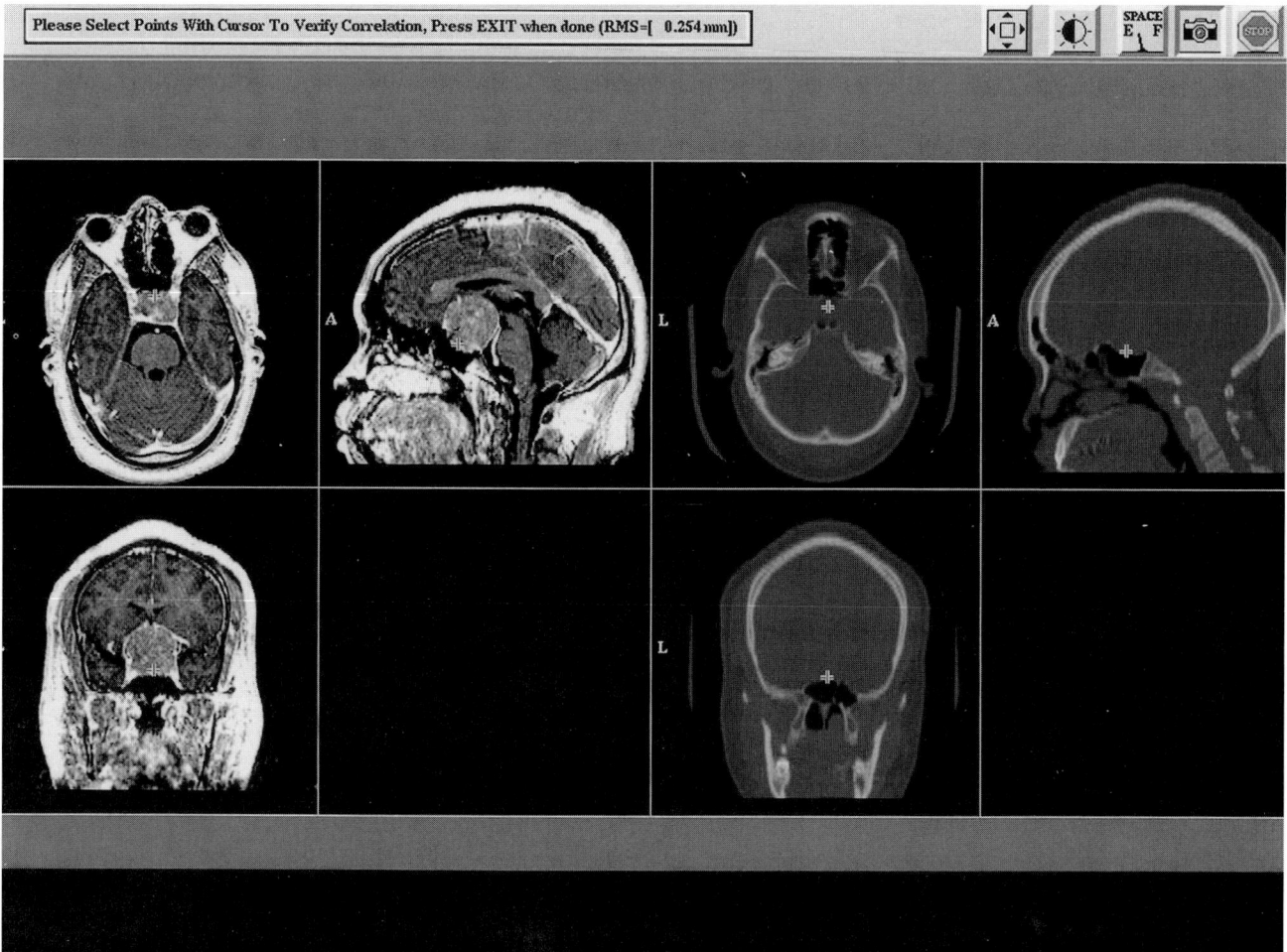

FIGURE 6-3. Image correlation of magnetic resonance imaging with computed tomographic data set.

Comparison magnetic/optic systems

Over the past 2 years we have conducted a study comparing the accuracy of a magnetic system (the Cygnus-PFS) with that of an optical tracking system (the Stealth-Station, Medtronic Surgical Navigation Technologies, Louisville, CO). Using a customized bracket, both systems were attached to the surgical head holder simultaneously in over 50 patients. Calculated accuracy at registration and true surgical accuracy were assessed and will be the subject of a detailed report elsewhere. For this chapter, the issue of true surgical accuracy is of the greatest interest. In the first 50 patients of the study, excellent true surgical accuracy was noted in 42 cases. Accuracy was poor with magnetic, but not with optical, tracking in three cases. Conversely, poor accuracy was noted with optical, but not with magnetic, tracking in three other cases. Both magnetic and optical systems had poor accuracy in the other two cases. Reasons for lack of surgical accuracy were unclear except in the two cases where inaccuracy was found using both systems. In these cases, poor accuracy was explained by the prone position, as discussed later in this chapter. With regard to the possibility of inaccuracies introduced into the magnetic field by metallic objects during surgery, we did not find this to be a problem. The introduction of a Budde Halo retractor system (OMI, Cincinnati, OH) during surgery did not seem to adversely affect the Cygnus-PFS. We did see some interference with the magnetic field when several large, self-retaining retractors were placed within an incision. This was easily corrected by removing all but one retractor, or by replacing retractors by traction sutures.

Overall, magnetic tracking and optical tracking appear to be comparable in terms of surgical accuracy.

■ Applications

The Cygnus-PFS has a number of practical applications in cranial surgery and can well be used by neurosur-

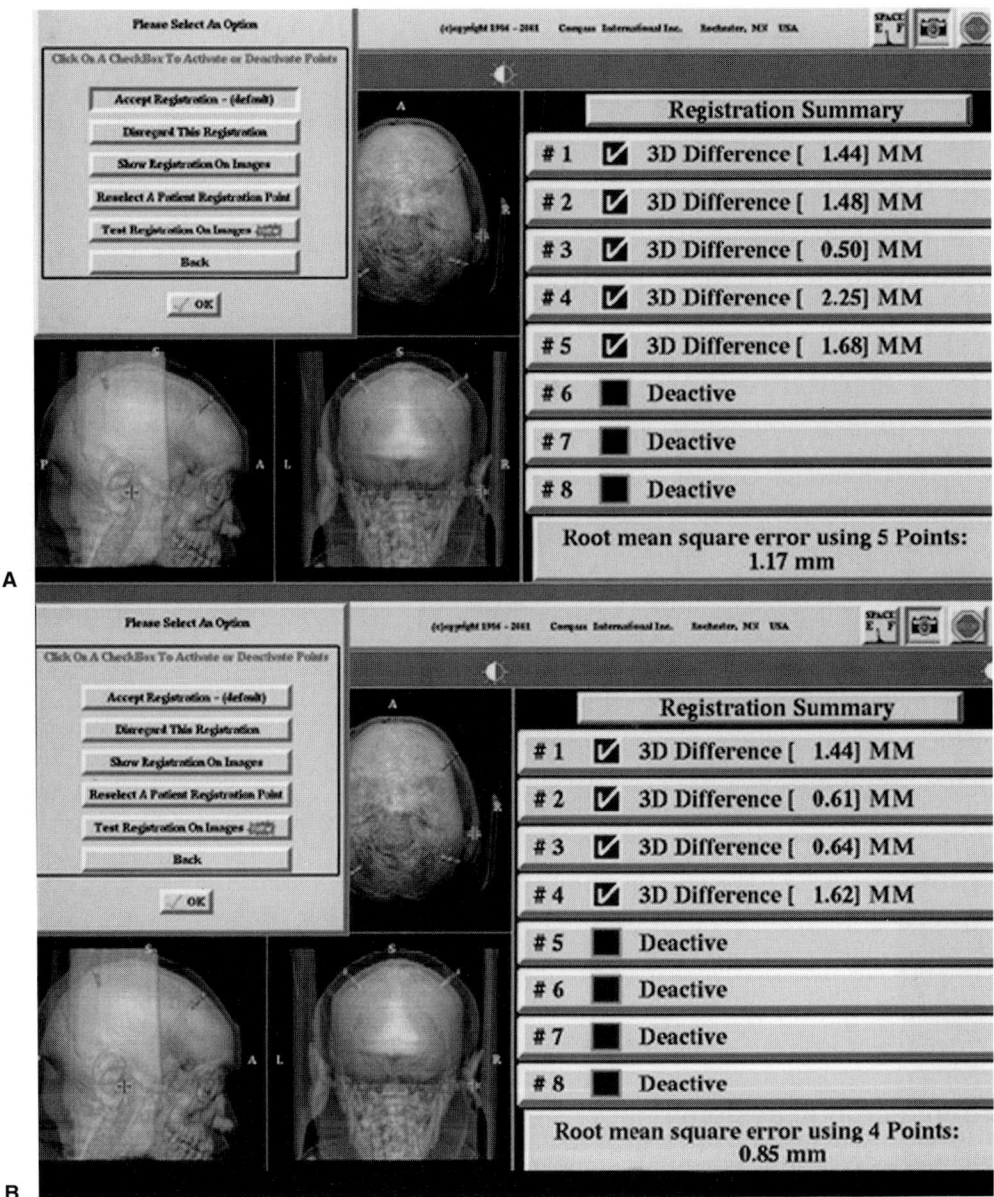

FIGURE 6–4. Registration readout screen using five points (A). Modified registration of the same patient after deactivating one point (B). The high calculated accuracy is a reflection of the use of implanted skull fiducials.

geons, ophthalmological surgeons, and ear, nose, and throat surgeons.

■ Neurosurgery

Tumors

The most obvious and common application of frameless stereotaxis in cranial surgery is for brain tumors. Regardless of the system that is employed, the principles and applications are similar. Preoperative planning can help determine the best surgical approach prior to surgery. In the operating theater, following registration, frameless stereotaxis can help center the incision and bone flap. Dural opening can be image guided as well as the approach and trajectory to deep-seated lesions.

Supratentorial

For small lesions, the advantages of image guidance for localization are obvious. This is particularly evident for small metastatic tumors, which are often not visible on the cortical surface. Because there is no frame, performing multiple small craniotomies for multiple metastatic lesions becomes more feasible. For particularly small lesions, deep locations, or posterior head regions, we would

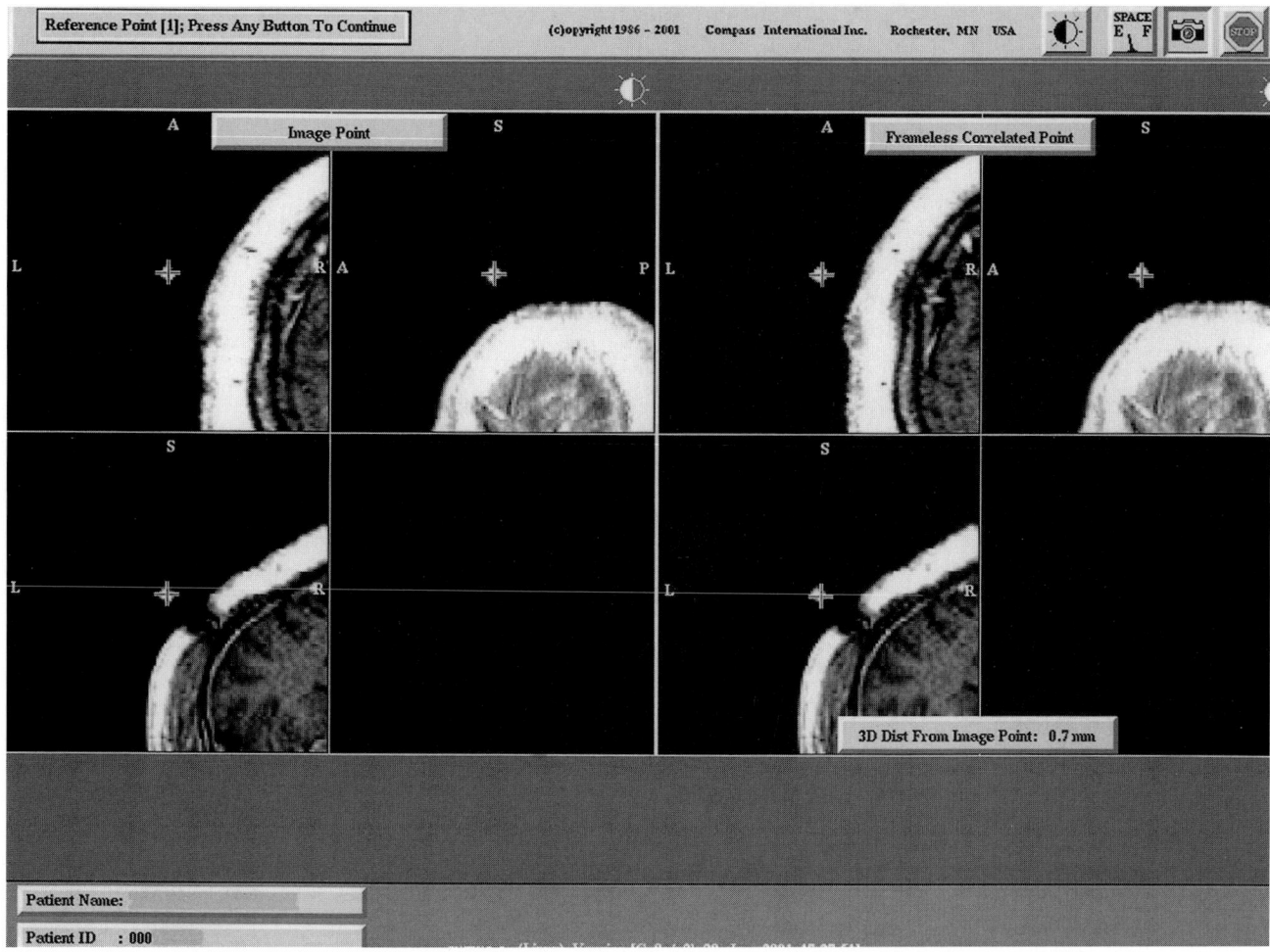

FIGURE 6–5. Screen shot of "Display Registration on Images" feature. The left side of the screen shows registration in image space. The right side of the screen graphically estimates the error in real space of each registration point and displays a corresponding image.

strongly recommend implanting skull fiducial screws, which, in our hands, results in framelike precision.

To preserve accurate image guidance, we usually try to keep tumor intact for as long as possible. In large tumors of softer consistency, this may not be possible. In these cases, internal decompression of tumor, while replacing the resected mass with cotton balls (our preference being Merocel surgical patties, Xomed Surgical Products, Jacksonville, FL) retains a reasonable degree of stereotactic accuracy. It is in this situation that the Cygnus-PFS suction probes have a particular advantage, giving constant imaging feedback. This can be illustrated with a recent case of a recurrent temporal lobe glioma where the deep aspects of the enhancing tumor were causing considerable shift of the midbrain and basal ganglia. Although we normally see no particular advantage to speed at surgery, the patient in question had an onset of pronounced electrocardiogram changes noted by the anesthesiologist shortly after dural opening. Urgent closure was discussed in view of a possible myocardial infarct. Prior to closure, a 5-minute temporal lobectomy and tumor debulking were performed with bipolar cautery and image-guided suction. Without changing instruments, we were able to ascertain depth of resection of the tumor in an essentially emergent situation. Postoperative imaging confirmed a 95% resection of enhancing tumor volume, which matched our intraoperative impression. Using another image-guidance system under similar time constraints would not have been realistic.

Infratentorial

We initially had very poor surgical accuracy in posterior fossa approaches, both with magnetic and with optical tracking systems, despite good calculated accuracies. Further study demonstrated a significant displacement of skin markers, which are imaged with the patient supine. With a prone or three-quarter prone surgical position, we were unable to obtain acceptable surgical accuracy until we resorted to systematic implantation

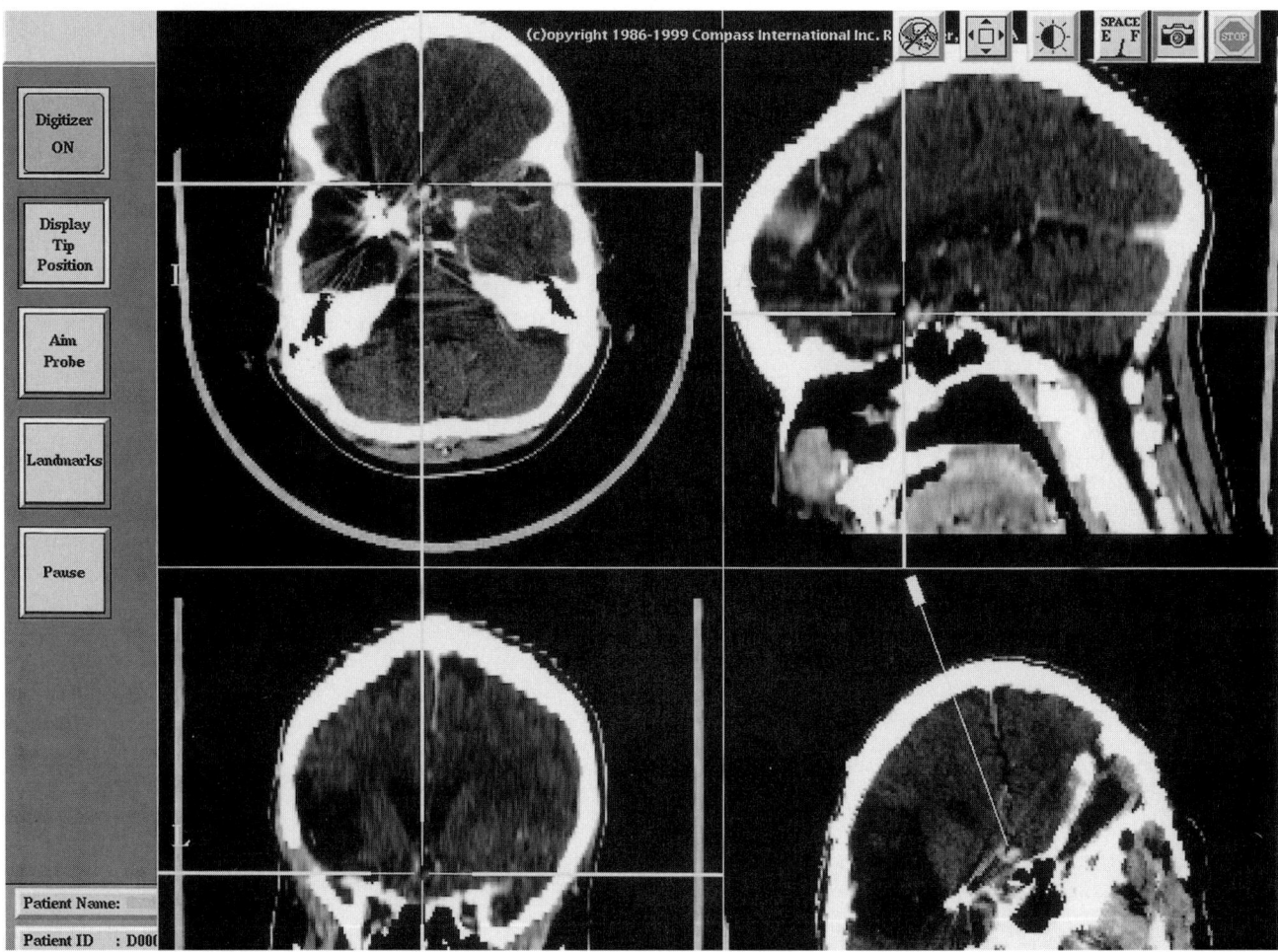

FIGURE 6–6. Intraoperative illustration of an interhemispheric approach to an unruptured anterior communicating artery aneurysm (ACom). The patient had prior surgery of a ruptured left middle cerebral artery (MCA) aneurysm with an ensuing left MCA stroke and aphasia that resolved over 1 year. The interhemispheric approach to the ACom artery was selected to avoid compromise of potentially tenuous speech cortex. The trajectory view is seen on the lower right.

of skull markers (fiducials) for all posterior fossa approaches.

Skull base

It may seem superfluous to employ image guidance for skull-base lesions. We have never regretted having image guidance available for these cases, however. Uses include defining the extent of a bone flap, determining the extent of skull-base bone drilling, and the avoidance of important structures such as arteries and nerves. We have also been using image guidance in lieu of fluoroscopy for transphenoidal approaches.

Vascular

Arterovenous malformations

We have used image guidance to ascertain the extent and depth of an arterovenous malformations (AVM) nidus has proven very useful. Stereotactic accuracy is usually maintained throughout the case because AVMs are best resected in one piece. Large feeding arteries and draining veins provide excellent intraoperative anatomical landmarks.

Cavernous angiomas

Cavernous angiomas are analogous to tumors when discussing the usefulness of image guidance. Guidance for localization is an issue for small or deep cavernomas, and again we recommend skull-implanted markers for these cases regardless of the type of image-guidance system used. For larger lesions, volumetric feedback is useful during surgery as with large tumors.

Aneurysms

Image guidance is rarely used during aneurysm surgery. We have found a number of indications that have proven useful and are linked to the advantages of the Cygnus-PFS magnetic system. Most vascular neurosurgeons would rightly consider image-guidance systems to be a cumbersome addition to aneurysm surgery. The Cygnus has a definite advantage here because of its ease of setup and unobtrusiveness during surgery. We have found image guidance to be particularly useful during interhemispheric approaches to anterior communicating artery aneurysms. In this situation, it is often difficult to assess the distance to the aneurysm despite the landmarks of the pericallosal and callosomarginal arteries (see Fig. 6–6). We have also employed image guidance to locate middle cerebral artery (MCA) aneurysms within the Sylvian fissure and to approach distal posterior inferior cerebellar artery (PICA) aneurysms.

Epilepsy

We have used image guidance extensively for lesional and nonlesional epilepsy surgery. In nonlesional cases, image guidance has been very helpful in defining a trajectory to find the temporal horn of the lateral ventricle in the context of selective amygdalo-hippocampectomies. The posterior extent of hippocampal resection and the superomedial extent of amygdalar resection can also be verified. Image guidance has also been a useful adjunct during functional hemispherectomies[13] and in defining the extent of corpus callosotomies. We have used the Cygnus to place intraoperative depth electrodes and are currently developing instrumentation for placement of chronically implanted depth electrodes as has been described using other image-guidance systems.[3,14]

Catheter placement

Placement of ventricular catheters with image guidance is not uncommon. The unobtrusiveness of the magnetic system has led us to use it relatively frequently to optimize routine shunt placement and also for placement of Omaya reservoirs.

■ Ear, Nose, and Throat

In combination with our ENT colleagues, we have used image guidance for approaches to the sphenoid and maxillary sinuses.

■ Ophthalmology

With our ophthalmological surgeons, we have used the Cygnus-PFS for image guidance during resections of orbital tumors with extraorbital invasion. They have also used the Cygnus for imaging feedback during lateral orbital decompressions for proptosis.

■ Conclusions

The Cygnus-PFS (Compass International, Rochester, MN) is a dedicated cranial image-guided system. It is particularly unobtrusive and lends itself to a number of cranial applications where other image-guidance systems would often be too cumbersome. The accuracy of the magnetic system has been shown to be comparable to that of an optical tracking system.

■ Acknowledgments

The author is grateful to Eugenie M. Donnelly, R.N., C.N.O.R. for proofreading.

REFERENCES

1. Gildenberg PL, Tasker RR, eds. *Textbook of Stereotactic and Functional Neurosurgery.* New York: McGraw-Hill; 1998.
2. Guthrie BL, Adler JR Jr. Computer-assisted preoperative planning, interactive surgery and frameless stereotaxy. *Clin Neurosurg* 1992;38:112–131.
3. Olivier A, Germano IM, Cukiert A, Peters T. Frameless stereotaxy for surgery of the epilepsies: preliminary experience [technical note]. *J Neurosurg* 1994;81(4):629–633.
4. Barnett H, Kormos DW, Steiner CP, Weisenberger J. Intraoperative localization using an armless, frameless stereotactic wand. *J Neurosurg* 1993;78:510–514.
5. Reinhardt H, Meyer H, Amrein E. A computer-assisted device for the intraoperative CT-correlated localization of brain tumors. *Eur Surg Res* 1988;20:51–58.
6. Roberts DW, Strohbehn JW, Hatch J, Murray W, Kettenberger H. A frameless stereotactic integration of computerized tomographic imaging and the operating microscope. *J Neurosurg* 1986;65(4):545–549.
7. Smith KR, Frank KJ, Bucholz RD. The NeuroStation: a highly accurate minimally invasive solution to frameless stereotactic neurosurgery. *Compu Med Imaging Graph* 1994;18(4):247–256.
8. Gumprecht HK, Widenka DC, Lumenta CB. BrainLab VectorVision Neuronavigation System: technology and clinical experience in 131 cases. *Neurosurgery* 1999;44:97–104.
9. Mascott CR. The Compass Cygnus-PFS Image-Guided System. *Neurosurgery* 2000;46:235–238.
10. Rousu J, Kohls PE, Kall B, Kelly PJ. Computer-assisted image-guided surgery using the Regulus Navigator. *Medicine Meets Virtual Rseality* 1998;50:103–109.
11. Maciunas RJ, Galloway RL Jr., Latimer J, et al. An independent application accuracy evaluation of stereotactic frame systems. *Stereotact Funct Neurosurg* 1992;58:103–107.
12. Maurer CR Jr., Aboutanos GB, Dawant BM, et al. Effect of geometrical distortion correction in MR on image registration accuracy. *J Comput Assist Tomogr* 1996;20(4):666–679.
13. Villemure JG, Mascott CR. Peri-insular hemispherotomy: surgical principles and anatomy. *Neurosurgery* 1995;37:975–981.
14. Mascott CR, Bizzi J, Tekkok I, Oliver A. Frameless stereotactic placement of depth electrodes for investigation of epilepsy. Poster presented at: Meeting of the American Association of Neurological Surgeons, April 22–27, 1995; Orlando, FL.

7

The Passive Navigational System
Application and Procedure for Use in the Operating Room

LISA TANSEY, DAVID DEAN, AND ROBERT J. MACIUNAS

The world of image-guided neurosurgery is constantly changing and evolving. Several companies are marketing surgical navigation systems; each employs similar steps to bring usable image guidance into the operating room. These steps include preoperative imaging, surgical planning, surgical registration, intraoperative localization, and intraoperative navigation.[1-2] Optically tracked systems are generally grouped into two categories with regard to the way in which they localize. The first group uses active localization. This group uses either light emitting diodes (LEDs) that flash, emitting light or ultrasonic wave pulses, which are triangulated by the camera.[3] The second group uses passive optical navigation. In this group specially designed reference surfaces reflect light. The light source in the passive group usually comes from the camera or camera system and it bathes the entire field looking for reflections.[1,4] This chapter describes the theory behind each step involved in the surgical navigational system and discusses an implementation procedure for the BrainLAB VectorVision neuronavigation system (BrainLAB USA, Redwood City, CA). The BrainLAB system uses a passive reference frame for image localization and navigation.[5]

■ Description of Components

The BrainLAB VectorVision neuronavigation system is a frameless, intraoperative, image-guided, localization system. It consists of three main components: a computer planning station, an intraoperative localization camera, and an intraoperative computer display.[5]

The computer planning station, consisting of a docking station and a laptop, is the location of all the surgical planning. The docking station is the site of network connection and allows for an initial site for image transfer and a constant battery supply. The laptop is an Intel Pentium III processor running Windows NT.[5]

The intraoperative localization camera and intraoperative computer display make up the single VectorVision intraoperative, image-guided navigation system (Fig. 7–1). Both the camera and the computer screen are mounted to individual arms that allow for flexible positioning in the operating room. The camera system consists of two infrared emitting cameras arranged at a fixed distance of 48 cm apart. The camera works by passively detecting reflections of infrared flashes. The infrared flashes are reflected by passive marker spheres that are located in a fixed orientation in relation to the patient's head. The spheres are 8 mm in diameter. The markers must be gas-sterilized and can be reused as long as the reflective covering is intact. The spheres are simply screwed onto different adapters that are used in the field.[1,5]

■ Fiducial Placement

Proper fiducial placement can greatly increase the registration accuracy in the operating room. For the patient to be registered during surgery at least four fiducial markers must be visible by the camera.[5] Therefore it is useful to know where the surgeon is planning to make

Patient positioning is also important to keep in mind. Not only can it be difficult to see the fiducial markers, but also registration accuracy can change with positioning of the head. If the patient is scanned supine and the case is going to be performed in the prone position the surgeon risks a greater error in registration due to the normal shifting of the brain in response to gravity.[6-7]

■ Image Acquisition

There are several ways in which images can be used in the operating room. At least one set of images must be used as the registration image. The images can be registered using the standard registration system (fiducial markers), landmark registration, or Z-touch (BrainLAB USA, Redwood City, CA) registration (Fig. 7–2). The fiducial registration system uses 5 to 6 marker sockets attached to the surface of the head. These markers must be on and visible during the scanning process and must remain in the same location until the patient is ready for surgery. Neither the landmark or Z-touch registration systems require patient preparation prior to the operating room. The landmark registration system recognizes user-defined landmarks on the patient to register the images in the operating room. Z-touch uses an infrared laser beam that scans across the structures of the face acquiring reference points that are used by the system for calibration.[5]

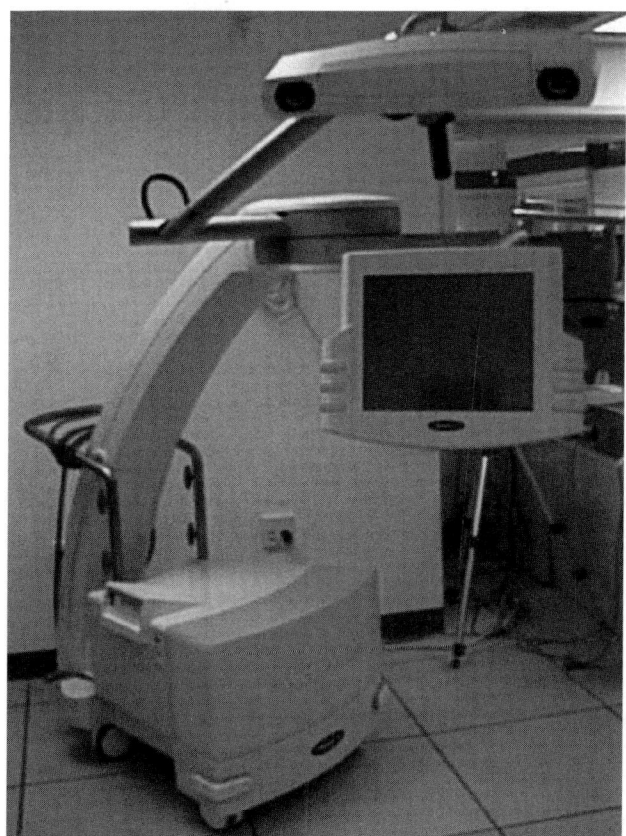

FIGURE 7–1. BrainLAB VectorVision Navigation System (Redwood City, CA). This device is the interface between the image transfer and planning process and the operating room. The computer is housed in the base of the machine, which is also the point of zip disk insertion and processing. As shown in the image, both the touch screen interface and camera are on separate adjustable arms that allow for the greatest mobility in the operating room. The touch screen can be used nonsterile by a circulator or technician or can be made sterile with the use of a specially designed plastic drape. This feature allows the surgeon to use image guidance without assistance.

the incision and to localize the fiducial markers where they are most likely to be visible in the operating room.

We have found it is best to use at least six fiducial markers per patient. Less than five or six markers provide reduced registration accuracy. Skin fiducial markers are by nature more mobile than bone implanted markers. For this reason it is important to place markers in locations where the skin is least likely to be deformed or shifted during scanning. Accuracy can be greatly improved by localizing fiducials around the midline and away from muscles.[6] In a general case the fiducials are spread out over the head, placing two on the forehead, two straddling the midline near the top of the head, and two behind the ears, but avoiding any muscular tissue of the mastoid.

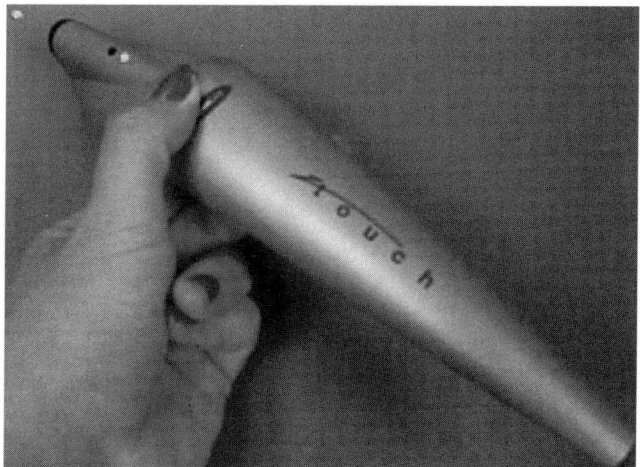

FIGURE 7–2. Z-touch registration instrument (BrainLAB, Redwood City, CA). This instrument can be used to register a patient in the operating room to images that do not have fiducial registration markers. The red laser beam emits an infrared beam of light that can be seen by the camera when the button (shown here) is pushed all the way down. This beam of light traces the structural features of the face, primarily picking out the bridge of the nose and the structures around the eye.

The BrainLAB neuronavigation system allows for image transfer of computed tomography (CT), magnetic resonance imaging (MRI), x-ray, single photon emmission computed tomography (SPECT), and positron emssion tomography (PET) imaging techniques. For preoperative imaging, we have been most successful in using a base image set from either MRI or CT. Before each scan using the standard registration procedure, the skin fiducials must be affixed to the patient's head. Each fiducial consists of a plastic socket and one of three different inserts. The sockets are glued to the head of the patient using double-adhesive tape. The markers must be affixed directly to the skin of the patient, which frequently requires shaving a small spot of hair, large enough to place the marker.

The insert in the socket depends on what imaging technique is being used and where the patient is at in the surgery process. The green, organic, oil-based markers are for MRI. They are spherical in shape and completely disposable. The CT markers are also spherical, but they are blue and made of aluminum. They can easily be cleaned and reused. The last set of markers is the red registration markers. These markers are for registering the patient in the operating room. They are made of aluminum and are colored red. Their hemispherical shape allows the computer to automatically triangulate the center of the sphere and thus provide the highest registration accuracy.[5]

Both the MRI and CT scanning techniques require a base volumetric scan. Additional images can be fused to the base image later using different protocols. Slice orientation for MRI is preferably axial with slice thickness of 1 mm and no gap between images. Oblique images are only acceptable within 10 degrees of angulation. The protocol for CT is similar although image slices of 2 mm are usually used. Contrast medium can be used with both imaging techniques if desirable.[1,5]

■ Surgical Planning

After scanning, the images are sent via the network to the planning station. Each planning station is networked with the radiology scanners to receive DICOM image data. To successfully transfer the image to the planning station it must be passed through PatXfer. PatXfer is a Windows-based program that carries the user step by step through the transfer process. It allows for the selection of the imaging modality and the individual patient that is to be transferred. It also allows for the selection of specific image sets contained in the patient's folder.

Following data transfer, the user will either open @Target, if using a framed localizer and stereotactic arc, or open the Planning software for fiducial registration and surgical planning. Both software suites allow for the simultaneous use of multiple sets of image data from one operating room registration procedure via image fusion. Image fusion is calculated by the computer to match multiple sets of data to one another. In this way the image sets can be registered off one base set and then navigation can occur on all of the images.[8] The Planning and @Target software are Windows-based programs that are intuitively designed and easy to use. The Planning software allows the user to pre-operatively select the six fiducial markers using the Automatic Marker Detection and set both a target and and entry point for the surgery. The images in this program allow for reconstruction in a triplanar format (axial, sagittal, and coronal), as well as three-dimensional reconstruction. The patient's image data is saved on a zip disk that can easily be transported to the VectorVision navigation system in the operating room.

■ Operating Room Positioning and Setup

In the operating room, the patient is positioned for surgery. The head is fixed in a stationary position using the Mayfield headrest. The VectorVision navigational system is positioned in the room so as to give the surgeons maneuverability while achieving the optimum camera view of the patient's head. The preferred distance for the camera is approximately 1.4 m (4.5 feet) from the patient's head.[5] Then the patient's data is loaded onto the navigation station via zip disk transfer from the planning station. The touch screen on the computer allows for easy access to imaging displays. Triplanar views are available. In addition it is possible to view the images from the Probes eye view and to view inline with the instrument in use, as well as three-dimensional reconstructions.

Reference frame instrumentation

Attached to the Mayfield headrest is a stainless steel clamp. The clamp allows for the attachment of a reference star. The reference star is actually a three-pronged adapter with reflective marker spheres on each arm that the computer recognizes as a point of reference within the field (Fig. 7–3). This instrument must remain in the same orientation to the head from the time of registration forward. Clamping the reference star to the Mayfield headrest allows the surgeon to move the patient around while maintaining registration because the reference star moves along with the head.[4,5]

Passive Navigational System 71

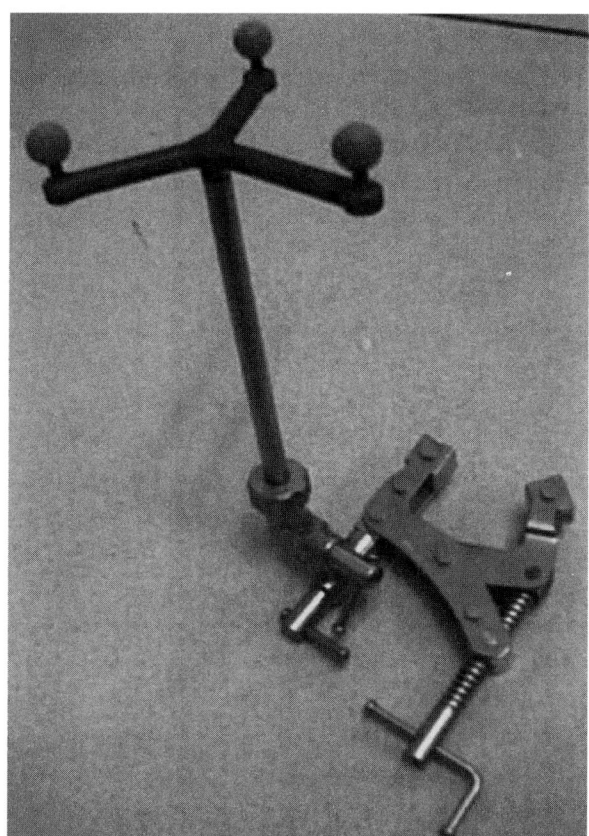

FIGURE 7–3. Mayfield clamp and reference star. This figure shows how the stainless steal clamp to the Mayfield head holder fits together with the reference star. The clamp tightens directly to the Mayfield head holder and must remain in the same reference frame in relation to the patient throughout the procedure. The reference star is completely detachable from the clamp so that the identical nonsterile and sterile stars can be substituted during the surgery. The three silver spheres on the three arms of the reference star are reflecting spheres. They cause reflection of the infrared light source that is detected by the cameras.

Pointer

What is most convenient about the BrainLAB VectorVision Navigation System is its ability to link a freehand pointer to the image-guidance system using tracking from a passive marker sensor system. A nonsterile version of the pointer is used for registration, and an identical sterile version can be used for navigation throughout the surgery. The pointer has two reflective spheres attached to it that are coaxial with the tip of the instrument. The computer recognizes this known geometry and can project the location of the pointer's trajectory.[4–5]

Registration

For standard registration the conical registration markers replace the spherical MRI or CT markers. Registration is carried out under nonsterile conditions. The computer instructs the user to touch the tip of the pointer to the center of each of the conical registration markers, in any order. If the computer is having difficulties calculating an accurate registration it will ask the user to reregister the patient by touching each fiducial marker in a specified order. The computer will calculate the error and allow the user to proceed with navigation if the error is less than 5 mm. Upon completion of the registration process, the skin incision can be outlined on the scalp and the surgical approach can be determined. Defining the borders of the lesion assures the surgeon that the most minimally invasive procedure is performed.

Patient draping

Following the completion of registration the fiducial markers should be removed from the head. They can remain on the patient during surgery, but are no longer viable for re-registration because they will be covered up by the sterile drapes. Removing them after registration keeps them out of the surgeon's way, and they can be cleaned and put away for reuse.

Before the surgeon begins the patient's cleaning and sterilization, the nonsterile reference star should be detached from the clamp. The patient then undergoes draping as usual, with the stainless steel reference clamp kept readily accessible under the drape. After complete draping, the reference star is replaced with a sterile copy. This is done by cutting a small incision in the drapes and sliding the sterile reference star into the clamp. To avoid contamination, a sterile cloth is wrapped around the bottom of the reference star, assuring the surgeon that the clamp stays underneath the sterile field.

■ Intraoperative Three-Dimensional Guidance

Once the patient has been draped and the incision made, both a sterile reference star and a pointer are to be used for the duration of the surgery. Other instruments can also be used for navigation. A set of four instrument adapters is included in each kit of varying sizes. Any instrument can be registered by touching the tip into the center of the calibration cone of the reference star. The computer calculates the distance from the instrument adapter to the center of the cone. It is important to understand that this calculation is a straight-line distance. Although the calibration is possible with curved instruments, it only guarantees exact placement of the tip of the instrument and can say nothing about the trajectory.

The location of the tip of the instrument is constantly being updated by the VectorVision system. Any instrument can be virtually extended to project the direction of the approach toward the lesion. In addition, the distance to the target lesion can be measured from the end of the instrument.[5]

■ Patients

From the time of its installation in March 2001 until August 2001, the BrainLAB system has been consistently used in approximately five cases per week. Cases range from brain biopsies and craniotomies to transphenoidals and deep brain stimulations. The biopsies and craniotomies usually prefer the standard registration implementation, whereas the transphenoidals prefer Z-touch, and the deep brain stimulations use a stereotactic arc and arc settings from the @Target software.

Many patients found the fiducial markers uncomfortable to wear and difficult to keep attached to their head for more than a few hours. In response to this we begin removing the markers from the head after the preoperative scan and marking the outline of the socket location with a blue sharpie marker. This procedure increases the opportunity for error in replacement of the markers, but, in return, increases the probability that we will have four usable markers for registration.

The operating room is governed by the ability to be flexible and mobile. The BrainLAB VectorVision system allows for constant adjustment throughout the surgery. In the event of accidental power loss or blockage of the camera's view, the system can easily be unplugged and moved about the room while still maintaining registration accuracy. The battery life is approximately 7 minutes.[5] This has proved to be especially helpful when using bulky instruments such as the microscope.

■ Conclusions

The BrainLAB VectorVision neuronavigation system has proven to be a reliable and user-friendly tool in the operating room.[9] The system is adaptable to many different pathological conditions and surgical procedures. Image guidance may increase the preparation time in the operating room, but it decreases the overall surgical time due to more direct approaches and smaller incisions.

The BrainLAB system's greatest advantages are its use of wireless instruments and adapters and the system's mobility while maintaining registration. Capabilities that would be useful additions would include the ability to continually update the registration image by fusing it to new intraoperative MRI images.[10] Currently, once the skull is opened accuracy decreases because the brain naturally shifts to release pressure. This becomes extremely important when resecting a large tumor. The brain may shift so much as to make the preoperative image no longer viable.[7]

■ Acknowledgments

TR contributed to this chapter while supported by the National Science Foundation under Grant No. EIA-0104114. David Dean and Robert J. Maciunas acknowledge the support of the Research Foundation of the Department of Neurological Surgery and the Research Institute of University Hospitals of Cleveland.

REFERENCES

1. Gumprecht HK, Widenka DC, Lumenta CB. BrainLAB VectorVision neuronavigation system: technology and clinical experiences in 131 cases. *Neurosurgery* 1999;44:97–105.
2. Spetzger U, Laborde G, Gilsbach JM. Frameless neuronavigation in modern neurosurgery. *Minimally Invasive Neurosurgery* 1995;38:163–166.
3. Barnett GH, Kromos DW, Steiner CP, Weisenberger J. Use of a frameless, armless stereotactic wand for brain tumor localization with two-dimensional and three-dimensional neuroimaging. *Neurosurgery* 1993;33:674–678.
4. Khadem R, Yeh CC, Sadeghi-Tehrani M, et al. Comparative tracking error analysis of five different optical tracking systems. *Computer Aided Surgery* 2000;5:98–107.
5. *Clinical User Guide, Revision 1.1: VectorVision².* Germany: BrainLAB AG; 2001.
6. West JB, Fitzpatrick JM, Toms SA, Maurer CR, Maciunas RJ. Fiducial point placement and the accuracy of point-based, rigid body registration. *Neurosurgery* 2001;48:810–817.
7. Nabavi A, Black PM, Gering DT, et al. Serial intraoperative magnetic resonance imaging of brain shift. *Neurosurgery* 2001;48:787–798.
8. Jannin P, Fleig OJ, Seigneuret E, Grova C, Morandi X, Scarabin JM. A data fusion environment for multimodal and multi-informational neuronavigation. *Computer Aided Surgery* 2000;5:1–10.
9. Maciunas RJ. Craniotomy for deep-seated gliomas guided by optical tracking. In: Alexander E, Maciunas RJ, *Advanced Neurosurgical Navigation.* New York: Thieme; 1999:373–396.
10. Hadani, M, Spegelman R, Feldman Z, Berkenstadt H, Ram Z. Novel, compact, intraoperative magnetic resonance imaging-guided system for conventional neurosurgical operating rooms. *Neurosurgery* 2001;48:799–809.

8

Image-Guided Neurosurgery Combining Mechanical Arm and Optical Digitizer

WILLIAM D. TOBLER

The decade of the 1990s was a transition time for technological innovation in neurosurgery. Computer-assisted surgery was introduced into the operating room, and by the end of the decade it had become a mainstream technology adopted by neurosurgeons worldwide. The term *frameless stereotaxy* was casually applied to the use of image-guided navigational systems in surgical procedures. Initially these systems were used as navigational instruments to follow the progress of tumor resection in open craniotomies. Recently, there has been widespread promotion by the spine implant companies to market these systems for use in the placement of pedicle screws, another form of open navigation. Today these systems continue to be used as open navigational tools in the great majority of cases. There has been minimal activity regarding the use of these systems for true stereotactic procedures; thus the term *frameless stereotaxy* is a misnomer.

This chapter is devoted to an image-guided system capable of advanced stereotactic applications in image-guided surgery. The Mayfield ACCISS system (Ohio Medical Instrument Company, Cincinnati, OH) was developed with innovative hardware and software components to successfully carry out and verify the precision of frameless stereotactic image-guided procedures.

■ History and Development of Digitizers for Image-Guided Surgery

The concept of surgical navigation was introduced by linking computer systems and digitizing instruments. These early computers had the capacity to process and render a three-dimensional model of the magnetic resonance imaging (MRI) or computed tomographic (CT) image of the patient's cranium. The digitizing instruments use multiple technologies to locate a point in three-dimensional physical space and to process that information in the computer.[1] These digitizers include sonic emitting probes, mechanical arms, infrared optical camera systems to track surgical probes embedded with light-emitting diodes (LEDs), and probes moving through electromagnetic fields.[2–10] Using one of these forms of digitizer, the surgeon matches or registers identifiable points on the patient to the same points on the patient's MRI or CT image reconstructed by the workstation. When this registration is successfully completed, one can navigate around and within the patient's anatomy using the digitizing probe and see the virtual representation of the probe move about with respect to the pertinent image in the workstation.

■ Development of Digitizing Technology

The decade of the 1990s saw an evolution of this digitizing technology and the continual development of faster, more powerful, and less expensive computers. It became apparent that each type of digitizing instrument possesses certain drawbacks that make its use as a surgical instrument somewhat difficult at times. Sonic digitizers, because of ambient noise interference in the operating room, never achieved practical utility.[2] Mechanical arms enjoyed a brief period of popularity in the early part of the decade, but the systems available at that time fell into disuse because of their cumbersome size and weight, which made them difficult to use in surgery.[4-9] They were also criticized because they had to be attached to the table or headrest and this tethering was undesirable. In spite of the opinion that mechanical arm digitizers may be the most robust and accurate of all digitizers, they were displaced by optical tracking systems. Electromagnetic systems have not gained widespread acceptance because of the apparent inaccuracies caused by contamination of the electromagnetic field by all other necessary instrumentation in the surgical field. Recent developments in this technology suggest that electromagnetic tracking may overcome these problems and has the potential to displace optical tracking in popularity because it eliminates the major drawbacks of optical tracking.[11] Specifically, with electromagnetic tracking there is no camera, and the need to maintain open optical pathways is eliminated.

Optical tracking systems are currently the most popular form of digitizer accepted and promoted in the marketplace in spite of significant drawbacks to their use. It is difficult to maintain an optical path free of interference in a usually crowded environment around the operating table. Placement of the camera in a strategic position over the field so that it can "see" the encoders on the digitizing instrument at all times presents a constant challenge. Turning or angling the probe out of the camera's range disrupts the tracking process, and the image and the probe's position on the computer screen are disrupted until the probe is returned to the position so that it can be "seen" again and the image restored. Other interference is encountered by drapes and IV poles and the movement of the hands and arms of assistants passing instruments. Introducing the microscope into the operating field makes the unrestricted use of optical tracking very challenging.

Many improvements have been introduced into optical tracking technology. The original probes required a wire to electrically power the LEDs. Recently, wireless probes have been introduced that contain a small nickel-cadmium battery powering the wireless LED-containing probes. Alternatively, passive optical tracking technology was introduced. Multiple large reflecting spheres can be attached to any pointing instrument, and an infrared light source placed on the camera allows the camera to "see" the reflection of the light from the spheres. This passive technology eliminates the power cord and enables the tracking of many different instruments, which may be especially attractive for spinal applications. Nonetheless, in spite of these improvements interference in the optical pathways in a restricted and crowded operating environment presents a continuous annoyance.

Other problems associated with optical tracking include the need to maintain the integrity and working order of all of the LEDs and to ensure that the reflective spheres are clear of blood and debris, which can diminish their ability to provide an accurate reflection. Troubleshooting an optical system that is not functioning properly when needed, usually after the operation has commenced, can be time-consuming and frustrating and may occasionally require discontinuation of the procedure if an alternative digitizing technique is not available.

Common Applications of Image-Guided Surgical Navigation Systems

Image-guided surgery is most widely utilized in the brain and spine for tracking the probe's position with respect to the anatomy involved. These applications are fairly straightforward. Commonly image-guided surgery is used for locating a small craniotomy flap strategically placed over a small tumor. It is used to track the progress during open resection of intra-axial neoplasms such as gliomas and extra-axial lesions such as meningiomas and acoustic neuromas.[12,13] In the spine the most common application is for the placement of lumbar pedicle screws. More difficult and challenging applications for open navigational procedures include the use of image-guided surgery for the resection of pituitary adenomas and the placement of thoracic pedicle screws and transarticular screws at the C1–C2 level.

The Concept of Frameless Stereotaxis

The term *frameless stereotaxis* was used early to refer to this new technology. More accurately described, these devices are computer-assisted, image-guided surgical navigation systems. The initial belief was that this technology would replace and make obsolete frame-based stereotaxis. That has not happened and these systems are still used largely as navigational devices for open surgical procedures. Enthusiasm for the term *frameless stereotaxis* may have reflected a hope to eliminate the current method of frame-based stereotaxis. In frame-based stereotaxis a bulky mechanical device surrounding the cranial vault is affixed to the patient by screwing four pins under high pressure while the patient is awake and aware of what is being done. This technology requires the patient to wear the device until the procedure is completed. More recently, some surgeons have attempted to perform true point-in-space stereotactic procedures by using image-guided systems and adapting existing hardware to facilitate this more complex level of application of image-guided surgery and, thus, eliminating the stereotactic frame.[14-16] Some image-guided man-

Image-Guided Neurosurgery Combining Mechanical Arm and Optical Digitizer 75

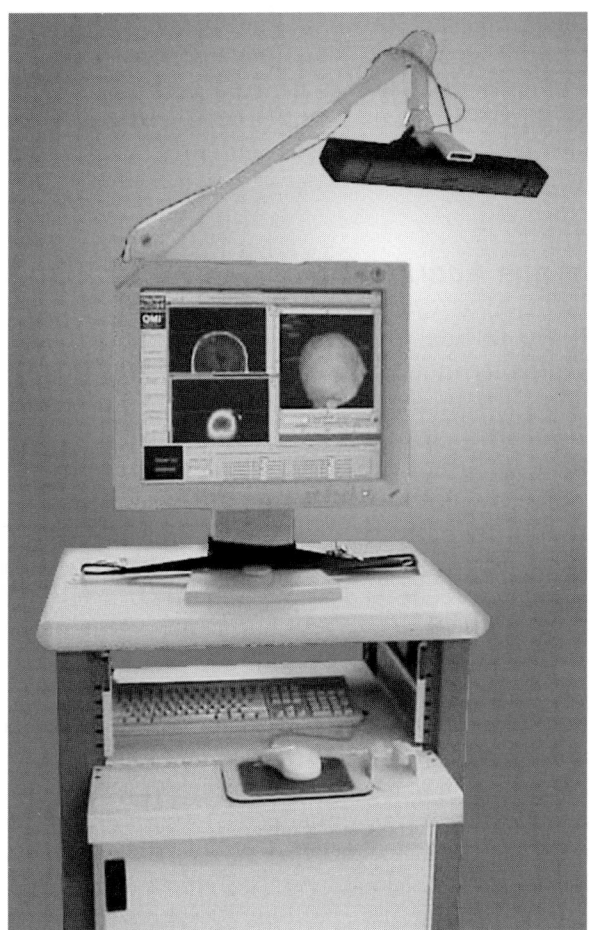

FIGURE 8–1. The standard cabinet for the Mayfield ACCISS system (Ohio Medical Instrument Co., Cincinnati, OH) houses the computer system and the flat screen monitor.

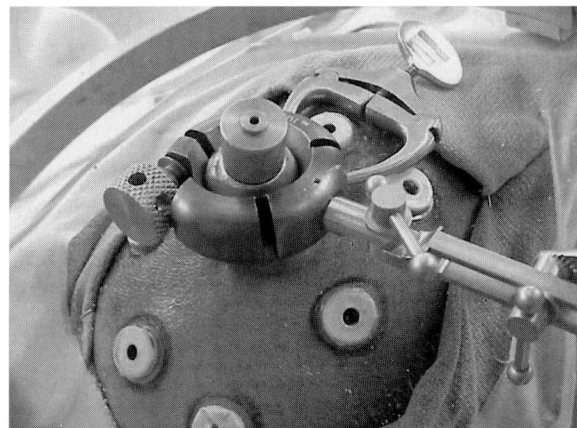

FIGURE 8–2. The AccuPoint sphere (Ohio Medical Instruments, Cincinnati, OH) rests in a housing that can be brought to the entry point and affixed rigidly into position once the trajectory to the tumor is determined. The biopsy catheter is passed through the collar, and the trajectory is rigidly held throughout the duration of the procedure.

ufacturers are adapting their computer programs to integrate stereotactic frames as if to indicate that true frameless stereotaxis may not be achievable. There may be widespread belief that image-guided systems cannot match the level of accuracy believed to be inherently present in stereotactic frames.

The Mayfield ACCISS, an image-guided, computer-assisted surgical navigation system (Fig. 8–1), has both the software capabilities and the custom-designed hardware required for point-in-space stereotactic surgery that eliminates the need to use traditional stereotactic frames.[12,13] Unlike other systems, which have tried to adapt an existing gooseneck-style Greenberg retractor arm to hold a stereotactic probe,[14] the Mayfield ACCISS system uses a custom-made device, the AccuPoint sphere (Ohio Medical Instrument Company, Cincinnati, OH). This sphere is capable of maintaining rigid fixation for a stereotactic trajectory for the duration of the stereotactic procedure (Fig. 8–2). The author has used the Mayfield ACCISS in more than 100 stereotactic procedures with demonstrable evidence of equivalence in accuracy and outcomes to any published experience using frame-based stereotaxis.

The image-guided workstation

The initial development of the Mayfield ACCISS workstation began in 1992. Its current configuration uses a 733 MHz, 128 MB RAM Pentium III PC running the Windows NT operating system. This combination provides rapid and powerful computing capacity in a form most familiar and easy to use for surgeons. The computer can be run by the operating surgeon and does not require the assistance of a dedicated technician.

The Mayfield ACCISS system was originally developed with a mechanical arm, which continues to be an important component of the system. This arm was developed to eliminate the undesirable characteristics of the early mechanical arm systems. The Mayfield mechanical arm is lightweight (13.5 oz) and small. It is anchored to the Budde Halo retractor system (Ohio Medical Instrument Company) and brought into the immediate vicinity of the operative field, minimizing the sense of tethering (Fig. 8–3). These features of the Mayfield ACCISS mechanical arm, along with its robustness and dependability, make it a very attractive digitizing tool. There are no line-of-sight issues when using the mechanical arm, and it is most proficiently used when the microscope is brought into the operating field. For surgeons who prefer to use optical tracking technology or in clinical situations in which optical tracking is preferred, the Mayfield ACCISS system employs both active and passive optical tracking instruments. An important advantage of the

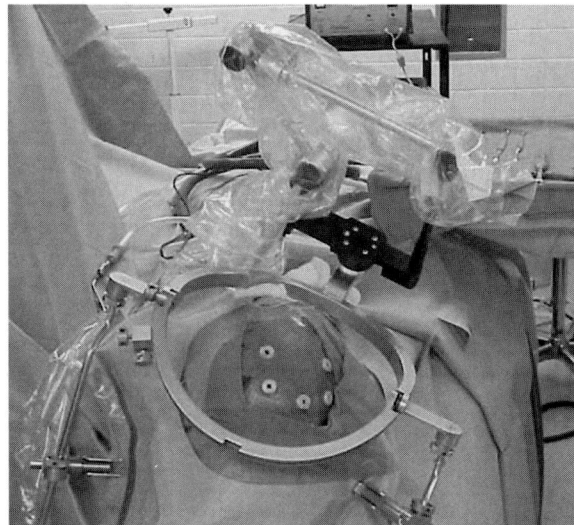

FIGURE 8–3. The Mayfield ACCISS mechanical arm (Ohio Medical Instruments, Cincinnati, OH) is placed within the operative field and anchored to the Budde Halo.

dual digitizing system lies in the fact that when the optical system fails to function properly, the mechanical arm functions in a fail-safe way, eliminating lengthy delays that can occur during surgery. This virtually ensures that the image-guided procedure will never need to be abandoned because of failures of the optical system.

Stereotactic components of the image-guided system

Rigid fixation is the key to achieving point-in-space stereotactic capabilities with an image-guided system and must be maintained through the many steps necessary to successfully complete the stereotactic procedure. These steps include moving the targeting device into position at the chosen entry point, generating the trajectory to the target with the digitizer placed in the stereotactic targeting device, making the opening through a standard burr hole or via a twist drill, and passing the stereotactic probe to complete the procedure. The AccuPoint sphere has been designed specifically to meet the requirements of stereotactic surgery. It is a stainless-steel sphere that rotates in a socket that can be fixed rigidly once the trajectory to the target has been established (see Fig. 8–2). The trajectory is determined by simulating the procedure on the patient and simultaneously at the workstation, where the computer becomes the electronic "phantom." The AccuPoint sphere can be attached to the Budde Halo retractor system, to the Mayfield headrest, or directly to the skull by placing it in a ring and securing it with self-tapping screws to the skull. These three different techniques can be used to satisfy the requirements of the most demanding stereotactic procedures. All intracranial targets can be accessed because there is no frame or set of posts associated with traditional frames, which can block access to certain entry or target points.

■ Image Acquisition and Surgical Planning

Adhesive fiducial markers are used ordinarily, although implantable fiducial markers are available. The experience reported in this chapter has been acquired with adhesive markers in most cases, supporting the notion that satisfactory accuracy can be achieved without invasive markers. Usually the author prefers to place five to seven markers around the region of interest and to prep those markers into the operative field so that accuracy can be checked and rechecked throughout the procedure (Fig. 8–4). The Mayfield ACCISS has a software feature that allows one to eliminate individually any fiducial marker from the registration paradigm that demonstrates an unsatisfactory registration error. Often excellent registration can be achieved with as few as three or four fiducial registration markers.

Volumetric contrast-enhanced TI-weighted images are the standard MRI sequences used. Occasionally T2-weighted or flair sequences are helpful in more extensively delineating the pathology, especially in glial lesions that exhibit poor enhancement characteristics. CT scanning with contrast enhancement using 3 mm contiguous slices with a 0 degree gantry tilt is required for reconstruction in the workstation. Occasionally 1.5 mm slices are used for improved accuracy. Images can be transferred from the scanner to the image-guided work-

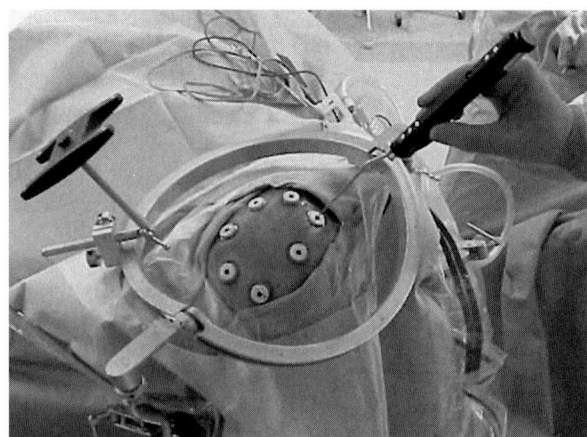

FIGURE 8–4. Rechecking the registration accuracy with the optical probe is easily accomplished when the fiducial markers are prepped into the field.

station by ethernet connections or by any other suitable media such as DAT tape or optical disc.

■ Evaluation of the Postoperative Image Sequence

With the Mayfield ACCISS workstation one has the capacity to co-register multiple images. Co-registration is performed by registration of one image to the other. An MRI can be co-registered to a CT scan; TI- and T2-weighted images can be co-registered. Co-registered images appear side-by-side on the computer screen. A point placed on one image appears at the same stereotactic point on the co-registered image. Surgical navigation can be carried out simultaneously with multimodal co-registered images. As one navigates with the digitizing probe, the virtual probe tip appears at the stereotactic point on each of the co-registered images. For stereotactic surgical procedures the co-registration feature enables the surgeon to co-register the preoperative image to the postoperative image (Fig. 8–5). Typically a preoperative MRI is co-registered to a postoperative CT to evaluate the accuracy of a stereotactic biopsy. The stereotactic target chosen for the biopsy can be annotated on the preoperative MRI, and its corresponding stereotactic point appears on the co-registered post-

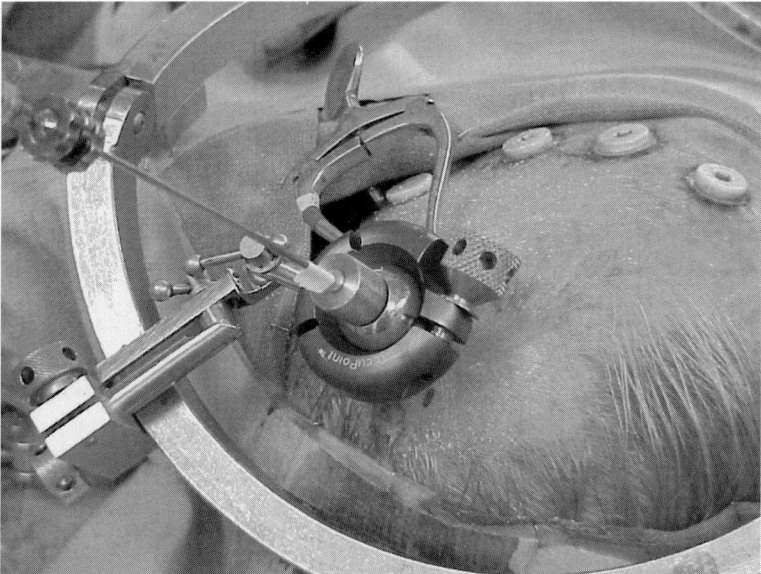

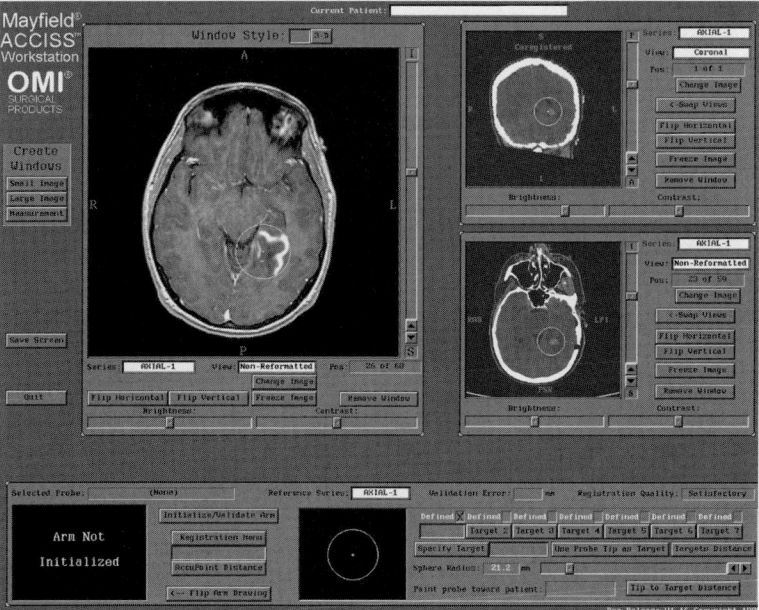

FIGURE 8–5. (A). Co-registered preoperative magnetic resonance imaging. (B). Postoperative biopsy computed tomographic scans. The intended biopsy target is marked. A small hemorrhage blush appears at the target site on the postbiopsy images. The distance from the intended target to the focal point of hemorrhage can be measured.

biopsy CT. The image-guided computer can reproduce the same image slice by slice on the pre- and postoperative scans in both standard orthogonal and nonorthogonal views. If the post-biopsy CT scans show an air bubble or hemorrhagic blush, its location in relation to the intended target can be measured (see Fig. 8–5). This co-registration capability has not been possible with frame-based stereotaxy. The Mayfield ACCISS workstation enables one to evaluate the accuracy of stereotactic targeting in a manner never before possible.

■ Stereotactic Experience with the Image-Guided System

A total of 110 stereotactic targeting procedures have been performed at this time using the Mayfield ACCISS and the AccuPoint stereotactic sphere. Most of these procedures have been stereotactic biopsies in 82 patients. The other 28 cases involved stereotactic aspiration of intracerebral hematomas, cyst aspiration, and placement of ventricular catheters.

In 82 patients a total of 87 stereotactic targeting procedures were performed. In five patients two separate trajectories were made to different targets. Eleven of the cases demonstrated pathology other than neoplasia: there were eight abscesses, two cases of demyelination, and one infarct. Of the 71 patients in this series who had brain tumors, three of the biopsies were nondiagnostic. Two of these three pathology specimens showed hypercellularity in cases that are probably low-grade gliomas. The third nondiagnostic case showed normal brain, a very early case in this series of a nonenhancing temporal lobe glioblastoma, representing a failure of the neurosurgeon to choose the correct target rather than a failure of the image-guided system. The total nondiagnostic rate of the 82 patients undergoing stereotactic biopsy was 3.7%.

Complications occurred in three biopsy cases and these were all biopsy-related hemorrhages. One required a craniotomy; the other two resulted in increased motor deficits treated conservatively. There were no other complications and no mortality associated with these procedures. The overall complication rate for the entire series is 2.7%, or 3.7% when applied to the biopsy series alone.

■ Discussion

Stereotactic surgical procedures performed with image-guided surgical navigation systems represent a more sophisticated application of this new technology. The ability to eliminate the stereotactic frame provides a significant benefit to the patient and surgeon. Valuable operating time is saved early in the morning while the surgeon and staff are waiting for the scan to be completed. The frequent delays encountered while transporting the patient to the operating room are eliminated. The patient does not have to endure the pain and anxiety that accompanies the placement of a frame, and wait time with the frame in place is eliminated. Acquisition of the image before the day of surgery also allows for adequate evaluation of the quality of the image and avoids last-minute delays caused by the need to repeat images.

Once in surgery unrestricted access to any entry point or target is possible because there is no stereotactic frame or posts, which can often be problematic with frame-based stereotaxis. Additionally there are no issues for anesthesia with respect to sterility and draping, as often occurs with frame-based stereotactic procedures. The use of the AccuPoint sphere and stereotactic software allows one to adjust entry points and select the target with greater ease compared with frame-based procedures.

Finally, in this series of stereotactic biopsies the diagnostic and complication rates, which are the only measurable criteria of accuracy in frame-based stereotactic surgery in the literature, are equivalent or better than those reported for frame-based stereotaxis.[17–21] Visual demonstration of the accuracy of co-registered pre- and postoperative images obtained with image-guided stereotactic biopsy provides striking reassurance of the efficacy of this technique.

Further refinements in technology will surely increase the attractiveness of image-guided stereotactic surgery for all neurosurgeons. Mastery of the image-guided system, including hardware and software components, is required for success at this level of application of image-guided technology.

REFERENCES

1. Roberts DW, Strohbehn JW, Hatch J, Murray W, Kettenberger H. A frameless stereotactic integration of computerized tomographic imaging and the operating microscope. *J Neurosurg* 1986;65:545–549.
2. Barnett GH, Steiner CP, Roberts DW. Surgical navigation system technologies. In: Barnett GH, Roberts DW, Maciunas RJ, eds. *Image-Guided Neurosurgery*. St. Louis: Quality Medical Publishing, Inc.; 1998:17–32.
3. Barnett GH, Kormos DW, Steiner CP. Intraoperative localization using an armless, frameless, stereotactic wand. *J Neurosurg* 1993;78:510–514.
4. Guthrie BL. Graphic interactive cranial surgery. *Clin Neurosurg* 1993;41:489–516.
5. Guthrie BL, Adler JR. Computer-assisted preoperative planning, interactive surgery, and frameless stereotaxy. *Clin Neurosurg* 1992;38:112–131.
6. Guthrie BL, Adler JR. Frameless stereotaxy: computer interactive neurosurgery. *Perspect Neurol Surg* 1991;2(1):1–19.

7. Golfinos JG, Fitzpatrick BC, Smith LR, Spetzler RF. Clinical use of a frameless stereotactic arm: results in 325 cases. *J Neurosurg* 1995;83:197–205.
8. Olivier A, Germano IM, Cukiert A, Peters T. Frameless stereotaxy for surgery of the epilepsies: preliminary experience. *J Neurosurg* 1994;81:629–633.
9. Watanabe E, Watanabe T, Manake S. Three-dimensional digitizer (Neuronavigator): new equipment of CT-guided stereotaxy surgery. *Surg Neurol* 1987;27:543–547.
10. Sandeman DR, Nitin P, Chandler P, Nelson RJ, Coakham HB, Griffith HB. Advances in image-directed neurosurgery: preliminary experience with the ISG viewing wand compared with the Leksel G frame. *Br J Neurosurg* 1994;8:529–544.
11. Sedlmaier B, Schleich A, Hoell T, Ohnesorge I, Jovanovic S. NEN-ENT navigation system: first clinical application. Proceedings: Fourth European Congress of Head and Neck Surgery; May 17, 2000. Berlin, Germany. Bologna, Italy: Modduzzi Editore; 2000:1247–1251.
12. Tobler WD. Image-guided neurosurgery with the Mayfield ACCISS Workstation. Surgical Technology International VII. San Francisco: Universal Medical Press, Inc.; 1998:459–464.
13. Tobler WD. Surgical navigation with the Mayfield ACCISS OMI system. In: *The Handbook of Stereotactic and Functional Neurosurgery.* New York: Marcel Dekker, Inc. In Press.
14. Barnett GH, Miller DW, Weisenberger J. Frameless stereotaxy with scalp-applied fiducial markers for brain biopsy procedures: experience in 218 cases. *J Neurosurg* 1999;91:569–576.
15. Dorward NL, Alberti O, Palmer JD, Kitchen ND, Thomas DGT. Accuracy of true frameless stereotaxy: in vivo measurement and laboratory phantom studies. *J Neurosurg* 1999;90:160–168.
16. Germano IM, Queenan JV. Clinical experience with intracranial brain needle biopsy using frameless surgical navigation. *Comput Aid Surg* 1998;3:33–39.
17. Apuzzo MLJ, Chandrasoma PT, Cohen D, Zee CS, Zelamn V. Computed imaging stereotaxy: experience and perspective related to 500 procedures applied to brain masses. *Neurosurgery* 1987;20:930–937.
18. Mundinger F. CT stereotactic biopsy for optimizing therapy of intracranial processes. *Acta Neurochir Suppl* 1985;35:70–74.
19. Niizuma H, Otsuki T, Yonemitsu T. Experience with CT-guided stereotactic biopsies in 121 cases. *Acta Neurochir Suppl* 1988;42:157–160.
20. Ostertag CB, Mennel HD, Kiessling M. Stereotactic biopsy of brain tumors. *Surg Neurol* 1980;14:275–283.
21. Thomas DGT, Nouby RM. Experience in 300 cases of CT directed stereotactic surgery for lesion biopsy and aspiration of hematoma. *Br J Neurosurg* 1989;3:321–326.

9

Videotactic Surgery
A Volume as an Image-Guided Target

PHILIP L. GILDENBERG

When computed tomography (CT) and then magnetic resonance imaging (MRI) were introduced, it was only natural that such sophisticated imaging techniques be combined with stereotactic surgery to allow surgeons to target accurately in space any mass that could be visualized.[1] As computer graphics became more accessible, techniques for reconstructing three-dimensional (3-D) images of the brain and any mass therein allowed unprecedented visualization of brain structures. The use of sophisticated 3-D images for accurate localization in the operating room is only now evolving, in part because of the limited ability of 2-D computer displays to deliver complex 3-D graphic images to the surgeon.

The programs described below address the problems of (1) how to get the maximum amount of information to facilitate surgical judgment, (2) how to process this information to define the target for resection as a unified volume, rather than merely a series of single points in space, and (3) how to display this information to the surgeon in an intuitive and useful manner, incorporating the computer-generated guidance graphic into a real-time view of the operating field throughout the resection.

The Exoscope program was developed to provide a real-time image of the operating field with a superimposed, computer-generated image of the target volume, usually a tumor. This augmented reality guides the surgeon to the tumor and demonstrates graphically the preplanned resection line to facilitate accurate resection.[2]

■ Concepts of Defining a Target in Space

Since the advent of stereotactic surgery and then image-guided surgery, it has been standard procedure to use a point in space as the target. Stereotactic frames guide a probe to a specific point localized in three dimensions. Stereotactic procedures work because they superimpose that point with the intended target. A stereotactic frame is mechanically applied to the patient's skull so that any structure therein is registered to stereotactic space. The images are then acquired, and any target or structure on those images is likewise oriented stereotactically. Thus the target might be a point from a CT- or MRI-visualized mass to be biopsied, a point in an anatomical structure such as the globus pallidus to be lesioned, or a point at the center of a landmark such as the anterior or posterior commissure from which an ultimate target is indirectly localized. In all these cases, the target is one or several points in space.[3]

Point-in-space targeting

Frameless image-guided surgery also uses a point in space as a target, or, more commonly, a series of points.[4] Even though the display of a frameless system might show a beautifully rendered, 3-D picture of the volume of the patient's head and the tumor within, that impressive image is generally not as useful to the surgeon as images showing the position of a pointer's tip in space. The point is oriented to 3-D space by the simultaneous display of three CT or MRI reconstructed slices. Each 2-D slice demonstrates the position of the probe tip. The surgeon mentally combines the 2-D images to appreciate the 3-D position of the tip of the pointer. By identifying a number of points in space in this fashion, the surgeon builds a mental picture of the edge of the tumor and consequently the volume within.[5–6]

Stereotactic frames can be used to define the outline of a volume in a similar fashion. A series of points are selected on the CT or MRI console or on the surgical planning workstation so that they represent the edge of the volume, whether it is a tumor or a line of resection around the tumor. Three-dimensional stereotactic coordinates [anteroposterior (AP), lateral, vertical] are determined for each point. By readjusting the stereotactic frame repeatedly, each of those points can be defined in the surgical field, and thus an approximation of the target volume can be obtained.

This principle can be illustrated by defining the volume of a cube in space. If you know it is a cube and you define one point on each of the six surfaces, the volume of that cube is accurately contained within those six points. A similar technique using six points can be employed to approximate the volume of a tumor, although errors are introduced because of irregularities in the shape of the tumor.

Volume-in-space targeting

Even though it is possible to build or develop a 3-D volume as a virtual target, there remains the problem of delivering that information to the surgeon in the simplest and most useful fashion. Such 3-D volumetric targeting is necessarily used in stereotactic radiosurgery, where the treatment volume must be defined. The actual targeting is done by displaying individual slices through the target volume, and the target or surface of the volume is designed slice by slice. The target volume or isodose volume may be displayed as a translucent rendered picture or on a 2-D display to provide the surgeon with the perception of seeing either a 3-D volume or a series of 2-D slices.[7–8]

Presenting three-dimensional information to the surgeon

How can 3-D volumetric information be presented to the surgeon during an image-guided procedure in the simplest and most useful manner? Because computer displays are 2-D, one possibility is to present the images in multiple views and allow the surgeon to mentally reconstruct the volume. Although this technique is simple enough for point-in-space targeting, there is too much information for even a neurosurgeon to process efficiently.

Another possibility is to present the information stereoscopically, to provide the surgeon with the perception of seeing a 3-D image. The problem then becomes how to register that perception to its location in the surgical field because it is a volume that is intuitively reconstructed in the human brain and not necessarily a true reflection of a solid. Such perceptions result from presenting two 2-D pictures taken from a perspective several degrees apart as viewed by each eye individually. That is the basis for the nineteenth-century stereopticon and the 3-D horror movies of the 1950s. One must be careful that the pictures were taken from the same perspectives as each of the viewer's eyes, or the depth will be either foreshortened or elongated.

The classical application of well-controlled stereoscopic vision is in the operating microscope, where a magnified 3-D picture of the surgical field is visualized. Not only does it permit an excellent view of the surgical field, it is also possible to inject a superimposed image in the surgeon's line of sight with a so-called heads-up display. (Certain military aircraft have flight or target information projected onto the windshield so that pilots can receive the information without looking down to the control panel—heads up). Such displays are 2-D, but the display can consist of a series of slices that form a volume when stacked one on the other.[9–10]

History

Kelly et al first introduced the concept of 3-D volumetric image-guided neurosurgery in the mid-1980s.[11] Kelly's Compass system at that time consisted of a large computer workstation that allowed the surgeon to define the tumor volume in three dimensions and a stereotactic frame that made it possible to localize that volume in stereotactic space.[12] The surgeon outlined the border of the mass in each CT or MRI slice. The computer stacked the slices to define the volume and then interpolated between slices to render the surface so the picture of a volume could be seen on the console. Because the images were taken with the stereotactic frame in place, it was possible to localize the volume accurately within the head. The biggest problem was to present that information to the surgeon. Kelly solved the problem by mounting a cylindrical retractor on the stereotactic frame so it pointed directly at the tumor. The computer displayed the outline of the tumor and also a surrounding circle to represent the retractor. When the operating microscope was properly aligned, the outline of the tumor was seen superimposed on the view of the surgical field. There were problems in that the retractor restricted access, so most resection had to be done with a carbon dioxide (CO_2) laser. Most gliomas are larger than the retractor diameter, so it was necessary to use several targets and shift the retractor during the resection. The vertical dimension or depth along the surgeon's line of sight was not initially indicated, but later versions outlined only part of the tumor at a time to provide the third dimension.[12-13]

Other systems have built on this concept and display the targeting information through an operating microscope. The Zeiss MKM system (Thornwood, NY) has used similar display techniques but with more refinement.[10] The position of the microscope in space is identified using frameless localizing techniques, so it is not necessary to use a stereotactic frame. The outline of the tumor is updated as resection progresses, and only the outline at a given depth is displayed.

Other systems, such as the StealthStation (Medtronic Surgical Navigation Technologies, Louisville, CO), incorporate a heads-up display through a microscope localized in space through frameless technology, with slice-by-slice visualization of the outline of the tumor. (The recently introduced Mach 4 software incorporates some of the concepts from the Exoscope described in the following text, such as projecting the outline of the mass on the scalp or bone surface, and defining the depth under display by positioning a pointer in the resection field.)

One must recognize, however, that most glioma surgery involves a target larger than is conveniently addressed through an operating microscope, and most glioma surgery is probably done without operating microscope magnification.

The concept presented herein uses a video camera to display a real-time image of the operative field showing the tissues and the instruments at work. The surgeon can look at the video monitor for guidance during the surgery, just as one would do while performing endoscopic surgery. Because the original device had an endoscope stereotactically mounted on a frame outside the tissue, rather than within, the device was originally called an Exoscope (Fig. 9–1). The combination of the video image of the surgery overlain with a computer-generated image of the target volume provides the augmented reality that has long been sought in neurosurgery.

The version under development uses a frameless system to identify the location of the video camera and thereby register the video image to the computer graphic of the volume to be resected. Portions of the videotactic software have already been integrated into the StealthStation operating microscope program.

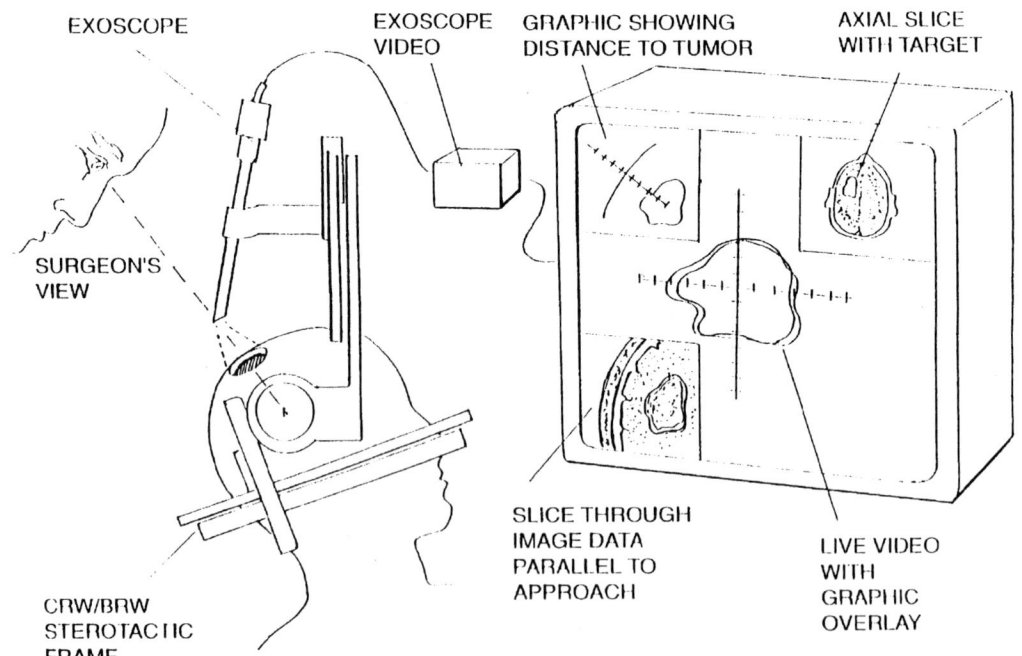

FIGURE 9–1. The original Exoscope consisted of an endoscope mounted on a Cosman-Robert-Wells (CRW) stereotactic frame so the surgical field was visualized. Superimposed on that view was a computer-generated graphic outlining the target tumor volume.

The Exoscope procedure

The Exoscope program allows the surgeon to look at an image that merges a real-time view of the operative field with a computer graphic to guide the extent of tumor resection.[14] The video view is enhanced by a superimposed view of the edge of the mass to be resected, as defined preoperatively by the surgeon. Magnification, orientation, and perspective are defined automatically, and the depth as the resection proceeds is defined by the surgeon updating the image. The surgeon resects along the border of the tumor while looking at the video display, just as in an endoscopic procedure. The surgeon can then look directly at the field to deal with tissue resection and hemostasis. Any conventional resection technique can be employed, so the Exoscope image is used as an adjunct to the surgeon's usual technique, rather than forcing the surgeon to modify the surgery to conform to the requirements of the guidance system. Retraction can be obtained by self-retaining retractors as resection involves deeper layers. The problems inherent with brain shift are present in the Exoscope program, as in any image-guided surgery, and must be minimized by the use of standard techniques, estimated and dealt with accordingly.

Scanning

The Exoscope program was originally developed for use with the Cosman-Robert-Wells (CRW) stereotactic frame. The head ring is secured to the patient's head in the usual fashion. A CT or MRI scan is taken, using whichever technique best defines the tumor boundary and the stereotactic fiducials (and depending on what was previously used to demonstrate the tumor). The data are transferred to the computer workstation using the ethernet, tape, or disk, in the usual fashion.

Surgical planning

The Exoscope program is grafted onto the Radionics StereoPlan software (Radionics, Burlington, MA).[15] A 3-D reconstruction of the head is made by alignment of the fiducials. Each 3-D structure may be built by segmenting according to the radiodensity of the structure or by manually drawing the image on each slice on which it appears. As a rule, it is better to draw the target volume so the surgeon can make the best judgment about the line of resection. For instance, it would be best to define the margin of a metastatic tumor tightly against the enhancing border. On the other hand, it would often be best to extend the resection line generously away from the enhancing border when resecting an infiltrating glioma. If a border abuts an eloquent area, the resection line might coincide with the edge of enhancement, or in a vascular area it may be best to leave some of the enhancing tissue to be dealt with later with stereotactic radiosurgery or radiotherapy. After the resection line is drawn on each slice, the program uses that data to reconstruct a 3-D volume as the target.

It may be desirable to define other structures as well. A major blood vessel passing through the target volume can be defined in a contrasting color so it can be anticipated and avoided or controlled. The ventricular wall can be defined so the surgeon can tailor the resection to lie as close to the ventricle as possible without actually entering it. Other structures or an imaginary marker can be introduced to provide the surgeon with orientation.

A reference point is selected, usually within the target volume, and the 3-D Cartesian stereotactic coordinates of that point are noted. This provides the setting of the stereotactic frame so the arc-mounted video camera points as efficiently as possible to the target.

The StereoPlan software allows the surgeon to visualize the CRW arc. The arc is adjusted on the workstation in the same orientation the surgeon will use in the operating room while standing at the head of the patient. The arc can be aligned either transversely or in an AP orientation to provide the least interference with the surgical approach. The ring angle and slide angle are adjusted to provide an ideal "surgeon's-eye view" simulating the view the surgeon will have in the operating room. The angles and coordinates can be readjusted repeatedly until the surgeon is satisfied that the approach will provide efficient access to the tumor while avoiding eloquent areas. Final adjustments can be made in the operating room when the surgeon addresses the actual anatomy of the head, and the settings can be readjusted throughout the procedure to afford efficient access to all parts of the tumor. Once the ideal access to the tumor has been noted in the preplanning session, the arc settings are recorded so the apparatus can be adjusted accordingly.

The Exoscope program includes a video camera holder that is offset 30 degrees from the arc. Thus the arc is angled 30 degrees away from the surgeon's-eye view, which provides additional working area in the surgical field with less interference from the stereotactic frame. When the Exoscope program is entered, the surgeon is provided with the proper arc settings to maintain an identical approach with either the normal 0 degree arc offset or the 30 degree offset used during surgery, and both settings are recorded, even though the settings are retained in the StereoPlan program.

Surgery

The CRW head ring serves as a head holder, being attached to a standard Mayfield bracket, with the patient's head in the optimal orientation to the surgeon just as it was in the preplanning session. The video monitor is placed at a convenient location, similar to endoscopic surgery, so the surgeon has a reasonable, close, unobstructed view of the monitor. The computer workstation is placed next to the video monitor so the computer-generated image can be inserted into the video image and the keyboard is accessible to the computer assistant.

Because the incision will be smaller than the conventional craniotomy incision, a smaller area of the scalp is shaved and prepped. The proposed opening would be located at the highest point to minimize loss of spinal fluid and consequent brain shift, as in any image-guided surgery.

The CRW arc is secured to the head ring and set to the same settings that had been determined in the preplanning session, with the arc in appropriate orientation to the frame. The stereotactic coordinates are set on the frame, and the ring angle and slide angle are adjusted. The video camera is attached to the arc with the 30 degree offset camera holder. The Exoscope program is turned on.

The Exoscope program has three modules.[16] The first calibrates the position and orientation of the video camera by aligning a small frame-mounted bracket with the video outline of the bracket on the screen. The second, Project Anatome, mode provides an image of the entire tumor as seen from the perspective of the camera, which allows the surgeon to select the best approach prior to making any incision. The Operate mode is used during surgery and provides only the outline of the tumor at any desired depth, with a small window in the corner indicating what depth is being displayed.

After the camera is calibrated, the Project Anatome mode is turned on. The distance between the camera and the patient's head can be adjusted so the entire view of the tumor fits just within the screen display, with the camera closer for smaller lesions and further away for larger tumors. Additional adjustments are made in the approach by changing the ring angle or slide angle, care being taken that the actual settings correspond with the computer settings. The surgeon sees on the video screen the surface of the scalp with the superimposed image of the tumor within the brain. The outline of the tumor is drawn on the scalp, which is used to fashion the best incision. Because the opening need not be any larger than the tumor border, a straight or "lazy-s" incision is usually possible, and a flap is reserved only for particularly large tumors.

After the scalp incision is made, the anatome is again projected on the bone, and the smallest possible bone flap is designed. Again, it is often possible to provide excellent access through a small craniotomy rather than the usual oversized bone flap. Only the brain tissue through which the approach is made is exposed, so there is no exposure or trauma to any other cortex. My impression, and that of other surgeons employing minimally invasive techniques, is that such limited exposure provides for a smoother postoperative course with fewer neurological sequelae than conventional surgery.

Once the bone flap has been removed and the dura opened, the Exoscope is placed in the Operate mode (Fig. 9–2). A measuring rod is used to measure the depth at which the image is displayed. The distance from the camera to the surface of the brain is measured, and the depth of the nearest surface of the tumor can be displayed on the monitor and measured. As the resection progresses through the brain tissue, the distance from the camera to the depth of the resection cavity is repeatedly measured and the display updated.

When the plane that first intersects the edge of the tumor volume is seen, the image of the tumor first appears on the screen indicating where the tumor resection itself begins. Contrary to the techniques employed in conventional tumor resection, image-guided resection begins with the surgeon defining the resection boundary; otherwise the resection boundary would collapse into the resection cavity before it is marked. After the resection line is freed, the center of the tumor is gutted. For large tumors, this might be done in stages, each perhaps 10 to 15 mm successively deeper.

The Exoscope provides guidance as the resection boundary is defined. While looking at the video display, the surgeon "cuts along the [dotted] line" that reflects the edge of the tumor or the preselected resection line (Fig. 9–3). Once the resection boundary is made, the surgeon can look directly at the surgical field to remove the tumor tissue, using the same technique that would be employed conventionally.

As the resection proceeds deeper into the tumor, the boundary further from the surgeon is displayed, as indicated by an adjustment made with a depth gauge ruler. When the boundary disappears from the screen, the resection is finished.

The Exoscope has been used in 73 craniotomies for tumor resection. In all cases, it provided accurate localization of the anatomical structures, tumor boundary, and resection line as documented on postoperative MRI. In many cases it assured more accurate resection because it identified irregularities in the shape of the tumor, or "flanges" of the tumor, that might have been overlooked.

Videotactic Surgery—a module of the frameless neuronavigator

With the successful operation of the frame-based Exoscope system and the increased use of frameless systems, it was only logical to adapt the use of a video camera to frameless technology. It is anticipated that the Exoscope program will be incorporated into a frameless system, where it will be renamed Videotactic Surgery. Several of the concepts have already been incorporated

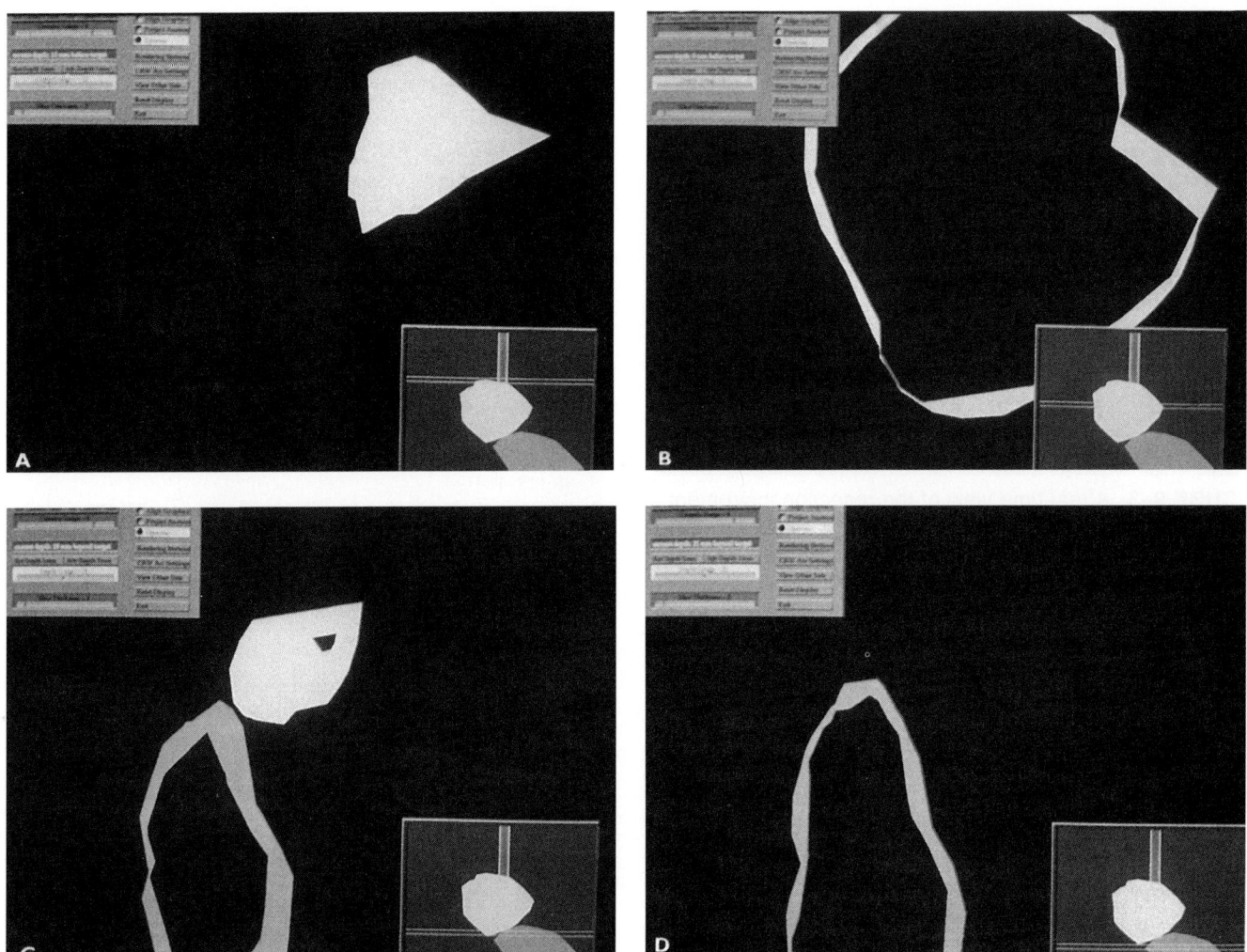

FIGURE 9–2. The outline of the tumor is displayed on the monitor. A window at the lower right displays the location of the demonstrated slice. The ventricle is also outlined for orientation. (A). The first contact with the tumor. (B). A slice near the center of the tumor at the midpoint of the resection. (C). The slice demonstrating the farthest or deepest point of the tumor. (D). The resection is completed. The tumor outline is gone, but the outline of the ventricle remains.

into the Mach IV Stealth software for use with the frameless operating microscope program. The profile of the volumetric target can be projected on the field, as in the Exoscope's Project Anatome module. The depth at which the volumetric target is outlined is selected by a frameless pointer, which might be the resection instrument, comparable to the depth gauge used in the Exoscope.

Positioning of the video camera with frameless localization has other advantages. The camera can be placed freely at the most convenient location so it is closely aligned with, but just out of, the surgeon's line of sight. The camera position can easily be changed as requirements may change during surgery. Fiducials mounted on the video camera identify the position of the camera, so it is not necessary to set the coordinates or angles on the frame and copy those settings to the computer—all settings are adjusted automatically. The position of the camera is known to the computer so it is possible to display the depth of resection by identifying the location of the tip of a pointer or resection instrument by frameless technology.

Fiducials are mounted on the video camera, which is held above the operating field on a flexible cable arm, similar to a system that holds self-retaining retractors. The computer workstation also provides the video display, either in the entire screen or in a smaller window. The video system is calibrated by successively centering on several calibration marks on the localizing arc. The video camera is then adjusted for the best line of sight, and the distance is selected so the volume of the target just fills the screen. A click of the foot pedal or mouse

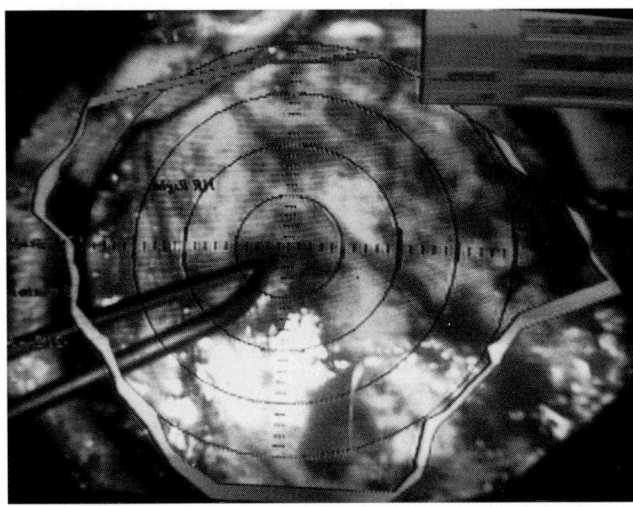

FIGURE 9–3. A real-time view of the resection instrument, a bipolar suction-coagulator, with the outline of the tumor displayed.

locks the camera in its perspective. The procedure is subsequently the same as for the Exoscope except that the depth to be displayed is indicated by a frameless localized pointer rather than the depth gauge. The resection is identical, with appropriate safeguards to minimize shift. The resection is completed when the image of the target disappears from the video screen.

The future

Additional improvements can be anticipated as new means are developed to visualize the computer screen. A head-mounted video display may provide the same information without the necessity of the surgeon looking away from the surgical field, but only by moving the eyes slightly upward (which may be an advantage for image-guided surgery in general). The use of two cameras and a different display in each eye may provide a true stereoscopic view of the target volume within the brain tissue. A heads-up display may be mounted on the surgeon's glasses, with the surgeon's head localized stereotactically.

Three-dimensional volumetric targeting continues to advance with more sophisticated techniques for defining volumes and the enhanced ability to segment by computer graphics various anatomical or pathological targets. The addition of holography to image guidance will allow the surgeon to see within the tissues even prior to resection. The use of video to provide a real-time image to merge with a computer-generated virtual target introduces enhanced reality into operative neurosurgery.

REFERENCES

1. Gildenberg PL. Whatever happened to stereotactic surgery? *Neurosurgery* 1987;20:983–987.
2. Gildenberg PL, Labuz J. Stereotactic craniotomy with the Exoscope. In: Alexander E III, Maciunas RJ, eds. *Advanced Neurosurgical Navigation*. New York: Thieme; 1999:301–309.
3. Gildenberg PL. General concepts of stereotactic surgery. In: Lunsford LD, ed. *Modern Stereotactic Neurosurgery*. Boston: Martinus Nijhoff; 1988:39–12.
4. Guthrie BL, Adler JRJ. Computer-assisted preoperative planning, interactive surgery, and frameless stereotaxy. *Clin Neurosurg* 1992;38:112–131.
5. Golfinos JG, Fitzpatrick BC, Smith LR, Spetzler RF. Clinical use of a frameless stereotactic arm: results of 325 cases. *J Neurosurg* 1995;83:197–205.
6. Barnett GH, Steiner CP, Weisenberger J. Intracranial meningioma resection using frameless stereotaxy. *J Image Guid Surg* 1995;1:46–52.
7. Flickinger JC, Lunsford LD, Kondziolka D. Dose prescription and dose-volume effects in radiosurgery. *Neurosurg Clin N Am* 1992;3:51–59.
8. Kooy HM, Nedzi LA, Loeffler JS, Alexander E III, Cheng CW, Mannarino EG. Treatment planning for stereotactic radiosurgery of intracranial lesions. *Int J Rad Oncol Biol Phys* 1991;21:683–693.
9. Roessler K, Ungersboeck K, Aichholzer M, Dietrich W, Goerzer H, Matula C. Frameless stereotactic lesion contour-guided surgery using a computer-navigated microscope. *Surg Neurol* 1998;49:282–288.
10. Levesque MF, Parker F. MKM-guided resection of diffuse brainstem neoplasms. *Stereotact Funct Neurosurg* 1999;73:15–18.
11. Kelly PJ, Kall B, Goerss S, Alker GJ Jr. Precision resection of intraaxial CNS lesions by CT-based stereotactic craniotomy and computer monitored CO_2 laser. *Acta Neurochir (Wien)* 1983;68:1–9.
12. Kelly PJ, Earnest F, Kall BA, Goerss SJ, Scheithauer B. Surgical options for patients with deep-seated brain tumors: computer-assisted stereotactic biopsy. *Mayo Clin Proc* 1985;60:223–229.
13. Kelly PJ, Kall BA, Goerss SJ. Computer-interactive stereotactic resection of deep-seated and centrally located intraaxial brain lesions. *Appl Neurophysiol* 1987;50:107–113.
14. Gildenberg PL, Ledoux R, Cosman E, Labuz J. The Exoscope: a frame-based video/graphics system for intraoperative guidance of surgical resection. *Stereotact Funct Neurosurg* 1994;63:23–25.
15. Pillay PK, Gildenberg PL, Labuz J. Computer workstation applications: StereoPlan, virtual reality, and the Gildenberg Exoscope. In: Pell MF, Thomas DGT, eds. *Handbook of Stereotaxy Using the CRW Apparatus*. Baltimore: Williams & Wilkins; 1994:219–233.
16. Gildenberg PL. The Exoscope system for 3-D craniotomy. In: Gildenberg PL, Tasker RR, eds. *Textbook of Stereotactic and Functional Neurosurgery*. New York: McGraw-Hill; 1998:485–490.

10

Endoscopic Image-Guided Surgery

AMIT Y. SCHWARTZ AND WESLEY A. KING

Learning neuroendoscopy begins with familiarizing oneself with the equipment. Early frustration often results from lack of understanding of the various neuroendoscopic components. A complete system includes the endoscope, light source, camera, image-recording device, monitor, and transendoscopic instruments. Although the specifics regarding the various equipment options are beyond the scope of this chapter, the authors cannot overemphasize the importance of becoming so acquainted with the various components and that working with the setup become second nature.

This chapter focuses on the cranial disorders in which endoscopy plays a significant role. Some of the techniques discussed here require significant experience before one can perform them safely, whereas other uses for the endoscope can be more broadly applied using basic skills.

■ Hydrocephalus

Shunt placement

Although ventricular shunting is a common procedure, a fair percentage of catheters are suboptimally placed. Poor placement may result in poor cerebrospinal fluid (CSF) outflow necessitating repeated transparenchymal passes or may contribute to early shunt failure. Theodosopoulos et al[1] have shown that endoscopic ventricular catheter placement significantly increases the percentage of optimally placed catheters over the conventional technique (100% vs 53%, $P < 0.001$).

In brief, the patient is positioned with the head turned to the opposite side and a shoulder roll placed ipsilaterally. The entry site is prepared in the standard fashion. A ventricular catheter with an opening at the tip is loaded onto the endoscope. The appropriate trajectory is chosen and the catheter is passed into the ventricle. Once the position of the catheter tip is confirmed, the endoscope is removed and the shunt procedure is completed. One must keep in mind that, because the catheter is free to move within the ventricle, the ultimate position of its tip is determined by the entry point and the trajectory. Consequently, endoscopic "guidance" of the catheter tip must be minimized.

Multiloculated hydrocephalus

Multiloculated hydrocephalus results from fibrous septations formed in response to infection or hemorrhage. Such patients may require multiple shunts to adequately drain the CSF spaces. Reducing the patient's dependency to one catheter minimizes the failure rate and long-term morbidity.

Workup of these patients should include a computed tomographic (CT) ventriculogram to identify the communications between the loculations. Magnetic resonance imaging (MRI) may demonstrate the septations, but it would not provide information regarding the CSF flow dynamics. If the studies demonstrate adequate communication of most of the loculi with distention of just one, it is reasonable to fenestrate the appropriate cyst and attempt to leave the patient shunt free. Approximately 30% of patients with loculated hydrocephalus will not require extracranial CSF diversion following a fenestration procedure.[2]

Although fenestration of the loculations may be accomplished via a transcortical or transcallosal craniotomy, endoscopy offers a significantly less invasive option. The patient is positioned for either a frontal or occipital approach depending on the location of the loculations. The endoscope is inserted through a burr hole into the ventricular system. Ideally, the scope should first enter a normal ventricle to allow for identification of normal structures. A thin-walled, avascular site is chosen for fenestration. Septal perforation can be performed bluntly with the transendoscopic forceps or with a laser. The communication is enlarged to approximately a 1 cm diameter with the use of a balloon catheter pulled retrograde through the perforation. Bleeding can usually be controlled with irrigation, although occasionally cautery may be needed. Shunting can then be limited to a single intraventricular catheter positioned in the frontal horn.

Lewis and Keiper[3] reported a series of 34 patients with uni- or multiloculated hydrocephalus who underwent endoscopic fenestration using a steerable fiberscope and laser fiber. During a mean 26-month follow-up period, cyst fenestration reduced the shunt revision rate from 3.04 per year to 0.25 per year. Patients with multiloculated hydrocephalus were at increased risk for shunt malfunction and cyst recurrence versus patients with uniloculated hydrocephalus. Furthermore, patients who underwent a shunting procedure prior to endoscopy were more likely to require a repeat endoscopic procedure. Compared with craniotomy, endoscopy offers a less invasive approach to treating patients with loculated hydrocephalus, simplifying their shunt system and reducing the rate of shunt failure.

Third ventriculostomy

Despite continued advancements in shunting hardware, extracranial CSF diversion is associated with a significant infection and failure rate that increases with each procedure. Performing a third vetriculostomy is a minimally invasive way of "internally" shunting patients with occlusive hydrocephalus and obviating the need for hardware placement.

Patients with radiological studies consistent with obstructive hydrocephalus are the ideal candidates. However, patients with a combined communicating and noncommunicating picture may also benefit. The arachnoid villi are capable of increasing their absorptive capacity in response to an increase in CSF load. CSF isotope clearance studies have been used to predict the absorptive capability of the arachnoid granulations but suffer from a significant false-negative rate.[2] In light of the benefits of third ventriculostomy and its low complication rate, we advocate performing the procedure in patients with an obstructive component to their hydrocephalus.

After induction of general anesthesia, the patient's head is placed in the vertical position on a doughnut. A frontal burr hole is placed 1 cm anterior to the coronal suture and 3 cm to the right of midline. The endoscope is passed transparenchymally into the lateral ventricle (Fig. 10–1). The third ventricle is entered through the foramen of Monro by following the choroid plexus and thalamostriate vein. A blunt forceps is used to perforate the tuber cinerum at the third ventricular floor between the infundibular recess and the mammillary bodies. The pulsation of the basilar artery can usually be identified through the transparent floor and is thus avoided. The perforation is then enlarged with a balloon catheter to maintain patency. The membrane of Liliequist must then be fenestrated to create a communication between the supratentorial and infratentorial cisterns.

Ventricular size does not necessarily correlate with clinical improvement.[4,5] Although an MR flow study may demonstrate a flow void at the floor of the third ventricle,[5] we elect to follow patients clinically. Patients who fail to improve despite patency of the third ventriculostomy undergo a standard shunting procedure.

Hopf et al[6] reported a series of 100 patients who underwent endoscopic third ventriculostomies. Of the 100 procedures, 98 were completed. The overall clinical success rate in the series, which included multiple etiologies, was 76%. The highest success rate was seen with benign space-occupying lesions, although resection of the lesion may have contributed to resolution of the hydrocephalus. Notably, 63% of patients whose etiology for the hydrocephalus was intraventricular hemorrhage responded to third ventriculostomy. The complication rate in this series was 6% with no mortalities. Others, however, report a lower long-term success rate[7] and the potential for devastating complications must be kept in mind.[5]

Third ventriculostomy also may be an alternative to shunt revision in the management of shunt failure in patients with obstructive hydrocephalus. Up to 76.7% of patients may become shunt independent.[8] Any preexisting shunt catheter should be removed or ligated to maximize CSF flow through the stoma and maintain its patency. Failures are usually manifest within days and a shunt revision is then performed.

■ Colloid Cysts

Colloid cysts are benign lesions that usually arise from the roof of the third ventricle near the foramen of Monro. They can be found, however, throughout the third ventricle, or they may involve the septum pellucidum or fornices.[9–12] They contain a gelatinous center

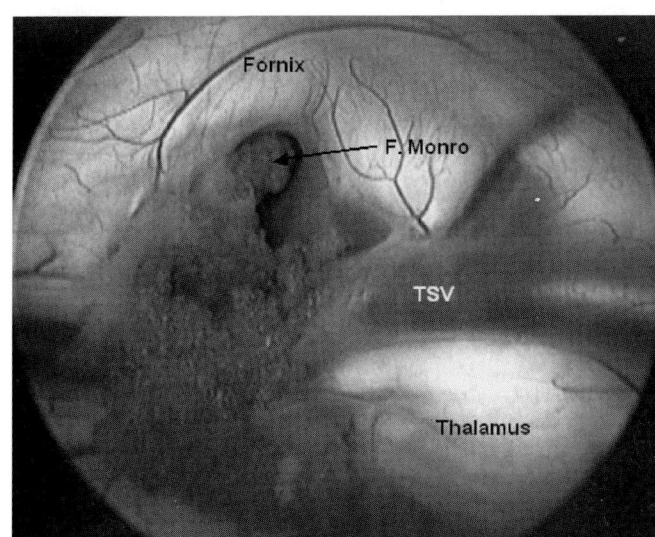 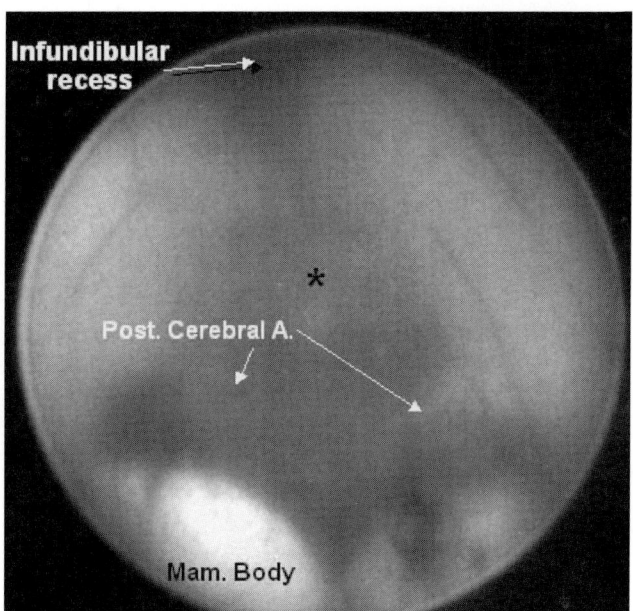

FIGURE 10–1. (A). Endoscopic view within the right lateral ventricle. The choroid plexus can be followed to the foramen of Monro. The thalamostriate vein (TSV) can also be identified. (B). Visualization of the floor of the third ventricle demonstrates the optimal site for performing an endoscopic third ventriculostomy (asterisk). The posterior cerebral arteries (arrows) and the mammillary bodies should be positively identified before penetrating the floor.

of variable viscosity. Although some patients present incidentally, most complain of headaches, nausea, vomiting, memory loss, personality changes, difficulty with gait, or visual deterioration.[13]

The treatment of asymptomatic patients remains controversial. Patients managed by conservative observation must be followed with frequent imaging and should be informed of the early warning signs of obstructive hydrocephalus. We recommend against such a course in patients with lesions greater than 1 cm and those with hydrocephalus. Symptomatic patients clearly require surgical intervention.

Surgical options include transfrontal or transcallosal craniotomy, stereotactic aspiration, ventricular shunting, or endoscopic resection.[14] Ventricular shunting is reserved for patients not medically fit to undergo a more definitive procedure. Minimally invasive techniques have been developed to reduce the operative morbidity associated with craniotomy. Stereotactic aspiration is initially effective, but the high recurrence rate has led to this procedure falling out of favor.[15]

Endoscopic resection of colloid cyst is a minimally invasive method of effecting a definitive treatment. Patients are positioned supine with the head secured in three-point fixation and flexed 15 degrees. A burr hole is placed 1 cm anterior to coronal suture and 4 cm off midline. The right side is chosen unless the left lateral ventricle is unilaterally dilated or the lesion is grossly asymmetrically deviated toward the left. An outer cannula is passed into the lateral ventricle and secured to the operating room table. The zero-degree endoscope is used to determine the relationship of the cyst to the foramen of Monro, choroid plexus, fornices, septum pellucidum, and third ventricle (Fig. 10–2). Small cysts can occasionally be grasped and removed entirely as a single specimen. Excessive traction, however, must be avoided to prevent vascular injury. Larger lesions are punctured and the cyst contents are evacuated via aspiration or intracystic irrigation. If the cyst wall does not separate easily, it is coagulated with bipolar cautery or neodymium:yttrium-aluminum-garnet laser and removed piecemeal using scissors and biopsy forceps. Gross total removal can be achieved in 85% of patients with a > 95% resection in the remainder where complete resection would unnecessarily risk vascular injury.[13] We routinely fenestrate the septum pellucidum with a grasping instrument and dilate the opening with a 3F Fogarty balloon catheter. Unlike others,[16] we do not leave a ventricular catheter in place. Patients are monitored overnight in the neurosurgical intensive care unit and transferred to the ward the following morning.

We believe that endoscopic resection should be considered the treatment of choice for patients with colloid cysts. Operative time is significantly reduced when compared with craniotomy. In addition, duration of hospital stay is reduced as is the time before returning to work.[14] In our series, there were no mortalities or permanent morbidities.[13] Furthermore, with a mean follow-up

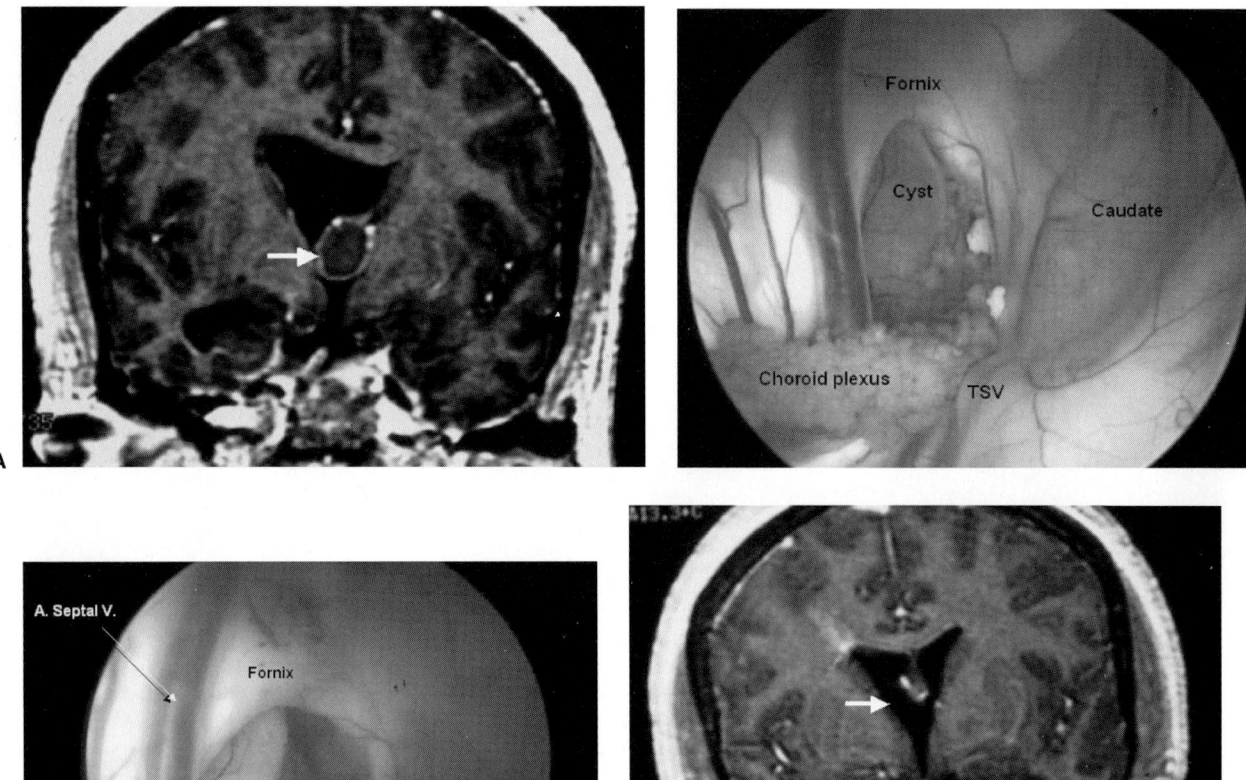

FIGURE 10–2. (A). Coronal magnetic resonance imaging (MRI) demonstrates a colloid cyst at the foramen of Monro (arrow). (B,C). Endoscopic exposure through the right lateral ventricle demonstrates the cyst, which can be excised in a piecemeal fashion. Care must be taken not to injure the thalamostriate vein (TSV) and anterior septal vein (A. Septal V.). (D). Postoperative MRI shows complete tumor removal (arrow).

greater than 4 years, there have been no recurrences even in patients with known residual cyst wall.

■ Arachnoid Cysts

Arachnoid cysts are intra-arachnoid CSF collections usually of congenital origin. They are often found incidentally, although they can produce mass effect and produce symptoms through neural compression.[17] Symptomatic cyst should be surgically treated barring medical contraindications. Although many surgical options have been described including stereotactic aspiration and cyst excision,[18] the more accepted treatments involve either shunting the cyst to the peritoneum or creating a communication between the cyst and another CSF compartment.

Prior to the advent of endoscopic surgery, shunting the cyst to the peritoneum offered a minimally invasive therapeutic option with a low morbidity. Fenestration required a craniotomy with its increased risk. However, with endoscopic techniques, the arachnoid cyst could be fenestrated with minimal morbidity thereby avoiding the need for shunt catheter placement. Although peritoneal shunting is effective, the shunt failure rate is as high as 10% and shunt dependency may occur.[19]

Middle fossa arachnoid cysts

The patient is placed in the supine position with the head turned to the contralateral side. A temporal burr hole is placed above the zygomatic arch. Care is taken when introducing the trocar and endoscope not to allow excessive egress of CSF because that would lead to cyst collapse and poor visualization. For orientation, one follows the Sylvian veins or middle cerebral artery toward the basal cisterns. A blunt forceps is used to puncture the arachnoid membrane between the frontal and temporal lobes at the most proximal extent of the Sylvian fissure. A Fogarty catheter is inserted into the cistocisternostomy to enlarge the fenestration. Partial resection of the cyst wall and arachnoid membrane may further prevent delayed occlusion and cyst recurrence. Some authors[17] advocate insertion of a fimbrial ventricular catheter to maintain patency.

Suprasellar arachnoid cysts

Patients are positioned supine and a right precoronal burr hole is placed. The right lateral ventricle is cannulated and the endoscope is passed through the foramen of Monro. If the third ventricle is preserved, the fenestration is performed with the blunt forceps through the bulging floor of the third ventricle anterior to the mamillary bodies. With large cysts that completely distort the third ventricle, a ventriculocystostomy is performed into the lateral ventricle and enlarged with a fogarty catheter. Caemaert et al[20] advocate additional fenestration of the cyst into the basal prepontine cisterns to prevent recurrences. In their series, all patients experienced initial symptomatic relief, but one of four patients required a second procedure for failure of the cyst to remain decompressed. Buxton et al[21] reported good results in three patients after performing a ventriculocystostomy alone. There were no recurrences after a 24- to 28-month follow-up. They believe that a second fenestration into the basal cisterns is risky and unnecessary. The authors advocate a single fenestration with efforts focused on maximally enlarging the opening to prevent recurrences.

Posterior fossa cysts

For cysts in the cerebellopontine angle the patient is placed in the supine position with the head maximally turned to the contralateral side. A retromastoid suboccipital burr hole is placed and the cyst is endoscopically inspected from within. A cystocisternostomy is performed into the prepontine cisterns between the cranial nerves. Patients with posterior midline arachnoid cyst are placed in the prone or semisitting position. Supracerebellar cyst can be fenestrated into the quadrigeminal cistern. More caudal cysts are fenestrated into the cisterna magna.

In the series reported by Choi et al,[22] 36 consecutive patients with congenital arachnoid cysts underwent endoscopic fenestration procedures. Seven patients early in their series underwent additional shunting procedures. Although one patient suffered an intraventricular hemorrhage, there were no permanent morbidities or mortalities. With a 4.2-year mean follow-up, there were no recurrences except for the patient who suffered the hemorrhage. This and other studies[23–25] have proven that endoscopic fenestration of arachnoid cysts is an effective minimally invasive technique that offers a low morbidity without the complications associated with permanent shunt catheter placement.

■ Intraventricular Lesions

Accessing intraventricular tumors through a microsurgical approach often requires significant brain dissection and retraction. Endoscopic surgery, however, provides excellent tumor visualization with no brain retraction. In addition to tumor removal, the associated hydrocephalus can often be treated during the same approach.

The ideal lesion is small, less vascularized, soft, and obstructs the CSF outflow producing ventriculomegaly. The enlarged ventricles provide the space necessary for endoscope insertion and instrument manipulation. Although tumor biopsy is often easily obtainable, complete tumor resection can become very time-consuming with increased tumor size. Gaab et al[26] advocate endoscopic tumor resection in tumors smaller than 2 cm because with larger lesions the benefits of endoscopic surgery are outweighed by the duration of the operation.

Lateral ventricular tumors

Frontal horn and ventricular body tumors are well visualized via the standard parasagittal burr hole 2 cm anterior to the coronal suture. Posterior lesions in the trigone are better approached through a burr hole placed 4 to 6 cm anterior to the coronal suture.

Orientation is achieved by examining the course of the choroid plexus. Following tumor inspection the attachment to the choroid plexus is coagulated. Tumor resection proceeds with intracapsular debulking via a piecemeal removal performed with the grasping and biopsy forceps. Visualized vessels are cauterized prior to resection. Hemostasis can usually be achieved with irrigation alone. If at the completion of the resection one foramen of Monro remains blocked, a septum pellucidotomy is performed to restore CSF flow.

Third ventricular tumors

Although many microsurgical approaches to the third ventricle have been described,[27–31] all involve significant brain dissection and retraction with risk to vital neural structures such as the corpus callosum, thalamus, and fornices. The endoscopic approach minimizes the risk of brain injury related to tumor exposure. Anterior third ventricular tumors are approached through a burr hole at the coronal suture, whereas more posterior lesions are approached through a more anteriorly located entrance. Following tumor resection, one must ensure that CSF outflow pathways are patent. Septum pellucidotomy, stenting of the Sylvian aqueduct, third ventriculostomy, or a combination of techniques may be employed to avert postoperative hydrocephalus.

Fourth ventricular tumors

Fourth ventricular tumors often cause obstructive hydrocephalus with enlargement of the lateral and third ventricles. Endoscopic third ventriculostomy may play a role in alleviating the hydrocephalus. On rare occasions, tumor-related obstruction leads to an isolated enlarged fourth ventricle, and tumor resection via an endoscopic approach through the foramen of Magendie becomes feasible.[32]

Gaab and Schroeder[33] reported a series of 30 patients with endoscopically treated intraventricular tumors. Two cases required conversion to microscopic resection secondary to the firm consistency of the tumor and their large size. They therefore do not advocate endoscopic resection in lesions larger than 2 cm. Hydrocephalus-related symptoms resolved in all 22 patients with CSF obstruction. Complications included one case of meningitis, one of mutism, two of memory loss, one of transient trochlear palsy, and one of transient confusion. There were no endoscopy-related deaths. With proper patient selection, minimally invasive techniques could be successfully employed in tumor resection and relief of hydrocephalus without the need for extracranial shunting.

■ Transsphenoidal Surgery

The sublabial–transseptal approach to transsphenoidal resection of sellar lesions is associated with local complications that include numbness of maxillary dentition, loss of nasal tip projection, and nasal perforation.[34] Patients may complain about recurrent nasal bleeding, breathing difficulty, and crust formation.[34] The transnasal approach has been developed to avoid some of these complications. The size of the nares may restrict the insertion of a nasal speculum necessary for microscopic resection through a transnasal approach. Furthermore, tumor out of the direct line of sight may be missed when relying on microscopic resection. Endoscopic resection addresses these issues.

After induction of general anesthesia cottonoids soaked with 4% cocaine are applied to the nasal cavity for 10 minutes. Under endoscopic guidance, the middle turbinate is bluntly lateralized. The nasal septum at the sphenoid rostrum is fractured and pushed contralaterally. The sphenoid ostium is enlarged with a Kerrison rongeur. The 0- and 30-degree endoscopes provide a panoramic view of the sphenoid sinus facilitating identification of the optic and carotid protuberances, clival indentation, and anterior sella. The sella and dura are then opened and the tumor is removed using pituitary curettes. The parasellar region along both cavernous sinuses as well as the suprasellar region can easily be inspected for residual tumor. At the completion of tumor resection, the sphenoid fossa is packed with gelfoam. A fat graft harvested from the abdomen together with fibrin glue is used to pack the sphenoid sinus whenever a CSF leak is seen during surgery. Nasal packing is not routinely used.

When compared with the sublabial approach, the endoscopic transnasal approach is associated with a shorter operative time[35,36]; absence of recurrent epistaxis, snoring, and denture problems; and a lower incidence of septal perforation, synechia, and crust formation.[35] Furthermore, the loss of nasal tip projection was only found in the group that underwent the sublabial technique. Some advocate the use of the endoscope for the approach alone, and following insertion of a speculum, proceed with standard microscopic resection.[34] The aforementioned benefits are realized while providing the surgeon a three-dimensional microscopic view for tumor resection.

Endoscopic tumor resection, however, provides for a more complete view of the sella contents and can effect a surgical cure.[37] In a series by Jarrahy et al,[38] residual tumor was found endoscopically in three of nine patients who underwent microscopic resection. Helal[39] reported finding residual tumor in 15 of 37 patients. In theory, the enhanced endoscopic view should allow for a more complete tumor resection, but there have been no randomized controlled studies to date demonstrating higher cure rates.

■ Acoustic Neuroma Surgery

Although microsurgery has allowed safe resection of acoustic neuromas with high rates of cranial nerve preservation, CSF leak has remained a significant morbidity with reported rates as high as 20%.[40–43] Additionally, residual tumor within the internal acoustic canal (IAC), not identified intraoperatively during a retrosigmoid approach, remains a problem. Neuroendoscopic techniques have been employed to address these two issues.

When the retrosigmoid approach is utilized, a suboccipital craniectomy is first performed in the standard fashion. Following microscopic tumor resection the rigid endoscope is brought into the field. The IAC is inspected with the 0- and 30-degree endoscope to look for residual tumor and exposed air cells not identified with the microscope. Any residual tumor is resected and bone wax is applied to the air cells. A muscle graft from the wound margins is then placed over the bony defect in the IAC.

Following a translabyrinthine approach, the endoscope aids in visualizing the undersurface of the stapes footplate to be certain that the stapes was not displaced from the oval window. Additionally, further inspection of the bony resection is performed to uncover open air cells not identified on microscopic examination. All air cells are sealed with bone wax, and fascia and fat are used to cover the bony defect. Similar inspection of the bone for open air cells can be performed following a middle cranial fossa approach.

In the series by Wackym et al,[44] the endoscope was utilized as an adjunct in 78 patients. There were no complications related to the endoscope. Following microsurgical resection, endoscopic inspection identified residual tumor in the fundus of the IAC in 11 patients and complete tumor resection was achieved in all. Endoscopic examination revealed exposed air cells not identified on microscopic examination in 24 cases. Those air cells were subsequently individually waxed. No displacement of the stapes footplate was identified in patients who underwent the translabyrinthine approach. Although two patients developed CSF leakage through the skin incision, there were no cases of CSF rhinorrhea. Other studies[40] have confirmed the lower CSF rhinorrhea rate with the adjunctive use of endoscopy.

■ Aneurysm Surgery

Inadequate clipping remains a problem associated with aneurysm surgery. Incomplete clipping occurs in approximately 5.9% of cases[45] leaving residual that may result in delayed aneurysm growth. Furthermore, inadvertent inclusion of perforating vessels within the clip may produce devastating neurological deficits (Figs. 10–3 and 10–4). Lastly, direct pressure of the aneurysm clip on vital neurological structures such as cranial nerves may lead to avoidable clinical deficits. Endoscopy provides additional information that may lower the incidence of the aforementioned complications.

Following microsurgical dissection of the appropriate vessels and surrounding structures, the endoscope provides a more detailed view allowing one to see around corners. After aneurysm clipping, the endoscope is once again introduced to confirm complete lesion obliteration and avoidance of normal vessels and surrounding neural structures. We prefer the 0- and 30-degree endoscopes when operating in narrow spaces adjacent to vital structures. Although some advocate the 70-degree scope,[46] we avoid its use in the skull base. Not visualizing structures in the direct line of the endoscope may lead to inadvertent injury. Even if the endoscope is introduced under microscopic view, gazing at the monitor and away from the microscope ocular creates a time interval during which the endoscope is held blindly in the surgical field. Picture-in-picture technology potentially curtails the blind moment thereby reducing the risk of accidental injury.

In a series of 48 patients operated upon for 54 cerebral aneurysms,[46] the endoscope provided additional information that further clarified the regional anatomy in 81.5% of cases. The aneurysm clip was reapplied on the basis of the endoscopic view in five cases (9.3%). These included two instances of incomplete neck obliteration, two cases of involvement of the perforating vessels within the clip, and one case where the clip compressed vital neural tissue. Additionally, there was a case where the surgical strategy was changed from clipping to wrapping after endoscopy demonstrated a perforating vessel tightly adherent to the aneurysm.

We have found the endoscope most useful in lesions involving the anterior communicating artery, basilar apex, and posterior circulation where neurovascular relations can be confusing and visualization of contralateral structures is essential. Although it is technically possible to clip aneurysms endoscopically, with the available technology we advocate using the endoscope as an adjunct to the operative microscope. Newer technologies such as an endoscopically equipped clip applicator[47] may in the future allow clipping under endoscopic view alone.

■ Stereotactic Endoscopic Surgery

The benefits of endoscopic surgery stem from its being minimally invasive to the brain. However, poor placement of the burr hole may necessitate traction on neural tissue to adequately visualize the target. Such maneuvers may lead to unintended injury. Stereotactic techniques have been adopted to more accurately plan the ideal trajectory.

Frame-based techniques

The Brown-Roberts-Wells and the Cosman-Roberts-Wells systems have both been modified to employ endoscopy.[48–50] All that is required is a guiding block and fixation device that accommodates the endoscope. The trajectory is established by choosing two points along the ideal path and extrapolating the trepanation point. For third ventriculostomies, target points are selected at the foramen of Monro and the floor of the third ven-

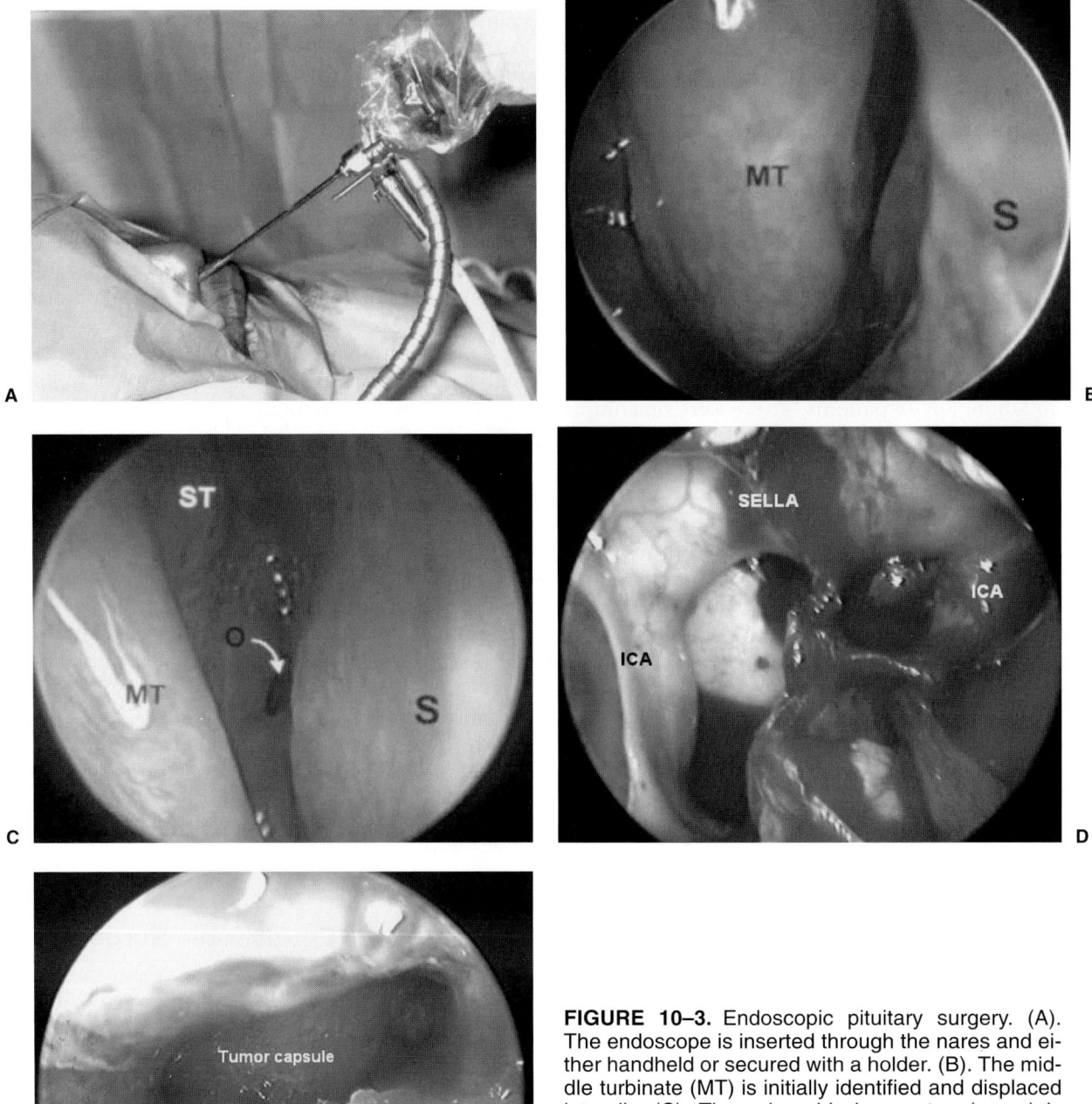

FIGURE 10–3. Endoscopic pituitary surgery. (A). The endoscope is inserted through the nares and either handheld or secured with a holder. (B). The middle turbinate (MT) is initially identified and displaced laterally. (C). The sphenoid sinus ostea (arrow) is usually seen adjacent to the superior turbinate (ST) and posterior nasal septum (S). (D). Within the sphenoid sinus the prominences of the optic canal, sella turcica, and internal carotid arteries (ICA) should be identified. (E). Once the tumor is excised the endoscope can be inserted into the tumor cavity to inspect for hidden residual fragments.

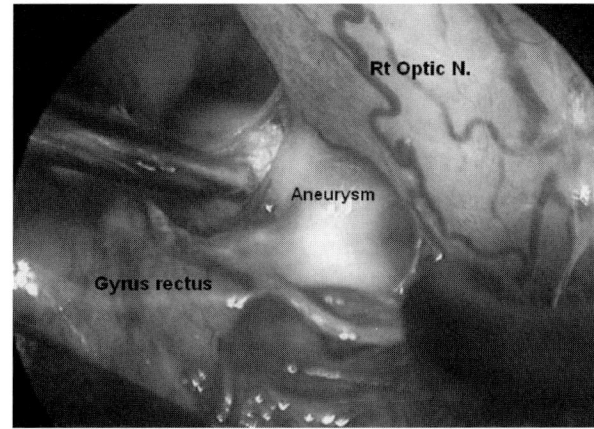
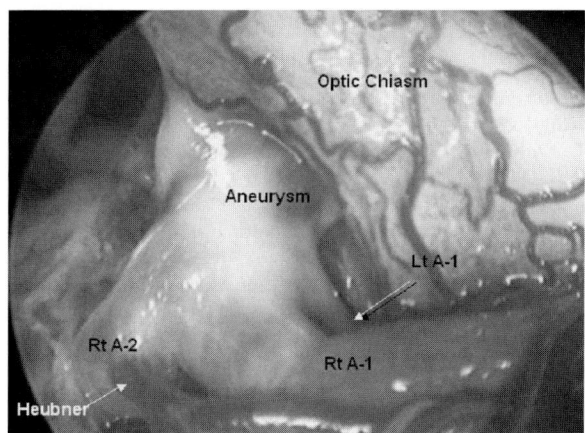
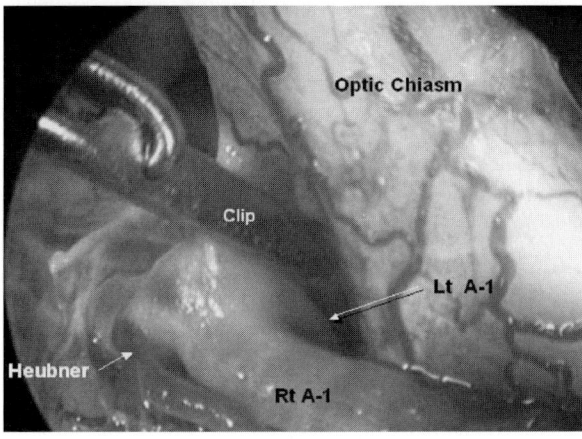

FIGURE 10–4. Endoscope-assisted aneurysm surgery. (A,B). Endoscopic view of an anterior communicating artery aneurysm through a right pterional approach. The A-1 and A-2 segments of the right anterior cerebral artery as well as the left A-1 segment and recurrent artery of Heubner are seen. (C). The endoscope can be used to confirm optimal clipping.

tricle just dorsal to the dorsum sellae and in front of the basilar artery. Burr hole placement in line with this trajectory minimizes endoscopic manipulation of the neural structure bordering the foramen of Monro and their potential injury. Frame-based techniques can similarly be applied during endoscopic biopsies.[50]

Frameless techniques

The specifics of the various systems available may vary, but the general concepts of the frameless stereotactic endoscopic systems remain similar. A camera system localizes the head and various instruments in three-dimensional space. By knowing the location of the tip of the surgical instrument relative to the attached markers, the computer can demonstrate the multiplanar MR views and their relation to the surgical instrument. Various adapter systems have been utilized to attach reference markers to the endoscope to allow for its localization in three-dimensional space.[51–54]

Frameless neuroendoscopic techniques have been employed for a variety of surgical interventions, including third ventriculostomies, tumor biopsy and resection, and multiloculated hydrocephalus. We and others[55] feel that for most endoscopic procedures in hydrocephalic ventricles, the freehand technique suffices. The dilated ventricular system provides room for maneuverability and well-known landmarks within the ventricles allows for proper orientation. Some feel that the frameless navigation system is helpful in maintaining orientation when the CSF turns bloody.[56] We prefer to continuously irrigate the CSF space and clear the endoscopic view rather than rely on the navigation system for orientation. Schroeder et al[55] found that the frameless system was most useful in patients with cystic lesions lacking clear anatomical landmarks such as loculated hydrocephalus, intraparenchymal cysts, cavum veli interpositum, and isolated fourth ventricle. One can plan the most appropriate trajectory and maintain orientation utilizing the navigation system. Furthermore, one can also more appropriately position the entry point when approaching the third ventricle through a small foramen of Monro. Stereotactic techniques applied to neuroendoscopy have not only served to enhance the safety of previously performed procedures but have also expanded the indications for minimally invasive endoscopic surgery.

REFERENCES

1. Theodosopoulos PV, Abosch A, McDermott MW. Intraoperative fiber-optic endoscopy for ventricular catheter insertion. *Can J Neurol Sci* 2001;28:56–60.
2. Teo C. Endoscopy for the treatment of hydrocephalus. In: King W, Frazee J, DeSalles A, eds. *Endoscopy of the Central and Peripheral Nervous System*. New York:Thieme Medical Publishers; 1998:59–67.
3. Lewis AI, Keiper GL Jr, Crone KR. Endoscopic treatment of loculated hydrocephalus. *J Neurosurg* 1995;82:780–785.
4. Jimenez D. Third ventriculostomy. In: Jimenez DF, AANS Publications Committee. *Intracranial Endoscopic Neurosurgery*. Park Ridge, IL: American Association of Neurological Surgeons; 1998:101–110.
5. Jones RFC, Brazier DH, Kwok BCT, Stening WA, Vonau M. Neuroendoscopic third ventriculostomy. *Minim Invasive Neurosurg* 1995;7:33–48.
6. Hopf NJ, Grunert P, Fries G, Resch KD, Perneczky A. Endoscopic third ventriculostomy: outcome analysis of 100 consecutive procedures. *Neurosurgery* 1999;44:795–804; discussion 804–806.
7. Tisell M, Almstrom O, Stephensen H, Tullberg M, Wikkelso C. How effective is endoscopic third ventriculostomy in treating adult hydrocephalus caused by primary aqueductal stenosis? *Neurosurgery* 2000;46:104–110; discussion 110–111.
8. Cinalli G, Salazar C, Mallucci C, Yada JZ, Zerah M, Sainte-Rose C. The role of endoscopic third ventriculostomy in the management of shunt malfunction. *Neurosurgery* 1998;43:1323–1327; discussion 1327–1329.
9. Antunes JL, Louis KM, Ganti SR. Colloid cysts of the third ventricle. *Neurosurgery* 1980;7:450–455.
10. Camacho A, Abernathey CD, Kelly PJ, Laws ER Jr. Colloid cysts: experience with the management of 84 cases since the introduction of computed tomography. *Neurosurgery* 1989;24:693–700.
11. Ciric I, Zivin I. Neuroepithelial (colloid) cysts of the septum pellucidum. *J Neurosurg* 1975;43:69–73.
12. Little JR, MacCarty CS. Colloid cysts of the third ventricle. *J Neurosurg* 1974;40:230–235.
13. King WA, Ullman JS, Frazee JG, Post KD, Bergsneider M. Endoscopic resection of colloid cysts: surgical considerations using the rigid endoscope. *Neurosurgery* 1999;44:1103–1109; discussion 1109–1111.
14. Lewis AI, Crone KR, Taha J, van Loveren HR, Yeh HS, Tew JM Jr. Surgical resection of third ventricle colloid cysts: preliminary results comparing transcallosal microsurgery with endoscopy. *J Neurosurg* 1994;81:174–178.
15. Mathiesen T, Grane P, Lindquist C, Holst H. High recurrence rate following aspiration of colloid cysts in the third ventricle. *J Neurosurg* 1993;78:748–752.
16. Rodziewicz GS, Smith MV, Hodge CJ Jr. Endoscopic colloid cyst surgery. *Neurosurgery* 2000;46:655–660; discussion 660–662.
17. Gaab MR, Schroeder HWS. Arachnoid cysts. In: King W, Frazee J, DeSalles A, eds. *Endoscopy of the Central and Peripheral Nervous System*. New York: Thieme Medical Publishers; 1998:137–147.
18. Schroeder HWS, Gaab MR. Neuroendoscopic treatment of arachnoid cysts. In: Jimenez DF, ed. *Intracranial Endoscopic Neurosurgery*. Park Ridge, IL: American Association of Neurological Surgeons; 1998:111–123.
19. Arai H, Sato K, Wachi A, Okuda O, Takeda N. Arachnoid cysts of the middle cranial fossa: experience with 77 patients who were treated with cystoperitoneal shunting. *Neurosurgery* 1996;39:1108–1112; discussion 1112–1113.
20. Caemaert J, Abdullah J, Calliauw L, Carton D, Dhooge C, Coster R. Endoscopic treatment of suprasellar arachnoid cysts. *Acta Neurochir* 1992;119:68–73.
21. Buxton N, Vloeberghs M, Punt J. Flexible neuroendoscopic treatment of suprasellar arachnoid cysts. *Br J Neurosurg* 1999;13:316–318.
22. Choi JU, Kim DS, Huh R. Endoscopic approach to arachnoid cyst. *Childs Nerv Syst* 1999;15:285–291.
23. Schroeder HW, Gaab MR, Niendorf WR. Neuroendoscopic approach to arachnoid cysts. *J Neurosurg* 1996;85:293–298.
24. Paladino J, Rotim K, Heinrich Z. Neuroendoscopic fenestration of arachnoid cysts. *Minim Invasive Neurosurg* 1998;41:137–140.
25. Gangemi M, Maiuri F, Donati P, Sigona L. Endoscopic ventricular fenestration of intracranial fluid cysts. *Minim Invasive Neurosurg* 1996;39:7–11.
26. Gaab MR, Schroeder HWS. Endoscopy for intraventricular lesions. In: King W, Frazee J, DeSalles A, eds. *Endoscopy of the Central and Peripheral Nervous System*. New York: Thieme Medical Publishers; 1998:68–77.
27. Camins MB, Schlesinger EB. Treatment of tumours of the posterior part of the third ventricle and the pineal region: a long-term follow-up. *Acta Neurochir* 1978;40:131–143.
28. Apuzzo ML, Chikovani OK, Gott PS, et al. Transcallosal, interfornicial approaches for lesions affecting the third ventricle: surgical considerations and consequences. *Neurosurgery* 1982;10:547–554.
29. Carmel PW. Tumours of the third ventricle. *Acta Neurochir* 1985;75:136–146.
30. Stein BM. The infratentorial supracerebellar approach to pineal lesions. *J Neurosurg* 1971;35:197–202.
31. Rhoton AL Jr, Yamamoto I, Peace DA. Microsurgery of the third ventricle, II: Operative approaches. *Neurosurgery* 1981;8:357–373.
32. Matula C, Reinprecht A, Roessler K, Tschabitscher M, Koos WT. Endoscopic exploration of the IVth ventricle. *Minim Invasive Neurosurg* 1996;39:86–92.
33. Gaab MR, Schroeder HW. Neuroendoscopic approach to intraventricular lesions. *J Neurosurg* 1998;88:496–505.
34. Yaniv E, Rappaport ZH. Endoscopic transseptal transsphenoidal surgery for pituitary tumors. *Neurosurgery* 1997;40:944–946.
35. Koren I, Hadar T, Rappaport ZH, Yaniv E. Endoscopic transnasal transsphenoidal microsurgery versus the sublabial approach for the treatment of pituitary tumors: endonasal complications. *Laryngoscope* 1999;109:1838–1840.
36. Sheehan MT, Atkinson JL, Kasperbauer JL, Erickson BJ, Nippoldt TB. Preliminary comparison of the endoscopic transnasal vs the sublabial transseptal approach for clinically nonfunctioning pituitary macroadenomas. *Mayo Clin Proc* 1999;74:661–670.
37. Jho HD, Carrau RL. Endoscopic endonasal transsphenoidal surgery: experience with 50 patients. *J Neurosurg* 1997;87:44–51.
38. Jarrahy R, Berci G, Shahinian HK. Assessment of the efficacy of endoscopy in pituitary adenoma resection. *Arch Otolaryngol Head Neck Surg* 2000;126:1487–1490.
39. Helal MZ. Combined micro-endoscopic trans-sphenoid excisions of pituitary macroadenomas. *Eur Arch Otorhinolaryngol* 1995;252:186–189.
40. Valtonen HJ, Poe DS, Heilman CB, Tarlov EC. Endoscopically assisted prevention of cerebrospinal fluid leak in suboccipital acoustic neuroma surgery. *Am J Otol* 1997;18:381–385.
41. Saim L, McKenna MJ, Nadol JB Jr. Tubal and tympanic openings of the peritubal cells: implications for cerebrospinal fluid otorhinorrhea. *Am J Otol* 1996;17:335–339.
42. Millen SJ, Meyer G. Surgical management of CSF otorhinorrhea following retrosigmoid removal of cerebellopontine angle tumors. *Am J Otol* 1993;14:585–589.
43. Hoffman RA. Cerebrospinal fluid leak following acoustic neuroma removal. *Laryngoscope* 1994;104:40–58.
44. Wackym PA, King WA, Poe DS, et al. Adjunctive use of endoscopy during acoustic neuroma surgery. *Laryngoscope* 1999;109:1193–1201.
45. Sindou M, Acevedo JC, Turjman F. Aneurysmal remnants after microsurgical clipping: classification and results from a prospective angiographic study (in a consecutive series of 305 operated intracranial aneurysms). *Acta Neurochir* 1998;140:1153–1159.

46. Taniguchi M, Takimoto H, Yoshimine T, et al. Application of a rigid endoscope to the microsurgical management of 54 cerebral aneurysms: results in 48 patients. *J Neurosurg* 1999;91:231–237.
47. Frank EH, Horgan M. An endoscopic aneurysm clip applicator: preliminary development. *Minim Invasive Neurosurg* 1999;42:89–91.
48. Duffner F, Dauber W, Skalej M, Grote EH. A new endoscopic tool for the CRW stereotactic system. *Stereotact Funct Neurosurg* 1996;67:213–217.
49. Deinsberger W, Boker DK, Bothe HW, Samii M. Stereotactic endoscopic treatment of colloid cysts of the third ventricle. *Acta Neurochir* 1994;131:260–264.
50. Grunert P, Hopf N, Perneczky A. Frame-based and frameless endoscopic procedures in the third ventricle. *Stereotact Funct Neurosurg* 1997;68:80–89.
51. Rhoten RL, Luciano MG, Barnett GH. Computer-assisted endoscopy for neurosurgical procedures: technical note. *Neurosurgery* 1997;40:632–637; discussion 638.
52. Rohde V, Reinges MH, Krombach GA, Gilsbach JM. The combined use of image-guided frameless stereotaxy and neuroendoscopy for the surgical management of occlusive hydrocephalus and intracranial cysts. *Br J Neurosurg* 1998;12:531–538.
53. Gumprecht H, Trost HA, Lumenta CB. Neuroendoscopy combined with frameless neuronavigation. *Br J Neurosurg* 2000;14:129–131.
54. Dorward NL, Alberti O, Zhao J, et al. Interactive image-guided neuroendoscopy: development and early clinical experience. *Minim Invasive Neurosurg* 1998;41:31–34.
55. Schroeder HW, Wagner W, Tschiltschke W, Gaab MR. Frameless neuronavigation in intracranial endoscopic neurosurgery. *J Neurosurg* 2001;94:72–79.
56. Muacevic A, Muller A. Image-guided endoscopic ventriculostomy with a new frameless armless neuronavigation system. *Comput Aided Surg* 1999;4:87–92.

11

Robotic Microscopes

ADNAN H. SIDDIQUI AND CHARLES J. HODGE

The ability to plan and perform complex neurosurgical procedures depends on the practical ability to navigate. Neuronavigation has progressed from a mental rendering of indirect anatomic reference points to a precise technology dependent on complex computational ability (i.e., computers). Like other types of navigation, neurosurgical navigation consists of two important elements. The first is the ability to plan a safe route from a starting point to a target destination. The second is the ability to determine current location in relation to the target and in relation to potential high-risk areas. In ocean navigation, the current location refers to the ship's position. In most neuronavigational systems, the current location refers to the tip of a pointer. When a navigational microscope is used, the current position refers to the tip of a virtual pointer, the location of which is at the focal point of the microscope optical system.

The progression of computer science has allowed frame-based stereotaxy to evolve into frameless methods[1,2] based on simple skin- or skull-based fiducial markers. Neural images, in the form of two-dimensional data such as computed tomographic (CT) scans, magnetic resonance imaging (MRI) scans, positron emission tomography (PET), or functional MRI (fMRI) can be obtained with a high degree of precision. These data can then be restructured into three-dimensional (3-D) views of the head and brain that can be registered for spatial orientation and manipulated by the surgeon. The surgeon can thus plan the starting point, target, and safest route prior to the actual surgery. This is equivalent to producing a navigational map for each procedure that can be individualized for the patient's particular anatomy and pathology.

A robot is a mechanical device that follows instructions to accomplish a task usually done by a human. Robots are particularly appropriate when repetitive actions or extreme precision is needed. The advantage of a robotic microscope combined with frameless stereotaxy is that a number of functions normally dependent on the operator can be performed by computer-driven mechanisms. These actions, such as moving to the planned starting position, following a planned course, focusing accurately on the target point, and avoiding a preplanned risk area can all be done automatically with great precision. Further, the robotic control mechanisms allow specific movement patterns such as rotating the microscope around a predetermined focal point or rotating the viewing axis around a preselected point along the optical axis thus maximizing the amount of visible area through a small opening. This chapter describes the design and use of robotic microscopes with particular emphasis on the multicoordinate manipulator (MKM) robotic microscope and navigational system developed by the Carl Zeiss Corporation.

■ Technical Features

The four principal components of a robotic stereotactic microscope system are the computer-based workstation, the robotic arm, the microscope itself, and the localizing system that allows monitoring of head or instrument location (Fig. 11–1).

At the heart of the system is the computer and workstation. It is the high-speed computer that allows manip-

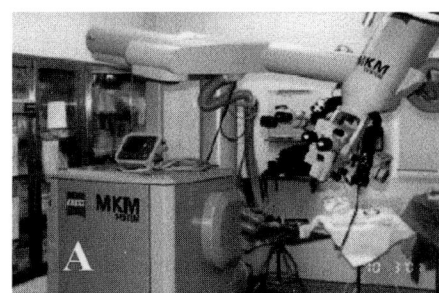
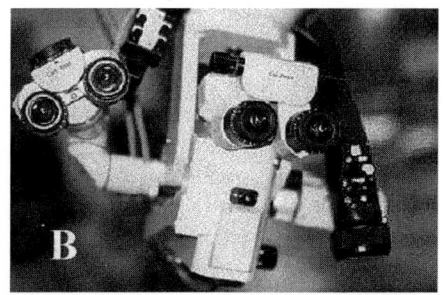
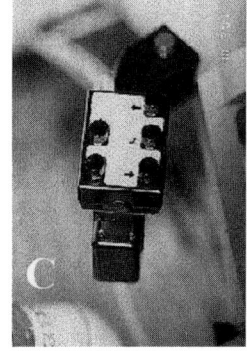
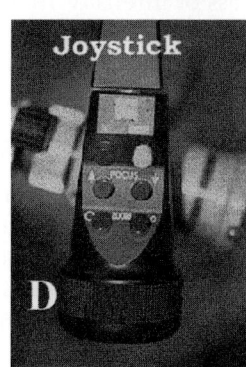

FIGURE 11–1. Some of the components of a robotic system. (A). The base of the microscope and the robotic arm used to position the microscope at the desired site. (B). The microscope, which is not unusual except for the two arms that are illustrated in C and D. (C). The left-hand grip of the robotic scope. This allows the user to leaf through many of the user menus, displayed in the heads-up display in the right ocular, without removing attention from the microscope. (D). The joystick, which allows operator movement of the microscope using the motors built into the robotic arm. Additionally, this handle contains a button that instructs the microscope to autofocus at the point of the crosshairs and buttons that allow operator-controlled focus and operator-controlled zoom (MKM Zeuss, Thornwood, NY).

ulation of the 3-D image data in relation to the microscope virtual pointer. Additionally, merging or fusion of different types of images can be done to take advantage of the differing kinds of information available through different imaging modalities (i.e., CT, MRI, fMRI, PET). The workstation allows image manipulation and thus determination of complex volumetric shapes and precise spatial definition of anatomy and pathology. Using this image-based information, anatomically safe approaches can be developed. The computational power of the MKM system is provided by a DEC Alpha workstation, running STP software (Leibinger, Freiburg, Germany), on a UNIX-based platform or a PC Windows-based system. These systems are equipped with digital audiotape (DAT) drives and optical drives thus allowing image data entry when direct line connection is unavailable.

The second component is the robotic mechanism. This is a positioning arm with six degrees of freedom (i.e., base rotation; translation in three primary axes: x, y, z; and two other rotational axes). The positioning mechanisms are motor driven and can be controlled either by an operator-maneuvered joystick or by computer-generated instructions. The operator-generated movements can be devolved into only orthogonal x, y, and z movements or only rotational movements centered on the focal point of the microscope system using permissive-selection buttons located on the joystick. The position of the arm is continually relayed back to the computer. The MKM microscope, base, and arm are motorized and internally encoded with an inherent accuracy of up to 0.75 mm. The robotic nature of the microscope also allows the scope to pivot around a point of focus, orient itself at any time along a planned trajectory, pivot around a cylinder (keyhole) to allow examination of a larger area when the surgical corridor is narrow, or go to any predetermined position under computer control.

The third component is the microscope itself, which is mounted on the robotic arm. The most important aspect of the microscope mechanism is the ability to accurately focus in response to operator-generated commands. This mechanism, based on laser matching, allows extremely precise and accurate focus. Currently, the Surgiscope by Leica (Allendale, NJ)[3] and the MKM by Zeiss (Thornwood, NY)[4] both use laser beams to provide the location of the focal point to their robotic microscopes. The MKM uses a Class I laser as its autofocus system with an accuracy of within 0.3 mm of its critical focus and with the 0.75 mm accuracy of the robotic arm gives an overall accuracy of 1.05 mm. The dynamic focus has a working range of 200 to 400 mm. This focal point location is relayed to the computer, which in turn computes the location of the area under focus and displays it on the monitor in the form of crosshairs on the three orthogonal planes of the image (CT or MRI) forming the navigational basis of the case as well as a 3-D rendering of the head. An added benefit is the ability to display the planned surgical approach, distance to target points, and outlines of predetermined important pathological or risk structures at the current plane of focus in one of the eyepieces as a heads-up display (HUD). This allows clear orientation for the surgeon without the need to continually look up from the point of surgical concentration. The microscope has a zoom ratio of 1:6. It is mounted with a stereo beam splitter to provide stereoscopic vision and 12.5× eyepieces. The microscope also has an attached microphone for verbal commands that can be programmed for up to 15 surgeons and allows manipulation of the microscope without removing either hand from the operative field. The microscope uses a xenon light source for constant temperature regardless of intensity. In addition to the microscope's manual controls, there are foot controls allowing another means of altering focus, zoom, and movement. All that is then required for the system to be functional is a constant, or at least measurable, spatial relation between the target and the robotic arm base. This is accomplished by fixing the position of the microscope base and registering the spatial location of the head using fiducial markers.

The fourth component is a localization system that will allow the locations of various tools to be determined and will also allow changes in head position to be determined. Several different types of systems are currently available to locate the fiducial markers and pointing devices. There are magnetic systems,[5,6] which develop a magnetic field around the head and, based upon its interference or modulation, reconstruct the 3-D localization data. However, they are subject to position degradation by nearby ferromagnetic materials such as most surgical instruments. Ultrasonic detectors[7] have been used in a similar capacity with emitters based around the microscope objective along with receivers that calculate the speed and modification of returned sound waves to reconstruct the area under observation and obtain localizing data. This methodology is also fraught with complicating factors such as interference with reflectors or other objects in the operative field. In addition, the temperature of the room and its relative humidity may influence sound velocity and, thereby, the computational accuracy of this system. The sound transmitters and receivers can be influenced by the draping methods around the microscope. Mechanical arms can also be used as pointer devices.[1,2,8,9] They rely on mechanical determination of position of the arm based on their articulated joint positions. Several systems are now available that rely on the optics of operating microscopes and their proximity to the intraoperative region of interest to generate localizing data that can be interpreted by the computing system and provide the surgeon with knowledge of his or her current position.[10–14] As in the microscope system we describe, localizing technologies are frequently combined and used to advantage.

Optical digitizers use information from light that can be emitted and then captured using infrared or laser cameras.[10,12–15] This avoids optical interference from ambient sources such as operating room lights. Infrared systems[10,12,15,16] utilize light-emitting diodes (LEDs), which emit pulsed infrared signals and are attached to the patient's head through the head clamp. This allows continuous monitoring of the head's position in space. Similar systems have been used with nonrobotic microscopes such as BrainLAB's VectorVision system.[10,12,16] The initial head position in relation to the microscope is determined by registering the fiducial markers placed on the scalp or implanted in the skull. The registration can be done using either the microscope focal point as the virtual pointer or a real pointer located with attached LEDs. Once registration is completed, the relative position of the microscope to the head in space and hence all the points in the images are known. Like other navigational systems, it is this spatial relation that allows accurate use of the stereotactic information.

■ Neuronavigation Procedure

Skin fiducials are placed on the patient's scalp on the afternoon or evening before surgery. Bone-based fiducials are also available and have the apparent advantage of slightly higher accuracy. Positioning the fiducials is important. There should be at least six and preferably eight fiducials placed. They should be as widely separated on the head as possible, remembering that if the microscope is to be used to register the fiducials, they must be in a visable position (i.e., the person placing the fiducials must be aware of the head position to be used during surgery). Fiducials should not be placed in the low suboccipital area because the patient will be lying on this part of the head during scanning and thus may distort the positions of the fiducials. At this point appropriate images are obtained. If fMRI routines are to be performed, they must be accomplished prior to contrast administration.

■ Imaging Protocols

At our institution we typically use MRI images for neuronavigation; only rarely do we supplement this with CT scans. MRI images are obtained as fast inversion recovery sequences in the form of gadolinium-enhanced 3-D gradient echo, axial images (TE $\sim$ 1–10 msec, TR $\sim$ 10 msec, and TI $\sim$ 400 msec). The slices are 1.2 mm thick without any gap. The entire head is scanned, usually requiring about 124 slices using a 256 × 256 matrix with a field of view of 24 × 24 cm. The average scan time is about 10 minutes. The most common functional scans we use are devised to activate either language cortex or sensorimotor hand cortex around the central sulcus. At times electrical stimulation of the median nerve, as in somatosensory evoked potential generation, will be used.[17]

Patient Setup

Following anesthesia induction, or sedation if awake mapping is to be done, the patient is positioned with the head fixed in a three-point head clamp. The MKM base is then moved into position and fixed by raising the retractable wheels. Minor changes in position are easiest to accomplish by moving the operating couch. A three-LED localizing array is connected to the head clamp so that changes in head position can be detected by the infrared camera system.

The surgeon will have numbered the fiducials on the images presented on the workstation. Additionally, the lesion will be outlined and important risk areas outlined (Figs. 11–2 and 11–3). At this time functionally important data such as the locations of language, motor, or sensory cortices are added using the fusion function. An entry point and at least one target point are identified. This defines a straight surgical trajectory to be followed. Alternatively, a multilegged course can be constructed.

The head is registered in space in relation to the microscope (Fig. 11–4). This is done by using the microscope focal point by autofocusing on the center of each fiducial under maximum magnification. This allows the workstation to perform a mathematical transformation of the microscope coordinates for each fiducial and match them with the location of the fiducials on the workstation images. This allows the workstation to create a spatial environment in which the patient's head, the microscope-based pointer, and all the additional information such as lesion and risk area locations are registered. The fiducials can also be registered using an optically tracked pointer. A mean deviation error is calculated based on the registered fiducial position compared with the positions expected from the fiducial locations selected on the images. This can then be reduced by selectively eliminating certain fiducial points that seem inaccurate. Once the surgeon is satisfied with the calculated error between the real and the image-based fiducial locations (usual range is between 1 and 3 mm) a landmark test is done. The surgeon focuses the microscope on some external structure on the patient's head, such as the tragus, and confirms that the area under focus is accurately depicted by the location of the crosshairs on the three orthogonal planes displayed at the workstation. The robotic aspects of the system are used to align the microscope with the planned trajectory so that an appropriately placed flap can be marked. The microscope can then be used as a simple pointing device to label the scalp structures or venous sinuses and to plan for tailored skin incision and craniotomy flap. If a head-tracking device is not used, internal fiducials using bone divots or small screws are placed immediately after the skin incision is made and recorded so that any head movement can be compensated for by re-registration. Once the operation has begun, the microscope can be used like any other microscope, albeit with the major advantage of having localizing data available both on the computer monitor (in the form of crosshairs on tripla-

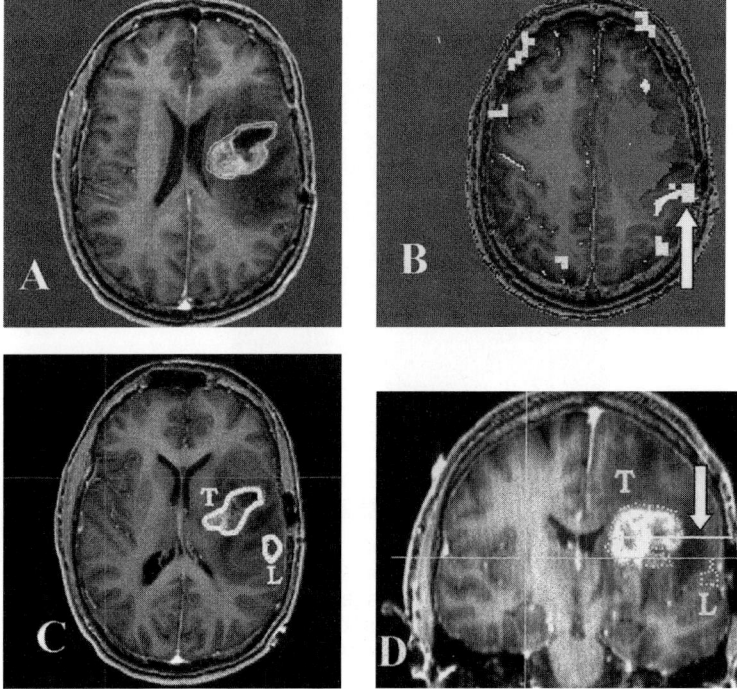

FIGURE 11–2. Images taken from the workstation illustrating the steps in developing a surgical plan. (A). An axial scan showing a left hemisphere tumor, the volume of which has been outlined by the surgeon. (B). An axial image with a functional magnetic resonance imaging scan merged with an anatomic scan. The vertical arrow points to language area in the posterior left temporal lobe, which can also be outlined by the operator for later identification. (C). An axial image that shows outlines of both the tumor (T) and language area (L). (D). A coronal image illustrating the tumor volume (T), a portion of the language area (L), and a surgical approach, which is indicated by the arrow.

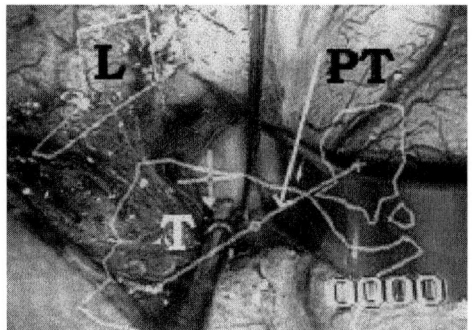
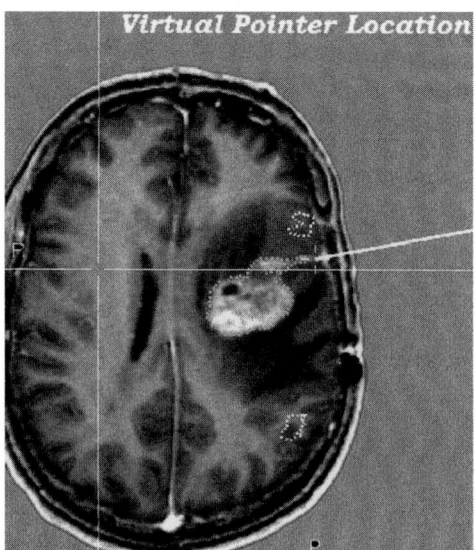

FIGURE 11–3. Operative procedure. (Left). The view through the microscope demonstrating the heads-up display outline of regions of interest. L is the outline of the language area determined by functional magnetic resonance imaging. T is the outline of the tumor at the depth of the exposure. PT is the planned trajectory for approach to this lesion. (Right). This axial scan shows the virtual pointer location indicated by the crosshairs over the right hemisphere. The planned trajectory is demonstrated by the oblique line pointing at the tumor.

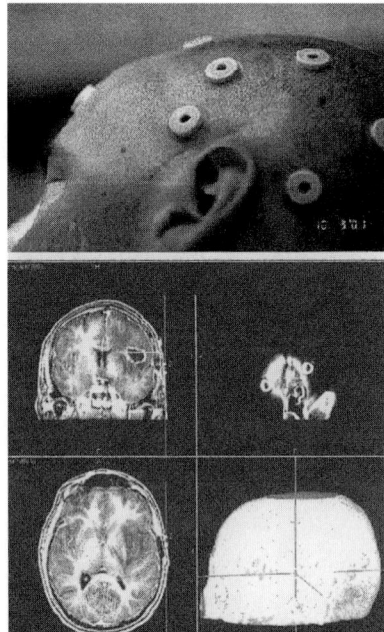

FIGURE 11–4. Registration using skin fiducial markers. (Upper). Fiducial markers placed on the operative side of the head. Note the wide spatial dispersion of the fiducials. (Lower). A triplanar image combination used to identify individual fiducial markers. The crosshairs indicate the focal point of the virtual pointer.

nar views) and as projected contours and point of focus information in the HUD. The current position of the virtual pointer is updated by pressing the autofocus button on the joystick hand piece.

Another robotic feature is that the microscope can be instructed to pivot around any point along the optical axis, which allows maximum visability of cavities through a small opening. At any time the autofocus function updates the surgeon's current location and allows the surgeon to refresh orientation without the need to remove eyes or hands from the operative field.

■ Accuracy

Frame-based neuronavigation has an accuracy error of 0.7 to 1.8 mm.[18,19] However, this accuracy comes at the cost of restricted surgical maneuverability and the added step of frame placement. Frameless system accuracy relies on three different components: the precision of radiographic data that are obtained, the precision of translation of skin fiducial markers into registration points, and the inherent accuracy of the system under use. This last component is determined by the accuracy of the robotic arms as well as the optical or other digitizing systems that form the hardware of the system. Based on fusion of pre- and postoperative images depicting biopsy sites, the mean error was 2.3 mm for CT-directed frameless stereotaxy compared with 2.6 mm for MR-derived images.[20] Using phantom accuracy models this error was 1.1 mm for CT-derived images versus 1.4 mm for MR-derived images.[20] The second component requisite for accuracy consists of the skin fiducial markers and their registration. Translation due to skin distortion can lead to inaccuracies, and some authors have suggested the routine use of bone-based fiducials to circumvent such error.[21] The placement of bone fiducials though adds to presurgical invasiveness of the procedure and has shown no consistent overall effect on the accuracy needed to perform surgery. An interesting study by Kaminsky et al[21] looked at the accuracy of the MKM system; as a part of their experiment they positioned the skin fiducials along a straight line, triangle, or square. They noted errors in the range of centimeters with the straight line, which were reduced to < 2 mm using a triangular or square pattern of fiducial placement. Accuracy increases as the distance between the registration points increases, and it declines with increased fiducial-target distances. The accuracy is in the range of 0.3 mm when the microscope is positioned over the center of the fiducial field and 1.2 mm when it is 200 mm away from center of the fiducial field. The final determinants of system accuracy are the hardware components of the system such as the robotic arm, which the manufacturer states is accurate to within 0.75 mm, and the laser-directed optical focusing system, which is accurate to within 0.3 mm. The laser-guided optical digitizer was noted to be accurate to 0.04 mm at maximum magnification and 0.1 mm at minimum magnification. The robotic arm was noted to be accurate to 0.4 mm at maximum magnification and minimum angular deviation of the microscope from perpendicular to the plane of the fiducials.[21] Increasing this angle increased the error measured.

In another study, the MKM system accuracy tested at 0.3 mm using a geometric model.[14] Similar testing for the MKM in cadaver skulls after 3-D CT-scan reconstruction yielded an accuracy of 0.6 to 0.7 mm.[22] Operative accuracy was reported to be 2.2 mm after gaining experience with fiducial placement and registration in a recently reported clinical series using the MKM.[23] In all, these figures are similar to frame-based systems. The difference between a 1 mm and a 2 mm error is of uncertain clinical significance. The underlying dilemma of intraoperative brain shift and failing accuracy with progression of surgery remains a concern with all current neuronavigation systems including the robotic microscopes. The solution appears to be intraoperative imaging and updating neuroradiographic data using implantable fiducials, brain surface landmarks, or even intraoperative scanning techniques. A recent study by Wirtz et al reported a mean accuracy of 0.8 mm after intraoperative re-registration using intraoperative MRI and the MKM microscope.[24]

■ Clinical Utility

Roessler et al[23] were one of the first groups to publish their series of patients on whom they used the MKM system for frameless stereotactic neuronavigation. The procedures were done primarily for tumor resection (64%) but were also done for resection of cavernomas and epileptic foci. They reported a learning curve in terms of fiducial placement and increased registration accuracy from 4.8 mm in their first 25 cases to 2.2 mm for their last 50 cases. They also reported the deterioration of accuracy as the cases progressed secondary to brain shift. The advantages of the system in their view included the ability to make smaller, tailored incisions and craniotomies, as well as utility of lesion contours projected into the eyepiece of the surgeon allowing a continuous view of the surgical bed. This enabled the surgeon to perform a more complete resection of gliomas, avoid eloquent areas during dissection, and minimize brain injury secondary to less retraction and more direct approach to deep-seated lesions.

Zamorano et al[25] presented their results on 15 patients with cavernomas where they used both infrared handheld pointers as well as the MKM robotic microscope. Their view was similar to Roessler's, in that deep-seated lesions could be approached in and around eloquent areas through more direct routes and with minimal brain retraction, which resulted in optimal neurological outcome. They did however perform awake craniotomies for patients with lesions in and around eloquent cortex. Ungersbock et al[26] compared MKM based resection of cavernomas with frame-based resections. They describe the difference between target-point stereotaxis and contour-guided stereotaxis. Thus, without loss of accuracy they had more surgical liberty in terms of patient positioning and approach, and the MKM system obviated the need for additional pointer devices to be introduced into the surgical bed for localization. Roessler et al[27] utilized pointer based systems as well as the MKM to locate small enhancing areas within nine large, presumed low-grade supratentorial gliomas to identify the heterogeneous nature of these lesions and to avoid undergrading of the tumor. They were equally successful with both methodologies and reported the utility of frameless stereotaxis to avoid sampling error in these lesions. Lévesque and Parker[28] operated using MKM on two diffuse brainstem neoplasms extending from the third to the fourth ventricle, a hemangioblastoma, and a malignant ependymoma in patients who were deemed to be inoperable after radiation and previous debulking and biopsy and were in a state of coma vigil. They were able to obtain gross radiographic resection in both patients with long-term survival and reversal of deficits. Nakamura et al[29] reported on four patients with deep-seated arteriovenous malformations (AVMs) that were resected using the MKM. They reported on the utility of the procedure with improved localization and directed approach. However, confirmation of the complete removal still required angiography.

■ Conclusions

Stereotactic navigation is now the standard of care for many types of intracranial neurosurgery. By the late 1980s frame-based stereotactic approaches were clearly superior to nonstereotactic surgery for deep-seated lesions.[19] Current large-volume studies establish that frameless stereotaxy is comparable to frame-based methods.[1,2] The last 10 years have seen the trial of multiple technological innovations to increase the operative efficiency and accuracy of frameless stereotaxy. These have been primarily directed at development of digitizers that transform the operative spatial environment onto preoperative neuroradiographic imagery to provide the surgeon with a 3-D view of the patient's intracranial anatomy. The available systems utilize magnetic fields,[5,6] ultrasound,[7] mechanical arms,[2,13] and optical digitizers using infrared[11,12] and laser[14,21,22] sources. These technologies were incorporated into pointer devices that could be placed on areas under question while the computer would display 3-D information on the screen. A logical next step has been the development of microscopes to complement digitizers, be it in construction of mechanical arms[8] or through conjunction with optical digitizers.[10,14–16] Adding robotics to these systems has been an important development affecting this rapidly changing field. The earliest attempts were with mechanical arms[8]; however, two current systems employ both mechanical arms and optical digitizers to enhance operability and accuracy.[3,4]

Germano et al[12] reported significantly shorter hospital stays for patients undergoing frameless stereotaxy versus conventional procedures. They speculated cases done with frameless techniques were less invasive due to smaller craniotomies and less retraction resulting in less perioperative morbidity and faster recuperation. In a study on operating time Alberti et al[30] reported that neuronavigation was time neutral for most conventional cases and actually time saving when used for biopsy procedures. These two considerations are a valuable indication that, more than just assisting the surgeon in the operation, neuronavigation results in possibly better economic and health based outcomes.

An interesting analysis of 208 cases using frameless stereotaxy by Roessler et al[31] showed that pointer based systems did not necessarily compete with microscope based systems. They used the EGN pointer (Phillips Medical Systems, the Netherlands) for 114 patients, including nine spinal cases, and the MKM for 92 cranial cases. It was their opinion that in cases where the lesions were deep seated and microscopes had to be used, MKM was clearly the choice. However, for cases such as cyst fenestrations or when the lesions were cortically based, such as meningiomas, the EGN system was very effective. It is therefore reasonable to state that microscope based systems and pointer based systems are complementary.

The benefits of any neuronavigational system are: (1) allowing for detailed preoperative planning including a tailored skin incision, craniotomy, and smaller corticectomy with minimal brain retraction and (2) allowing to use the most direct route to the lesion with avoidance of critical/eloquent areas. The major advantages of robotic microscopes include the precision made available by mechanical arms. The preoperative planning allows the surgeon to instruct the microscope in the planned trajectory, and this can be very useful in keyhole approaches when the surgeon is operating through a long, narrow corridor. The microscope can maneuver itself around either a focal point or a cylinder rim of the corridor to increase the operative viewing angles. The optical digitizing system within the microscope's optics obviates the need for introduction of additional instruments into the operative field for localization. The HUD allows the surgeon to maintain concentration on the microscopic field without turning toward the screen to obtain current position. The display updates the contours of predefined lesions and areas and the current focus information as well as distances to targets with either verbal or tactile commands. In addition the controls of the microscope, including menu options, can also be seen in the HUD. Other technologies that are currently becoming incorporated with robotic microscopes include endoscopes and radiation delivery systems.

The robotic microscopes are not as flexible as traditional microscopes,[9] and the special joystick controls of the MKM do require a learning period. Similarly, placement of fiducials, although fairly simple, is something that can result in errors, and again a learning curve is noted by many studies.[23,32] The neuronavigational system can fail due to technical problems, such as computer crashes, which were reported to occur in 2.6% of cases.[23] We have noted an improvement in crash occurrence with software updates that have taken place over the past several years. There can be differences in visual focus and laser auto focus that can lead to discrepancies,[21] and therefore the navigational tool has to use the autofocus and not the current visual focus of the surgeon. One of the biggest drawbacks of the current technology has to be accommodation of brain shift. Clearly this is a bigger problem for larger lesions causing mass effect than smaller ones. This deterioration was reported to be as great as 5 mm at the end of the case in up to 29% of patients.[23] This is worrisome, especially when the targeted goal is complete removal of a glioma or a large metastatic lesion. Some of these effects are countered by good surgical skills that are based on the surgeon's ability to distinguish tumor tissue from normal brain tissue based on texture and vascularity. In edematous brain this certainly becomes more difficult. Inaccuracies are compounded in these situations because the brain is more mobile, and it shifts after craniotomy due to altered intracranial pressure dynamics. The current neuronavigational technologies are all equally ineffective at ameliorating this drawback. The solution has to be real-time intraoperative re-registration. The intraoperative MRI or CT scan has recently been promoted for this reason. Intraoperative imaging and incorporation of ultrasound techniques are the only known solutions to the problem of brain shift. The current systems are fairly accurate for most discrete lesions; however, larger mass-producing lesions are clearly still problematic.

REFERENCES

1. Barnett GH, Miller DW, Weisenberger J. Frameless stereotaxy with scalp applied fiducial markers for brain biopsy procedures: experience in 218 cases. *J Neurosurg* 1999;91:569–576.
2. Golfinos JG, Fitzpatrick BC, Smith LR, Spetzler RF. Clinical use of a frameless stereotactic arm: results of 325 cases. *J Neurosurg* 1995;83:197–205.
3. Haase J. Neurosurgical tools and techniques: modern image-guided surgery. *Neurol Med Chir Suppl* 1998;38:303–307.
4. Kiya N, Dureza C, Fukushima T, Maroon JC. Computer navigational microscope for minimally invasive neurosurgery. *Minim Invas Neurosurg* 1997;40:110–115.
5. Marmulla R, Hibert M, Niederdellmann H. Intraoperative precision of mechanical, electromagnetic, infrared and laser-guided navigation systems in computer assisted surgery [German]. *Mund-, Kiefer- und Gesichtschirurgie* 1998; 2(suppl 1):S145–S148.
6. Rousu JS, Kohls PE, Kall B, Kelly PJ. Computer assisted image guided surgery using the Regulus navigator. In: Westwood JD, Hoffman HM, Stredney D, Weghorst SJ, eds. *Medicine Meets Virtual Reality*. Amsterdam: IOS Press and Ohmsha; 1998:103–109.
7. Barnett GH, Kormos DW, Steiner CP, Weisenberger J. Use of a frameless, armless stereotactic wand for brain tumor localization with two-dimensional and three-dimensional neuroimaging. *Neurosurg* 1993;33:674–678.
8. Giorgi C, Eisenberg H, Costi G, Gallo E, Garibotto G, Casolino DS. Robot assisted microscope for neurosurgery. *J Image Guid Surg* 1995;1:158–163.
9. Wirtz CR, Knauth M, Hassfeld S, et al. Neuronavigation: first experiences with three different commercially available systems. *Zentralbl Neurochir* 1998;59:14–22.
10. Gumprecht HK, Widenka DC, Lumenta CB. BrainLAB VectorVision Neuronavigation System: technology and clinical experiences in 131 cases. *Neurosurg* 1999;44:97–105.
11. Kaus M, Steinmeier R, Sporer T, Ganslandt O, Fahlbusch R. Technical accuracy of a neuronavigation system measured with a high-precision mechanical micromanipulator. *Neurosurg* 1997;41:1431–1437.
12. Germano IM, Villalobos H, Silvers A, Post KD. Clinical use of the optical digitizer for intracranial neuronavigation. *Neurosurg* 1999;45:261–270.
13. Takizawa T, Soto SH, Sanou A, Murakami Y. Frameless isocentric stereotactic laser beam guide for image-directed microsurgery. *Acta Neurochir* 2001;125:177–180.
14. Marmulla R, Hibert M, Niederdellmann H. Inherent precision of mechanical, infrared and laser-guided navigation systems for computer-assisted surgery. *Journal of Cranio-Maxillofacial Surgery* 1997; 25:192–197.
15. Westermann B, Trippel M, Reinhardt H. Optically-navigable operating microscope for image-guided surgery. *Minim Invas Neurosurg* 1995;38:112–116.
16. Gumprecht H, Lumenta CB. The operating microscope guided by a neuronavigation system: a technical note. *Minim Invas Neurosurg* 1998;41:141–143.
17. Boakye M, Huckins SC, Szeverenyi NM, Taskey BI, Hodge CJ. Functional magnetic resonance imaging of somatosensory cortex activity produced by electrical stimulation of the median nerve or tactile stimulation of the index finger. *J Neurosurg* 2000;93:774–783.
18. Goerss S, Kelly PJ, Kall B, Alker GJ. A computed tomographic stereotactic adaptation system. *Neurosurg* 1982;10:375–379.
19. Apuzzo MLJ, Chandrasoma PT, Cohen D, Zee C, Zelman V. Computed imaging stereotaxy: experience and perspective related to 500 procedures applied to brain masses. *Neurosurg* 1987;20:930–937.
20. Dorward NL, Alberti O, Kitchen ND, Palmer JD, Thomas DGT. Accuracy of true frameless stereotaxy: in vivo measurement and laboratory phantom studies. *J Neurosurg* 1999;90:160–168.
21. Kaminsky J, Brinker T, Samii A, Arango G, Vorkapic P, Samii M. Technical considerations regarding accuracy of the MKM navigation system: an experimental study on impact factors. *Neurol Res* 1999;21:420–424.
22. Brinker T, Arango G, Kaminsky J, et al. An experimental approach to image guided skull based surgery employing a microscope-based neuronavigation system. *Acta Neurochir* 1998;140:883–889.
23. Roessler K, Ungersboeck K, Aichholzer M, et al. Frameless stereotactic lesion contour-guided surgery using a computer-navigated microscope. *Surg Neurol* 1998;49:282–289.
24. Wirtz CR, Bonsanto MM, Knauth M, et al. Intraoperative magnetic resonance imaging to update interactive navigation in neurosurgery: method and preliminary experience. *Comp Aid Surg* 1997;2:172–179.
25. Zamorano L, Matter A, Saenz A, Buciuc R, Diaz F. Interactive image-guided resection of cerebral cavernous malformations. *Comp Aid Surg* 1997;2:327–332.
26. Ungersbock K, Aichholzer M, Gunthner M, Rossler K, Gorzer H, Koos WT. Cavernous malformations: from frame-based to frameless stereotactic localization. *Minim Invas Neurosurg* 1997;40:134–138.
27. Roessler K, Czech T, Dietrich W, et al. Frameless stereotactic-directed tissue sampling during surgery of low-grade gliomas to avoid histological undergrading. *Minim Invas Neurosurg* 1998;41:183–186.
28. Lévesque MF, Parker F. MKM-guided resection of diffuse brainstem neoplasms. *Stereotact Funct Neurosurg* 1999;73:15–18.
29. Nakamura M, Tamaki N, Tamura S, Yamashita H, Hara Y, Ehara K. Image-guided microsurgery with the Mehrkoordinaten manipulator system for cerebral arteriovenous malformations. *J Clin Neurosci* 2000;7(suppl 1):10–13.

30. Alberti O, Dorward NL, Kitchen ND, Thomas DGT. Neuronavigation: impact on operating time. *Stereotact Funct Neurosurg* 1997;68:44–48.
31. Roessler K, Ungerboeck K, Aichholzer M, et al. Image-guided neurosurgery comparing a pointer device system with a navigating microscope: a retrospective analysis of 208 cases. *Minim Invas Neurosurg* 1998;41:53–57.
32. Roessler K, Ungerboeck K, Czech T, et al. Contour-guided brain tumor surgery using a stereotactic navigating microscope. *Stereotact Funct Neurosurg* 1997;68:33–38.

12

Image-Guided Robotic Radiosurgery

STEVEN D. CHANG, IRIS C. GIBBS, DAVID P. MARTIN, AND JOHN R. ADLER JR.

Radiosurgery combines principles of stereotactic localization with multiple cross-fired beams from a highly collimated high energy radiation source.[1] This noninvasive technique has proven to be an effective alternative to conventional neurosurgery and irradiation for selected small cranial tumors and arteriovenous malformations. Because virtually all existing stereotactic techniques rely on rigid target fixation, almost all cases treated with radiosurgery to date have involved intracranial lesions. Recent improvements in high-speed computing, radiographic imaging, and lightweight linear accelerator design have led to the development of the Cyberknife: a frameless image-guided robotic stereotactic radiosurgical system. The Cyberknife has overcome many of the limitations of existing radiosurgical systems.

■ Constraints of Existing Radiosurgical Systems

Current stereotactic radiosurgery systems have several constraints. Existing cranial frame-based systems only allow access to intracranial or the highest cervical lesions. Previous attempts at extracranial stereotactic radiosurgery involved spinal tumors, and these have involved prototypes that require either open surgery[2] or transcutaneous placement of clamps[3] to fix bony processes. A more recent report reviewed 19 patients with spine metastases treated with modified linear accelerator radiosurgery using the surgical placement of metal clamps for rigid fixation.[4] However, this surgery, along with the necessary prolonged anesthesia, subjects a patient to potential complications (two wound infections noted in the above 19 patients) and a lengthy procedure when the open procedure is combined with the radiosurgical treatment. Fixed frames also limit the treatment degrees of freedom, and the metal components of current frames produce imaging artifacts on computed tomographic (CT) and magnetic resonance imaging (MRI) scans. Finally, the discomfort associated with skeletal fixation makes fractionation impractical and the treatment of children difficult.

Standard radiosurgical instruments such as the Gamma Knife (Elekta, Atlanta, GA) and conventional linear accelerators utilize a fixed isocenter to which all radiation beams converge. This design works well with spherical targets but is not ideal for complex or irregular shapes. To treat nonspherical lesions, these radiosurgery methods rely on multiple overlapping spherical dose volumes. The disadvantage of this approach is dose heterogeneity; some portions of the target are overdosed whereas other regions are underdosed. A system that involves both shape matching and increased dose homogeneity would improve treatment. Furthermore, a frameless stereotactic radiosurgery system with greater degrees of freedom would allow treatment of extracranial and even nonneural tumors.

To address these limitations, the Cyberknife, a radically new technology that uses high-speed computers, noninvasive image-guided localization, a lightweight high-energy radiation source, and a robotic delivery system has been developed by Accuray, Inc. (Sunnyvale, CA, USA). The Cyberknife has been used to treat all types of intracranial lesions, but more importantly, has expanded the use of radiosurgery to treat extracranial lesions within the spine, thorax, and abdomen.

■ The Cyberknife: Technical Characteristics

The Cyberknife (Accuray, Palo Alto, CA) (Fig. 12–1) combines three advanced technologies to deliver frameless conformal radiosurgical doses. The first is a lightweight 6 MV X-band linear accelerator (LINAC), designed especially for radiosurgery and mounted to a highly maneuverable robotic manipulator (GMFanuc, Auborn Hills, MI, USA). Because the Cyberknife operates at an RF frequency of about 7.5 GHz, compared with 2.9 GHz for a typical medical S-band LINAC, the dimensions of the 6 MV accelerator cavity are decreased by a factor of 2.5. Less shielding is required, and the collimators for narrow radiosurgical fields are much smaller than those required for large therapeutic fields. This leads to an X-band accelerator head that measures 25 cm by 45 cm by 70 cm and weighs only 130 kg. A LINAC of this size can be carried by the robotic arm, whereas the heavier clinical S-band accelerators are far beyond the load limits of robotic arms and require a substantial gantry mechanism, which limits their positioning capability. The robot can position and point the LINAC with six degrees of freedom and has a pointing precision of 0.3 mm.

The second innovation incorporated in the Cyberknife is real-time image guidance, which eliminates the need to position and rigidly immobilize the target via skeletal fixation (e.g., with a frame). This imaging system acquires radiographs of skeletal features associated with the treatment site, uses image registration techniques to determine the treatment site's coordinates with respect to the LINAC robot, and transmits the target coordinates to the robot, which then directs the beam to the treatment site. If the target moves, the process detects the change and corrects beam pointing. This process is rapid enough that the system reacts in near real time to changes in the patient's position.

The third innovation has been the development of amorphous-silicon detectors, which has allowed improved radiographic imaging. The Cyberknife localization method can in principle be used wherever radiopaque features are associated with an anatomic target, a concept that allows the extension of radiosurgical technique to extracranial sites. Frameless radiosurgery has already been used to treat sites within the cervical spine[5-8] prior to the use of amorphous silicon detectors. Earlier x-ray cameras were fluoroscopes consisting of a gadolinium oxysulfide screen viewed by a light-amplified video charge-couple device (CCD). Lens optics require that the CCD be 60 cm from the screen, which results in (1) poor signal-to-noise at low exposure levels, (2) low contrast, and (3) significant veiling glare. This design has made it difficult to obtain good-quality images of the skeletal anatomy within and around the thorax and abdomen. To overcome these limitations, the previous cameras in the Cyberknife have been replaced with flat-panel amorphous-silicon x-ray cameras (dpiX, Palo Alto, CA).[9] These devices have a pixel pitch of 0.125 mm and acquire flat images that avoid distortions inherent to

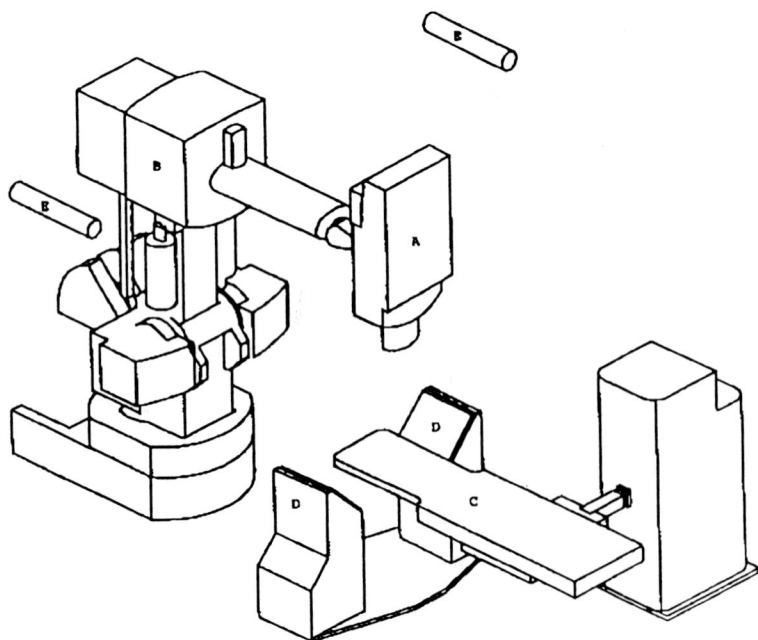

FIGURE 12–1. A schematic of the image-guided radiosurgery system, identifying the major system components. The 6 MV X-band linear accelerator (LINAC) (a) is mounted on the arm (b) of the robotic manipulator. The treatment couch (c) is positioned between the two x-ray cameras (d) and their respective diagnostic x-ray tubes (e) (Cyberknife, Accuray, Palo Alto, CA).

lensed or x-ray image intensifier techniques. When images from these sensors are processed by the new six-dimension registration software, a tenfold improvement in spatial resolution results. This imaging software and hardware have been specifically designed to provide variable fields of view and magnification ranges that can be adapted to multiple anatomic locations. For example, amorphous silicon x-ray sensors create a high-quality image of the lumbar spine using the typical Cyberknife imaging geometry (10 mAs, 75 kV x-ray exposure[9]). Such an exposure corresponds to a dose per image of approximately 25 mrads.

■ Target Localization

The components of the imaging system are fixed at known positions within the treatment room. This provides a stationary frame of reference for locating the patient's anatomy, which in turn has a known relationship to the reference frame of the robotic arm and LINAC. As with conventional forms of brain stereotaxy, this approach assumes a fixed relationship between the target and the skeletal system. Once the skeletal system has been located within the imaging system's coordinate frame, the position of the lesion is known. The Cyberknife determines the location of the skull or spine in the coordinate frame of the radiation delivery system by comparing digitally reconstructed radiographs (DRRs) derived from the treatment planning CT study with radiographs acquired by the real-time imaging system.

The DRRs are produced using a computer model that replicates the actual fluoroscope geometry and optics, so that if the patient's skeletal anatomy is positioned in the coordinate frame of the treatment room in precisely the same way as in the treatment planning CT study, the radiographs and the DRRs will be identical. If the positioning is not the same, the system calculates the differences using either of two different computational algorithms. One algorithm uses a large database of precomputed DRRs to simulate the full range of possible positions during treatment. The acquired radiographs are correlated with each of the precomputed DRRs to obtain a measure of their similarity. The degree of correlation with each DRR is used to interpolate to the most probable actual position of the cranium or spine in the imaging reference frame. DRRs are computed prior to the beginning of treatment; an array processor computes the correlation in near real time during treatment. This algorithm makes accurate measurements of the translational position but cannot determine all rotational effects. Consequently, a noninvasive head restraint maintains the patient's head and neck orientation when using this algorithm.

The latest Cyberknife software utilizes a more advanced algorithm[10] that measures both translation and rotation of the anatomy by iteratively changing the position of the anatomy in the DRR until an exact match of the two radiographs and two DRRs is achieved. This algorithm does not require the database of precomputed DRRs or the array processor and eliminates the need to fix the orientation of the patient during treatment.

Once the skeletal position has been determined, the coordinates are relayed to the robotic arm, which adjusts the pointing of the LINAC. The speed of the imaging process and the maneuverability of the lightweight LINAC on the robotic arm allow the system to detect and adjust to changes in target position in near real time (less than a second). With this capability, the rigid stereotactic frame is not needed as either a method of positioning the treatment site at a fixed beam isocenter or a patient restraint.

■ Treatment Methodology

The Cyberknife operates in a set sequence in which the LINAC is moved to a prescribed position, the imaging system acquires target position information, any necessary adjustments are made to beam pointing, and the radiation beam is turned on. A predetermined number of monitor units is delivered for a set time, and then the beam is turned off. The LINAC is then moved to a new position where the process is repeated. This treatment method accommodates two features of the system: (1) positioning images are optimally taken with the LINAC beam off, (2) the robot path from point to point is not sufficiently well defined to allow the beam to stay on while the LINAC is in motion.

A unique treatment planning process has been integrated into the treatment delivery system to take advantage of the point-and-shoot scenario used by the Cyberknife. The treatment site is taken to be near the center of a sphere of 80 cm radius. The sphere's center is fixed with respect to the patient's anatomy. Approximately 300 equally spaced points are defined on the surface of the sphere. The robotic arm moves the LINAC through space in such a way that the x-ray source stops at these particular points, which are called nodes. At each node the robot pauses, the beam is aimed at the treatment site, and irradiation begins as already described. Although the LINAC stops at fixed nodes on a sphere, the beam is not constrained to point at the center of the sphere but can be aimed anywhere within a volume around the center. Treatment planning consists of selecting from among the fixed nodes and developing a dose distribution involving beams from each of the selected nodes. Each node has variable dose intensity and beam direction, allowing for the delivery of nonisocentric treatment plans.

Programming the LINAC to visit only fixed nodes simplifies the problem of planning the robotic manipulator paths around the treatment site. The center of the nodal sphere is nominally located at a fixed point within the treatment room. Each node is then identified as a point that the robot can reach without collisions or interference from obstacles in the room. This reachability analysis needs to be done only once during system installation and is unaffected by details of individual treatment plans. The analysis recognizes that an actual treatment site, and thus the center of the nodal sphere during treatment, will not necessarily remain at a fixed point in the treatment room (given that there is no mechanical fixation of the patient to an isocenter and the patient can make small movements during treatment). To accommodate this possible variability in position the reachability analysis allows latitude for up to 2 cm translation and/or 5 degree rotation of the nodal sphere in any direction away from the nominal home position of the sphere. Thus the treatment plan is unaffected by small variations in patient position.

In the step-and-shoot patient treatment sequence, a change in target position during irradiation will not be detected and compensated for until the beginning of the next irradiation cycle. Because a minimum of 50 to 100 nodes are utilized, with positioning updates between each, only 1 to 2% of the total dose fraction is delivered before a pointing correction is made. Clinical experience has shown that in the vast majority of patients, movements are few in number and small in magnitude. Total treatment time depends on the complexity of the plan and delivery paths but approximates that of a standard LINAC treatment. The Cyberknife is capable of emulating a gantry-mounted LINAC or a Gamma Knife. It can also produce a wide array of dose distributions for complex-shaped lesions, which is unachievable with conventional radiosurgery systems. Critical structures adjacent to the target can be mapped out and accounted for during treatment planning, and, by selecting nodes and optimizing the weight of the radiation dose delivered from each node, these structures can be spared. Given that skeletal fixation is not required, fractionation is possible with minimal patient discomfort.

■ Accuracy of Dose Placement

The Cyberknife has a dose placement precision comparable to existing frame-based radiosurgery systems. Its dose placement accuracy has been measured in a series of tests that simulate both intracranial and spinal treatment scenarios.[11,12] The mean total radial error observed was 1.6 mm, with a mean positioning error along each coordinate axis of ± 0.9 mm. This accuracy incorporates all sources of error in the treatment process, including uncertainties in target localization during treatment planning, the pointing precision of the robotic arm, and the positioning accuracy of the image-guidance process. Similar measurements of the application accuracy of stereotactic frames show an overall probe targeting error of 1.2 to 2.7 mm that includes treatment planning error, frame flexure, and other mechanical tolerances in the use of the frame.[13–15]

■ Treatment Planning

The flexibility of the Cyberknife with respect to beam placement creates new opportunities for treatment planning. Because tumors vary in size and shape, as well as location with respect to critical structures, planning algorithms must be adaptable to a variety of treatment situations. Conventional radiosurgical systems (e.g., LINAC-based or the Gamma Knife) are limiting in that their restrictive kinematics allow only for isocentric based treatments whereby all radiation beams converge at a single point. Because the resulting region of high dose is necessarily spherical,[15–18] treatment of nonspherical lesions is problematic. The use of multiple isocenters results in some measure of both overtreatment in normal tissue and undertreatment within the target. The Cyberknife, however, enables the delivery of more complex treatments in which beams originate at arbitrary points in the workspace and target arbitrary points within the lesion. Such flexibility makes it possible to generate highly conformal treatment plans for irregularly shaped tumors.

The Cyberknife treatment planning system (TPS) was developed to take advantage of the kinematic flexibility of the system. This allows specification of the treatment-planning problem in terms of geometry (size, shape, and location of the tumor and critical structures), set of constraints on the dose distribution, and maximum number of allowable beams. The system's output is an optimal set of beam configurations that will produce a treatment plan that satisfies the input constraints. The system considers the geometric relationship among the tumor, critical structures, and beams of radiation in determining beam configurations. It does not rely on isocenter-based treatments, nor does it attempt to approximate the tumor shape with a few basic shapes.

Treatment planning with this system begins by outlining target volume and other critical structures on CT or MR images, and the amount of radiation that each can tolerate is specified. Next, the system uses the contour data to create a three-dimensional representation of the tumor geometry, and based on this the system defines an initial set of beam configurations such that the beams aim from random orientations at points that are evenly spaced over the surface of the tumor. Finally, optimization techniques are used to determine dose weighting of the beams to satisfy the specified dose constraints. If the constraints cannot be satisfied in the context of initial beam selection, information gained during optimization is used to select a new set of beam configurations more likely to satisfy the constraints. This iterative process of beam selection and optimization continues until the system finds a feasible set of beams and weights. The Cyberknife then calculates the dose distribution and presents the plan for review prior to patient treatment.

The Cyberknife's TPS has two features that enable it to generate conformal treatment plans for arbitrary tumor shapes. First, the TPS exploits the Cyberknife's flexibility in beam positioning to choose beams based on the specific geometry of the case being treated. The ability to generate conformal treatment plans is independent of tumor shape. It is not based on any a priori classification of the tumor into "typical" cases, such as spheres or ellipsoids. Second, the planner uses linear programming to evaluate the contribution of each beam to satisfy the dose constraints. It iteratively refines the set of beam configurations to contain only those beams important to the solution. The iterative nature of the algorithm allows the system to learn about a problem and eventually determine an appropriate set of beam configurations.

■ Clinical Experience— Intracranial Lesions

Treatment of intracranial tumors with the Cyberknife has been performed for over six years. As of January 2002, over 500 patients with intracranial tumors and arteriovenous malformations have been treated at Stanford with doses ranging between 12 and 26 Gy. Worldwide, over 1800 intracranial lesions have been treated at ten centers, and an additional 80 to 90 patients per month undergo treatment by the Cyberknife. Treatment outcome in terms of radiographic and clinical response closely parallels that achieved with standard radiosurgery.[19]

■ Clinical Experience—Spinal Lesions

Twenty-one patients with spinal tumors and arteriovenous malformations have been treated with the Cyberknife at Stanford University to date (Figs. 12–2 and 12–3). These include spinal hemangioblastomas ($n = 2$),

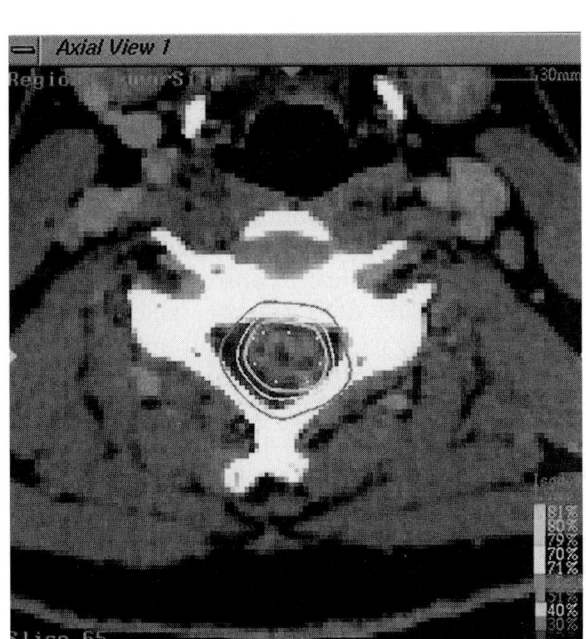
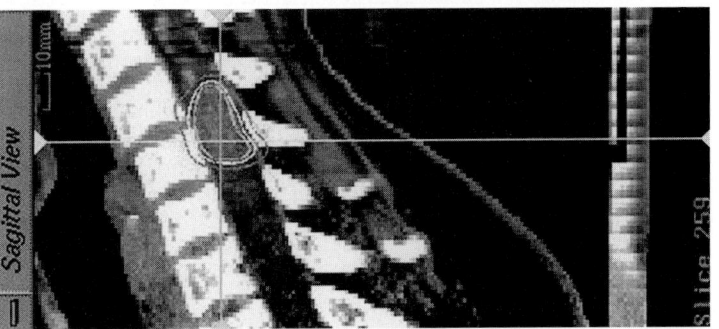
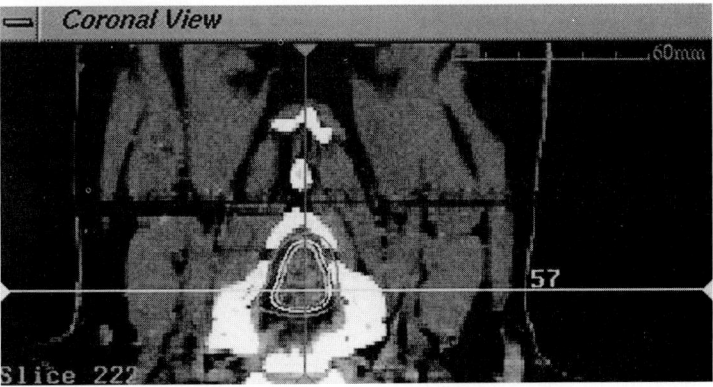

FIGURE 12–2. A 35-year-old male presented with onset of numbness and paresthesias in his upper extremities. Evaluation revealed a C5 cervical spinal cord arteriovenous malformation, which was considered to be unresectable using conventional neurosurgical techniques. The patient underwent Cyberknife stereotactic radiosurgery using a total dose of 21 Gy delivered in three 7 Gy fractions. The patient's treatment plan with 80, 70, and 50% isodose lines is shown in (A) axial, (B) sagittal, and (C) coronal views.

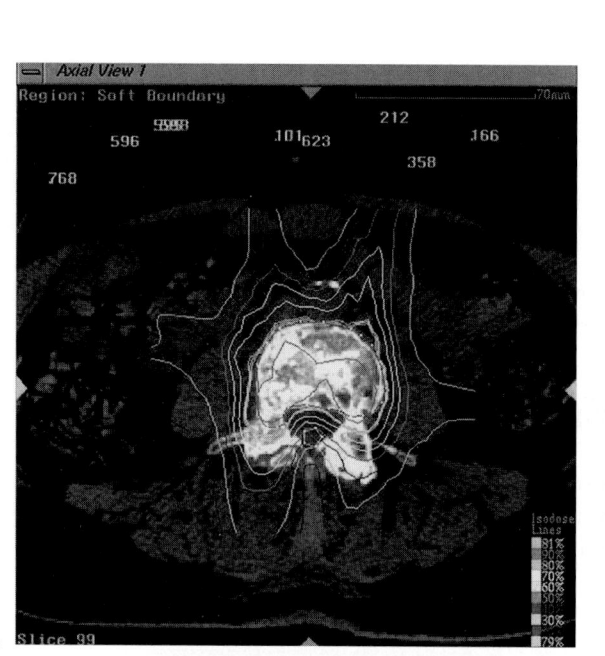
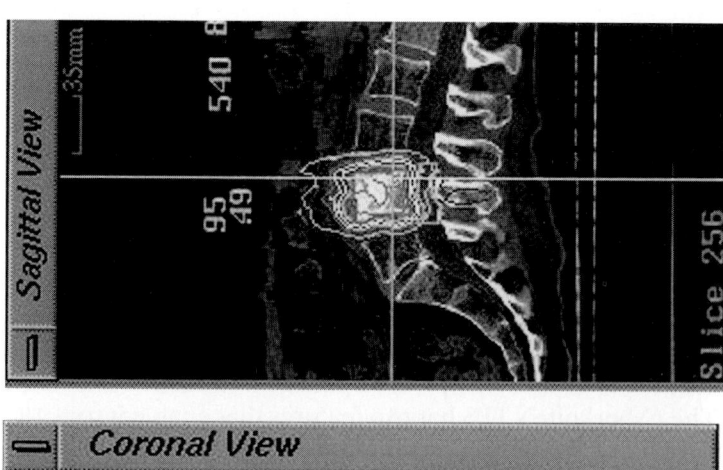
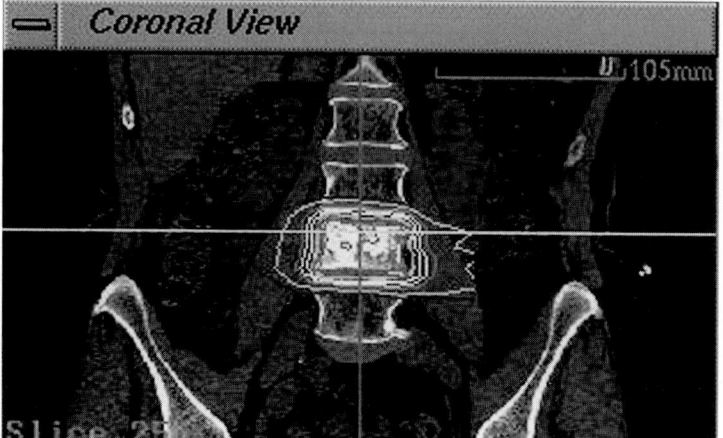

FIGURE 12–3. A 73-year-old female presented with back pain from a breast metastasis to the L4 vertebral body. She had received external beam radiotherapy to this site 6 years earlier, with pain relief for approximately 6 months. Over the past 5 years the pain increased in severity, and a positron emission tomography scan showed hypermetabolism at the L4 level. A percutaneous biopsy confirmed active adenocarcinoma. She was treated with Cyberknife stereotactic radiosurgery to the involved vertebral bone, with the treatment plan shown in (A) axial, (B) sagittal, and (C) coronal views. Six months following treatment, the patient had significant improvement in her back pain.

arteriovenous malformations ($n = 7$), metastases ($n = 7$), schwannoma ($n = 2$), chordoma ($n = 1$), meningioma ($n = 1$), and ependymoma ($n = 1$). Lesion location varied from C2 to S1. Results have been promising: no treated tumor with more than 6-month follow-up has increased in size, and some have shown dramatic decreases in volume. None of the spinal patients treated on the Cyberknife to date have exhibited clinical or radiographic evidence of radiation-induced complications.

■ Conclusions

The Cyberknife was developed to provide state-of-the-art radiosurgery. Whereas early results with intracranial tumors, arteriovenous malformations, and unresectable spinal lesions have been promising in themselves, they also demonstrate the technical feasibility of treating with image-guided stereotactic radiosurgery. Homogeneous irradiation of tumors with complex shapes, improved patient comfort, and the delivery of fractionated therapy are benefits of this robotically controlled system. Even though the Cyberknife does not use skeletal fixation, overall accuracy compares favorably with invasive stereotactic frames.

Decades of clinical experience has established radiosurgery as an important surgical tool for managing a diverse set of lesions. From a radiobiological or oncological perspective, there is no fundamental reason the same principles cannot be applied with equal efficacy to lesions outside the brain. The current status of radiosurgery comes about only by happenstance; precision localization (stereotaxis) was first developed by neurosurgeons for treating disorders of the brain where accuracy is of critical importance. Furthermore, the relative sophistication of brain imaging prior to the arrival of CT and a skeletal structure of the cranium that allows attachment of simple external frames of reference were critical factors in the development of stereotaxy. The

Cyberknife promises to radically change current notions of the types of tumors and body locations that can be treated with radiosurgery. In the future this technology will be applied to small tumors throughout the body including the spine, prostate, kidney, liver, and lung.

REFERENCES

1. Leksell L. The stereotactic method and radiosurgery of the brain. *Acta Chir Scand* 1951;102:316–319.
2. Nadvornik P. Woroschiloff's locating device for interventions on the spinal cord and its influence on spinal stereotaxis. *Appl Neurophysiol* 1985;48:247–251.
3. Hamilton AJ, Lulu BA, Fosmire H, et al. Preliminary clinical experience with linear accelerator-based spinal stereotactic radiosurgery. *Neurosurgery* 1995;36:311–319.
4. Takacs I, Hamilton AJ, Lulu B, et al. Frame-based stereotactic spinal radiosurgery: experience from the first 19 patients. Presented at: 1999 Quadrennial Meeting of the American Society for Stereotactic and Functional Neurosurgery; July, 1999; Snowbird, UT.
5. Chang SD, Murphy M, Geis P, et al. Clinical experience with image-guided robotic radiosurgery (the Cyberknife) in the treatment of brain and spinal cord tumors. *Neurol Med Chir* (Tokyo) 1998;38:780–783.
6. Chang SD, Murphy MJ, Tombropoulos R, et al. Robotic radiosurgery. In: Alexander E, Maciunas R, eds. *Advanced Neurosurgical Navigation*. New York: Thieme Medical Publishers; 1998:443–449.
7. Chang SD, Adler JR, Murphy MJ. Stereotactic radiosurgery of spinal lesions. In: Maciunas RJ, ed. *Advanced Techniques in Central Nervous System Metastasis*. Park Ridge, IL: American Association of Neurologic Surgeons; 1998:269–276.
8. Adler JR, Chang SD, Murphy MJ, et al. The Cyberknife: a frameless robotic system for radiosurgery. *Stereotact Func Neurosurg* 1998;69:124–128.
9. Antonuk LE, Yorkston J, Huang W, et al. A real time, flat panel, amorphous silicon, digital x-ray imager. *Radiographics* 1995;15:993–1000.
10. Murphy MJ, Cox RS. Frameless radiosurgery using real-time image correlation for beam targeting. *Medical Physics* 1996;25:1052.
11. Murphy MJ, Cox R. The accuracy of dose localization for an image-guided frameless radiosurgery system. *Medical Physics* 1996;23:2043–2049.
12. Adler JR, Murphy MJ, Chang SD, et al. Image-guided robotic radiosurgery. *Neurosurgery* 1999;44:1299–1307.
13. Maciunas RJ, Galloway RL Jr, Latimer JW. The application accuracy of stereotactic frames. *Neurosurgery* 1994;35:682–694; discussion 694–695.
14. Yeung D, Palta J, Fontanesi J, et al. Systematic analysis of errors in target localization and treatment delivery in stereotactic radiosurgery. *Int J Radiat Oncol Biol Phys* 1994;28:493–498.
15. Lutz W, Winston KR, Maleki N. A system for stereotactic radiosurgery with a linear accelerator. *Int J Radiat Oncol Biol Phys* 1988;14:373–381.
16. Nedzi LA, Kooy HM, Alexander ED, et al. Dynamic field shaping for stereotactic radiosurgery: a modeling study. *Int J Radiat Oncol Biol Phys* 1993;25:859–869.
17. Podgorsak EB, Olivier A, Pla M, et al. Physical aspects of dynamic stereotactic radiosurgery. *Appl Neurophysiol* 1987;50:263–268.
18. Podgorsak EB, Olivier A, Pla M, et al. Dynamic stereotactic radiosurgery. *Int J Radiat Oncol Biol Phys* 1988;14:115–126.
19. Chang SD, Murphy MJ, Martin DP, et al. Image-guided robotic radiosurgery: clinical and radiographic results with the Cyberknife. *Radiosurgery* 2000;3:23–33.

PART IIA

Cranial Applications

13

Image-Guided Brain Biopsy

GENE H. BARNETT

Over the past two decades, image-guided needle biopsy has become an indispensable tool in modern neurosurgical practice.[1-8] Just as image-guided stereotactic brain biopsy using reference frames largely replaced freehand techniques, biopsy using contemporary surgical navigation systems is gradually displacing frame technologies. This chapter reviews the principles of stereotactic needle biopsy, as well as advanced methodologies.

■ Image-Guided Freehand Stereotactic Brain Biopsy

The advent of computed tomography (CT) in the 1970s marked the beginning of the modern era of brain biopsy. Surgeons could for the first time directly "see" the lesion they wished to sample on an image rather than infer its location by displacement of cerebral vessels or ventricular structures. Early efforts to exploit this information generally relied on "freehand" methods, often performed in the CT suite.[9-11] A burr hole would be strategically placed and a biopsy instrument, sometimes just an angiocatheter, would be advanced to the target area while intermittently obtaining scans to check on its proximity to the target. On the rare occasion when the trajectory was within the plane of the image plane, this could be a relatively simple procedure, although the approach may not have been optimal with regard to intervening structures. When the approach crossed image slices, however, this could be a daunting, time consuming, and often hazardous procedure. Although the technique still has its advocates,[9,12] most practitioners were eager to adopt a technique that offered unambiguous, rigid guidance to the lesion.

■ Image-Guided Frame Stereotactic Brain Biopsy

In the late 1970s, it became recognized that CT scans harbored spatial information that could be mathematically extracted and applied to existing (or newly developed) stereotactic frames.[5,13] This process usually required that a frame would be rigidly applied to the patient's head prior to imaging, and would remain in place throughout the entire procedure, literally serving as a "frame of reference" for all that followed. Some type of adapter that served as a CT scan encoder was then secured to the frame in a stereotypical manner (Fig. 13–1), producing reference marks, or "fiducials," on each image slice. The pattern of fiducials on the slice of interest could then be decoded to derive a coordinate, usually in Cartesian space (i.e., x, y, z) with respect to the frame. A guidance jig could then be set to direct the biopsy instrument (or other device) to that coordinate, when affixed to the reference frame (Fig. 13–2). Image-guided frame stereotactic brain biopsy (IGFSBB) set new standards for low morbidity and diagnostic success for brain biopsy.[1,4,14–15] Also, the rationales for targeting and trajectory selection were established, better biopsy instruments developed, means of managing hemorrhage devised,[16] and target imaging extended to magnetic resonance imaging (MRI) and other imaging techniques.[17]

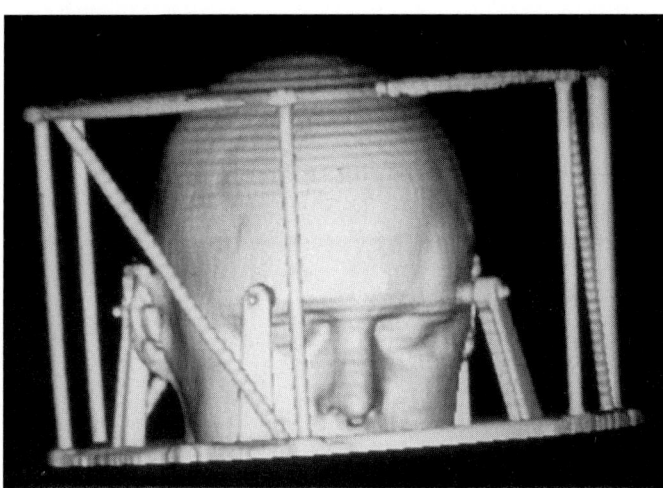

FIGURE 13–1. Three-dimensional surface rendering of Brown-Roberts-Wells (BRW) stereotactic localizer (Radionics, Burlington, MA), used to encode CT scans for stereotactic localization.

Despite the clear advance over freehand techniques,[11] IGFSBB was practiced by only a small fraction of neurosurgeons and became a niche procedure. Several reasons probably accounted for this, including that stereotactic frames were foreign to most practicing neurosurgeons and that the procedures were often logistically cumbersome, requiring frame application and imaging prior to the biopsy later that day, or use of invasive frames capable of reapplication.

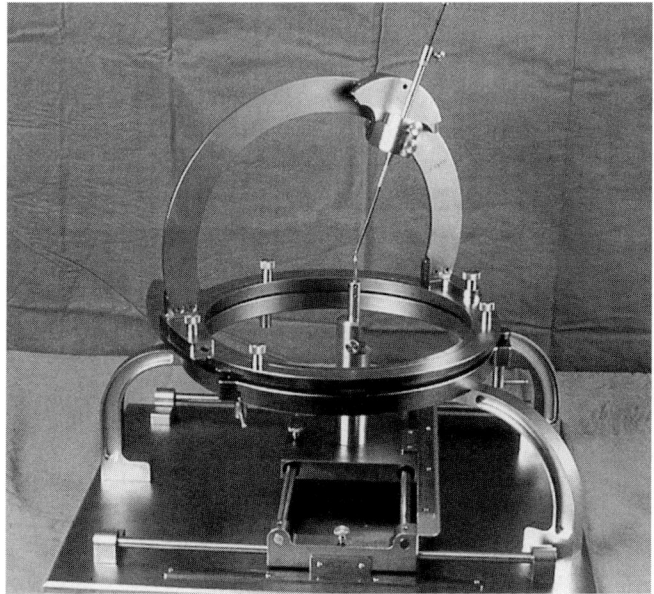

FIGURE 13–2. Brown-Roberts-Wells (BRW) frame atop its phantom.

■ Image-Guided Frameless Stereotactic Brain Biopsy

Almost a decade after the development of IGFSBB, three technological developments occurred that, together, allowed for accurate neurosurgical guidance without reliance on a stereotactic reference frame: (1) the three-dimensional (3-D) spatial accuracy of both CT and MRI substantially improved, allowing for *volumes,* not just slices, of image data to be used for guidance; (2) inexpensive, spatially accurate 3-D digitizers were becoming available using sonic or multiarticulated arm technologies; (3) high-speed, reasonably inexpensive computers became available that could accurately present the location and orientation of a pointing device on displays of the image volume data.[18–20]

The procedure remains largely unchanged from the original descriptions, although the technology has dramatically improved. A volume of image data is acquired that incorporates the target area as well as a reference region (which may be applied markers to the scalp or skull, anatomic landmarks, or surfaces with distinctive features). This imaging may be done days or weeks prior to the procedure as long as the reference region and target are not expected to change in that time frame. At surgery a pointing device that is part of a 3-D digitizer is used to inform the navigation system of the location of the patient's head in the operating room (Fig. 13–3). Most contemporary systems use passive or active infrared technology—a stereoscopic charge-couple device (CCD) camera "sees" reflective or infrared emitting diodes on the pointing device, which is of known configuration. As such, the navigation system can determine the location of the point and axis of the pointing device within the camera's field of view. When using applied or anatomic reference markers, they are frequently identified in the image volume, then physically touched with the pointing device. So-called matched-pair co-registration is among the most accurate ways of achieving registration of image and operating room space—indeed, when skull-applied fiducials are used the accuracy may exceed that achieved with stereotactic frames. This process is usually achieved in but a few minutes and thereafter allows for real-time display of the tip of the pointing device and its axis on the image set. Unless the digitizer is mechanically attached to the head (directly or indirectly), a "dynamic reference frame" with digitizer-compatible technology is generally affixed to the head holder to allow the navigation system to track and compensate for head motion.

The early capabilities of these systems lent themselves to use for open craniotomy navigation. It was not until various schemes evolved for target and trajectory guid-

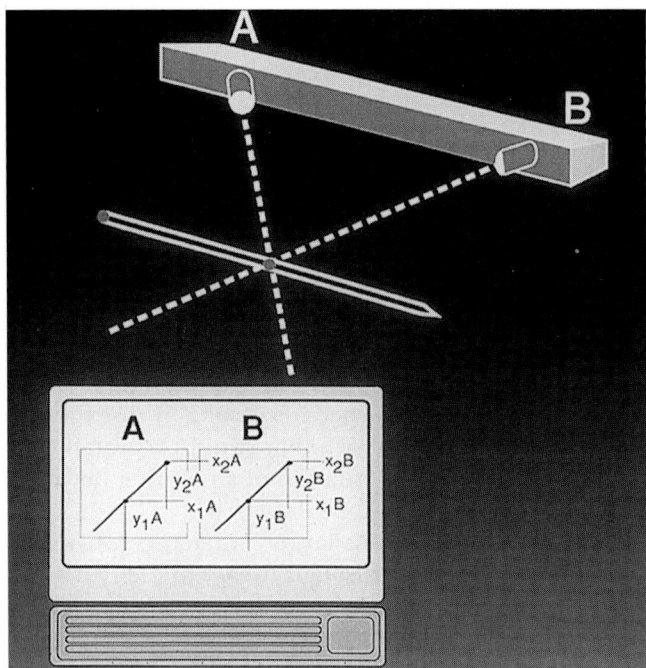

FIGURE 13–3. Representation of three-dimensional digitizer used with many surgical navigation systems. Active or passive infrared markers on a pointing device are "seen" by dual charge-coupled devices serving as a stereoscopic camera. As the physical dimensions of the pointer and camera are known, the computer can determine the location of the pointer and its orientation in space.

ance, however, that surgical navigation systems became practical as a means of image-directed brain biopsy.[21] In 1999 we published our series of brain biopsies using surgical navigation and scalp fiducials as reference marks.[2] The biopsy instrument was stabilized by a flexible instrument holder that is positioned using the SNS, then locked in place. This provided diagnostic results in 96.3% of cases while limiting sustained neurologic, infectious morbidity and death to 1.4%, 1.4%, and 1.0% respectively. Results for lesions in the posterior fossa, however, were substantially worse. It may be that use of skull fiducials, which provide accuracy superior to that of stereotactic frames,[22–23] may overcome this problem (Fig. 13–4).

When properly performed, frame or frameless stereotactic brain biopsy may be safely performed as an outpatient procedure when certain management guidelines are followed. For supratentorial brain biopsy, patients may be safely discharged if there was not excessive intraoperative bleeding, the postoperative neurological exam is unchanged compared with the preoperative exam, and there is absence of hemorrhage (> 1 cm) on a nonenhanced CT scan of the brain obtained 2 hours after the procedure.[24]

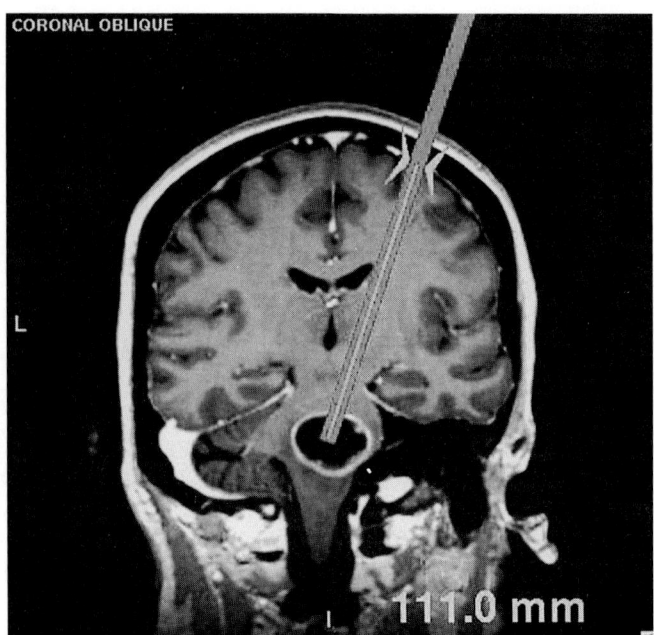

FIGURE 13–4. Biopsy of this deep-seated pontine metastasis was possible using ultra-accurate skull fiducials with surgical navigation.

■ Intraoperative Magnetic Resonance Imaging

The development of MRI systems for neurosurgical procedures allows for a new dimension in stereotactic brain biopsy.[17,25] Preoperative navigational scans are no longer required because they may be obtained intraoperatively. More importantly, the location of an MRI-compatible biopsy instrument can be visualized prior to obtaining tissue. This may prove valuable when the target is small and deep or when it is located near vascular structures. In this setting we have chosen to use a scalp-mounted guidance device (Navigus, Image-Guided Neurologics) that allows for biopsies through a simple scalp puncture and twist-drill hole (Fig. 13–5).[25] By attaching passive or active markers to the biopsy instrument, the plane(s) of image acquisition can be oriented to the wand, showing its orientation throughout its trajectory (Fig. 13–6).

■ Summary

Image-guided stereotactic brain biopsy continues to evolve, with the state of the art being navigation-based biopsy with MRI guidance and monitoring. Multimodality imaging may assist with optimum target definition using magnetic resonance spectroscopy (MRS), positron emission tomography, or other methods of physiological imaging combined with conventional anatomic data.

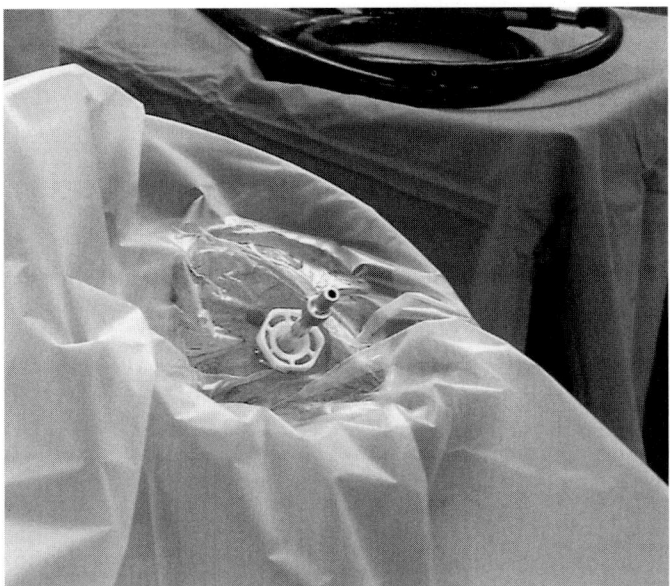

FIGURE 13–5. Navigus guidance device (Image-Guided Neurologics, Melbourne, FL) allows for guidance in intraoperative magnetic resonance imaging.

With adherence to proper guidelines, biopsy may often be safely performed in the outpatient setting.

■ Acknowledgment

The author thanks Ms. Martha Tobin for her assistance with manuscript preparation.

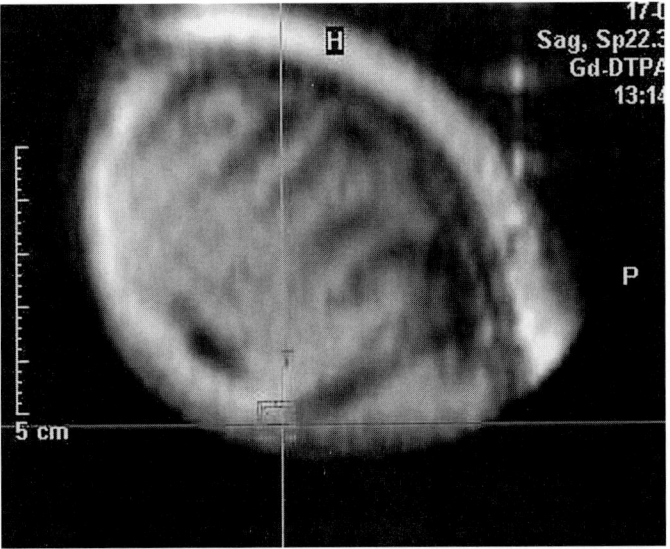

FIGURE 13–6. Intraoperative magnetic resonance imaging confirms location of biopsy instrument before sample is taken.

REFERENCES

1. Apuzzo MLJ, Chandrasoma PT, Cohen D, Zee C, Zelman V. Computed imaging stereotaxy: experience and perspective related to 500 procedures applied to brain masses. *Neurosurgery* 1987;20: 930–937.
2. Barnett GH, Miller DW, Weisenberger J. Brain biopsy using frameless stereotaxy with scalp-applied fiducials: experience in 218 cases. *J Neurosurg* 1999;91:569–576.
3. Bernstein M, Parent A. Complications of CT-guided stereotactic biopsy of intra-axial brain lesions. *J Neurosurg* 1994;81:165–168.
4. Gomez H, Barnett GH, Estes ML, Palmer J, Magdinec M. Stereotactic and computer-assisted neurosurgery at the Cleveland Clinic: review of 501 consecutive cases. *Cleve Clin Med* 1993;60:339–410.
5. Kelly PJ, Earnest F IV, Kall BA, Goerss SJ, Scheithauer B, Earnest F. Surgical options for patients with deep-seated brain tumors: computer-assisted stereotactic biopsy. *Mayo Clin Proc* 1985;60(4): 223–229.
6. Lunsford LD, Martinez AJ. Stereotactic exploration of the brain in the era of computed tomography. *Surg Neurol* 1984;22:222–230.
7. Whiting DM, Barnett GH, Estes ML, et al. Stereotactic biopsy of nonneoplastic lesions in adults. *Cleve Clin J Med* 1992;50:48–55.
8. Whittle IR, Denholm SW, Elshunnar K. CT-guided stereotactic neurosurgery using the Brown-Roberts-Wells system: experience with 125 procedures. *Aust N Z J Surg* 1991;61(12):919–928.
9. Goldstein S, Gumerlock MK, Neuwelt EA. Comparison of CT-guided and stereotactic cranial diagnostic needle biopsies. *J Neurosurg* 1987;67:341–348.
10. Hahn JF, Levy WJ, Weinstein MJ. Needle biopsy of intracranial lesions guided by computerized tomography. *Neurosurgery* 1979;5: 11–15.
11. Lee T, Kenny BG, Hitchock ER, et al. Supratentorial masses: stereotactic or freehand biopsy? *Br J Neurosurg* 1991;5(4):331–338.
12. Di Lorenzo N, Esposito V, Lunardi P, Delfini R, Fortuna A, Cantore G. A comparison of computerized tomography-guided stereotactic and ultrasound-guided techniques for brain biopsy [see comments]. *J Neurosurg* 1991;75(5):763–765.
13. Brown RA. A computerized tomography-computer graphics approach to stereotaxic localization. *J Neurosurg* 1979;50:715–720.
14. Chandrasoma PT, Smith MM, Apuzzo MLJ. Stereotactic biopsy in the diagnosis of brain masses: comparison of results of biopsy and resected surgical specimen. *Neurosurgery* 1989;24:160–165.
15. Kulkarni AV, Guha A, Lozano A, Bernstein M. Incidence of silent hemorrhage and delayed deterioration after stereotactic brain biopsy. *J Neurosurg* 1998;89:31–35.
16. Chimowitz MI, Barnett GH, Palmer J. Treatment of intractable arterial hemorrhage during stereotactic brain biopsy with thrombin: report of three patients. *J Neurosurg* 1991;74(2):301–303.
17. Black PM, Moriarty T, Alexander E III, et al. The development and implementation of intraoperative MRI and its neurosurgical applications. *Neurosurgery* 1997;41:831–842.
18. Barnett GH, Kormos DW, Steiner CP, Weisenberger J. Intraoperative localization using an armless, frameless stereotactic wand. *J Neurosurg* 1993;78:510–514.
19. Roberts DW, Strohbehn JW, Hatch JF, Murray W, Kettenberger H. A frameless stereotaxic integration of computerized tomographic imaging and the operating microscope. *J Neurosurg* 1986;65: 545–549.
20. Watanabe E, Watanabe T, Manaka S, Mayanagi Y, Takakura K. Three-dimensional digitizer (neuronavigator): new equipment for computed tomography-guided stereotaxic surgery. *Surg Neurol* 1987;27:543–547.
21. Barnett GH, Steiner CP, Weisenberger J. Target and trajectory guidance for interactive surgical navigation systems. *Stereotactic and Functional Neurosurgery* 1996;66:91–95.

22. Galloway RL, Maciunas RJ, Latimer JW. The accuracies of four stereotactic frame systems: an independent assessment. *Biomed Intrument Tech* 1991;25:457–460.
23. Wang MY, Maurer CR Jr, Fitzpatrick JM, Maciunas RJ. An automatic technique for finding and localizing externally attached markers in CT and MR volume images of the head. *IEEE Trans Biomed Eng* 1996;43:627–637.
24. Kaakaji W, Barnett GH, Bernhard D, Warble A, Valaitis K, Stamp S. Clinical and economic consequences of early discharge after supratentorial stereotactic brain biopsy. *J Neurosurg* 2001. In press.
25. Hall WA, Liu H, Truwit CL. Navigus trajectory guide. *Neurosurgery* 2000;46(2):502–504.

14

Cerebrovascular Applications of Image-Guided Surgery

JOSHUA BEDERSON

The majority of treatments for patients with cerebrovascular disease involve modern neuroimaging techniques. The term *image guidance* therefore has broad applications in the fields of cerebrovascular neurology and neurosurgery. The cerebrovascular applications of image guidance can be separated into four different categories. These include pretreatment evaluation and planning, surgical rehearsal, lesion localization, and intraoperative navigation.

This chapter focuses on selected conditions for which neurosurgical or endovascular treatments are being considered. These include intracranial aneurysms, cranial base lesions, cavernous angiomas, and arteriovenous malformations.

■ Pretreatment Evaluation of Intracranial Aneurysms

Radiological studies used in evaluating intracranial aneurysms include "invasive" studies: catheter cerebral angiography, rotational three-dimensional catheter angiography (3-DA), and "noninvasive" studies: computed tomographic angiography (CTA), magnetic resonance imaging (MRI), and magnetic resonance angiography (MRA).

Catheter cerebral angiography and 3-DA provide superior resolution of small vascular structures. Catheter cerebral angiography remains the gold standard for detection of intracranial aneurysms and is the study of choice for this purpose, whereas 3-DA provides detailed anatomical information about aneurysm morphology and the relationships between the lesion and adjacent normal vasculature. The level of detail that can be achieved by catheter cerebral angiography and 3-DA remains unrivaled by the noninvasive methods. However, catheter cerebral angiography also has disadvantages. The majority of patients find that despite all precautions the procedure is painful and uncomfortable. Many describe postprocedural pain at the femoral artery puncture site. Although serious complications are rare, catheter cerebral angiography is associated with a neurological complication rate of as much as 2.0%, leading to persistent neurological deficits in 0.07 to 0.8%, and nonneurological complications in 14.7% of patients.[1-3] The longer injection of intra-arterial contrast required by 3-DA adds additional discomfort and may therefore require heavy sedation that is frequently not tolerated by sensitive patients.

A number of investigators have recently reported on the considerable utility of 3-D reconstruction of CT, MR, and angiographic data for preoperative evaluation of patients with cerebrovascular disease.[1,4-24]

Case 1: Pretreatment evaluation of a posterior communicating artery aneurysm

Rationale
Surgical planning can be facilitated by visualizing the craniotomy necessary to expose the aneurysm. This is particularly valuable for residents and students who are less familiar with the surgical anatomy. In addition it may be helpful to understand the anticipated degree of

proximal control, and the vicinity of the aneurysm to the anterior clinoid process.

Case description
A 58-year-old female was evaluated for a new left third nerve paresis, and a left posterior communicating artery aneurysm was discovered (Fig. 14–1A). Preoperative CTA with 3-D reconstruction of the volume-rendered surface was manipulated to simulate the pterional craniotomy required to expose the aneurysm. The preoperative simulation in Figure 14–1B and C predicted the appearance of the aneurysm and adjacent structures found at surgery, and facilitated uneventful clipping (Figs. 14–1D and 14–1E).

Discussion
Preoperative simulation of the craniotomy is a useful tool for teaching neurosurgical residents and students. It can be helpful to surgeons in predicting the relevant surgical anatomy such as the degree of proximal control, the proximity of the anterior clinoid process, and the like.

Limitations
Important soft-tissue structures such as the dura of the tentorial edge, the optic and occulomotor nerves, and brain parenchyma are not visualized on the preoperative CTA. Estimating the amount of proximal internal carotid artery (ICA) control with the pterional exposure must take this into account.

Case 2: Pretreatment evaluation of a middle cerebral artery aneurysm

Deciding whether to clip or coil an intracranial aneurysm depends on several anatomical and clinical factors. In patients whose clinical status supports both treatment options the decision is based primarily on anatomical features such as the size, shape, and location of the aneurysm; its relation to surrounding anatomical structures; and the precise configuration of the parent and perforating vessels. For middle cerebral artery (MCA) aneurysms, long-term success rates for coiling are highest for small aneurysms with small necks, and lowest for large aneurysms with large necks. It is important to know the relationship of the aneurysm neck to the M1 and M2 segments, and for clipping, it is helpful to visualize the structures in relationship to the planned craniotomy.

Case description
A 50-year-old female was evaluated for an intracranial aneurysm discovered on MRI done to evaluate left-sided headaches. Catheter angiography revealed three aneurysms of the left MCA: a small lenticulostriate aneurysm, an anterior temporal artery aneurysm, and a large multi-lobulated MCA trifurcation aneurysm (Fig. 14–2A). Preoperative CTA with 3-D reconstruction and surface rendering defined the anatomy of the three aneurysms (Fig. 14–2B) and their relation to a standard pterional opening (Fig. 14–2C). The preoperative simulation in Figure 14–2C closely predicted the appearance of the aneurysm and related vasculature that was found at surgery (Fig. 14–2D) and facilitated uneventful clipping (Fig. 14–2E).

Discussion
In this case preoperative noninvasive imaging with 3-D reconstruction provided additional information about the anatomy of the aneurysms and their relationship to adjacent vascular and bony structures. Preoperative simulation gave an excellent estimation of the surgical appearance. However, limitations in the resolution of CTA using single-slice CT scanners mean that important vessels that are visible on catheter angiograms and at surgery, such as the anterior temporal artery, are not seen on the CTA. This limitation must be considered during surgical planning.

Case 3: Pretreatment evaluation of a paraclinoid aneurysm

Case description
A 27-year-old female was found to have a right paraclinoid aneurysm, demonstrated with a carotid angiogram (Fig. 14–3A). Preoperative CTA with 3-D reconstruction and surface rendering defined the anatomy of the aneurysm and its relation to the anterior clinoid process (Fig. 14–3B). The CTA predicted that only minimal drilling of the anterior clinoid would be required for exposure and proximal control. The preoperative simulation in Figure 14–3B closely predicted the appearance of the aneurysm and related vasculature that was found at surgery (Fig. 14–3C) and facilitated uneventful clipping (Fig. 14–3D).

Discussion
In this case preoperative imaging gave a good indication of how much drilling would be required for proximal control. Key features of the surgical anatomy (e.g., the optic nerve and the dura covering the clinoid process) were not visualized preoperatively.

Case 4: Pretreatment evaluation of a paraclinoid aneurysm

Case description
A 47-year-old female was evaluated for an intracranial aneurysm discovered on MRI done to evaluate left retro-orbital pain. Catheter angiography demonstrated a broad-based carotid-ophthalmic aneurysm projecting superiorly (Fig. 14–4A). Preoperative CTA with 3-D

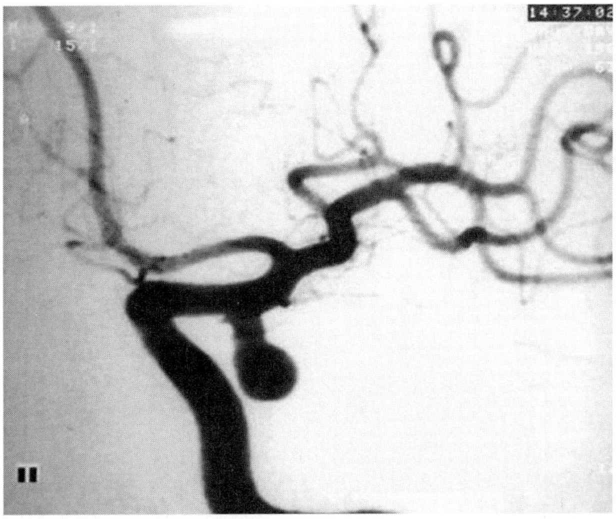

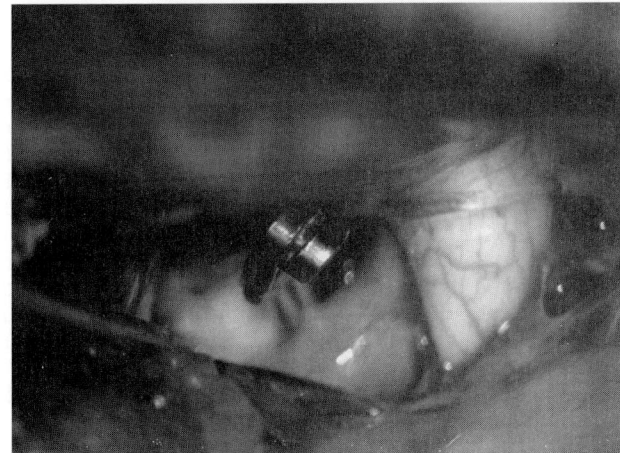

FIGURE 14–1. (A). Preoperative left carotid angiogram demonstrating an inferiorly projecting posterior communicating artery aneurysm. (B). Preoperative CTA with 3-D reconstruction and surface rendering. The anatomy of the aneurysm and its relationship to a simulated pterional craniotomy are shown. (C). The relationship of the aneurysm (a) to the internal carotid artery (b), the anterior clinoid process (c), and the posterior cerebral artery (d) is well defined by the reconstruction. (D). Intraoperative photo during exposure, demonstrating the surgical anatomy and the position of the clip (E).

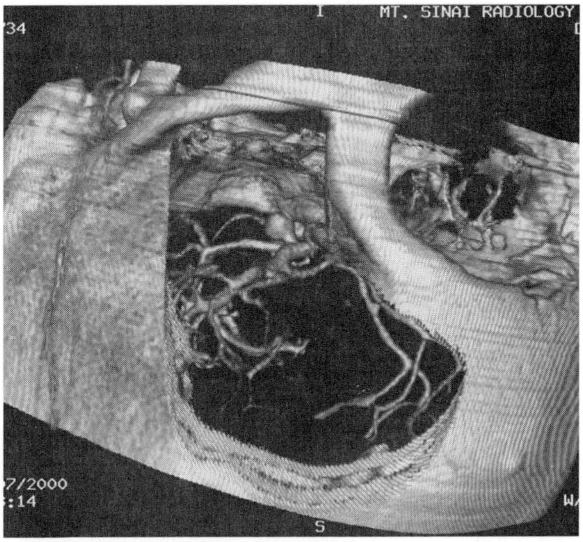

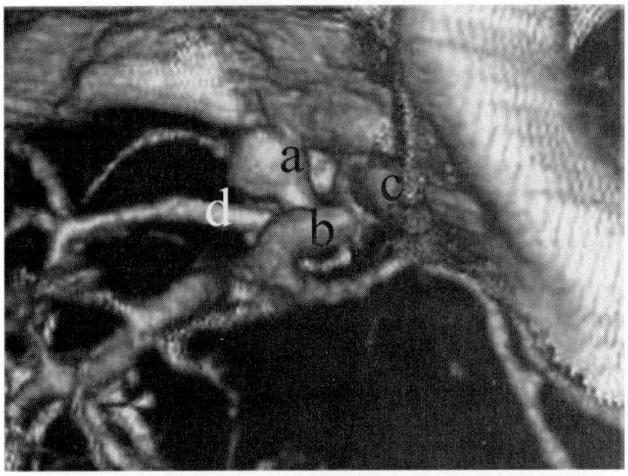

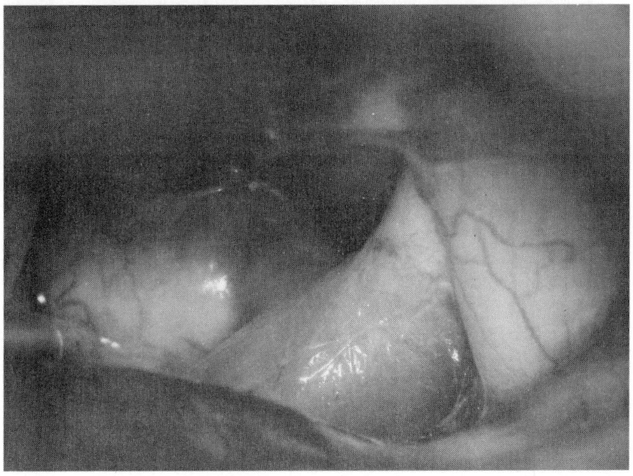

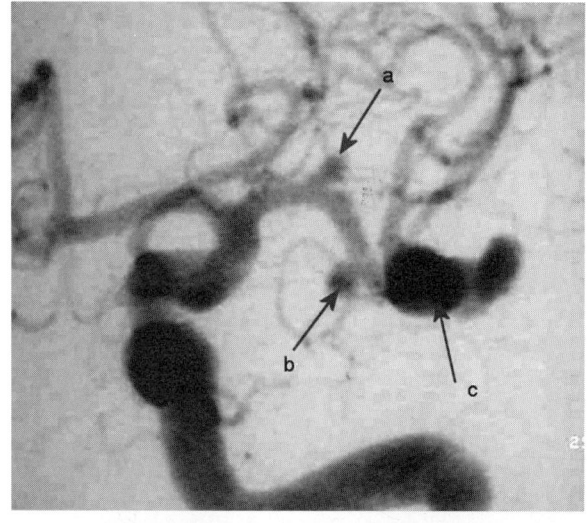
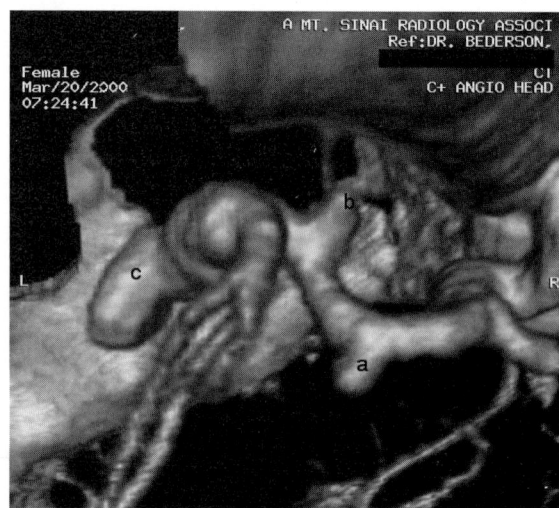
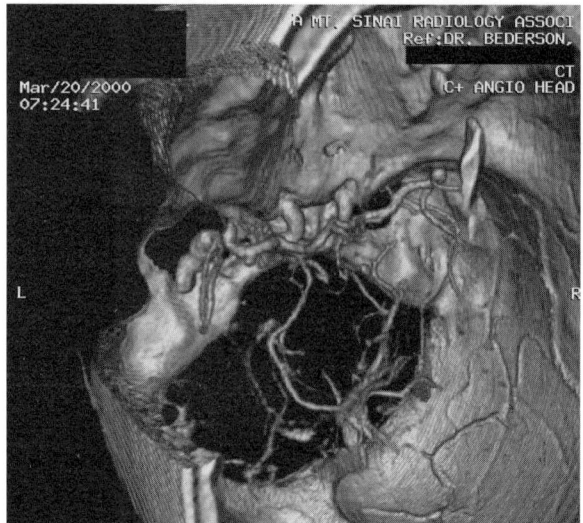
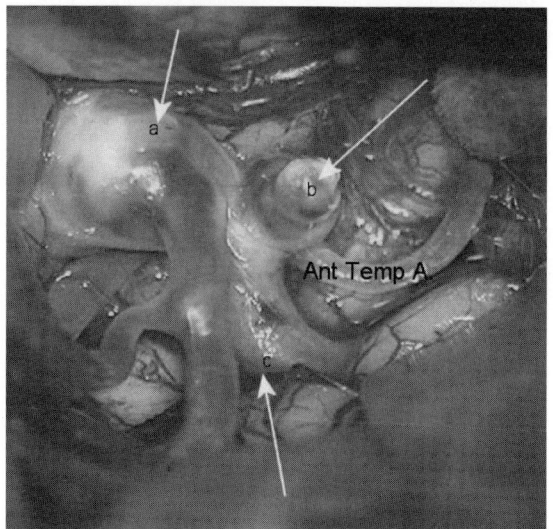
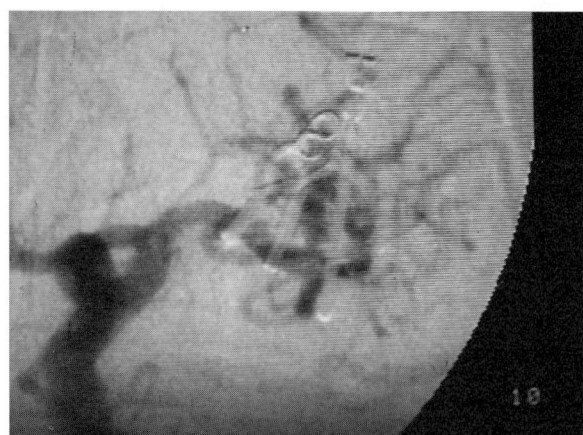

FIGURE 14–2. (A). Preoperative left carotid angiogram demonstrating three aneurysms of the middle cerebral artery (MCA): a small lenticulostriate aneurysm (a), an anterior temporal artery aneurysm (b), and a large multilobulated MCA trifurcation aneurysm (c). (B). Preoperative CTA with 3-D reconstruction and surface rendering. The anatomy of the three aneurysms (the labels a, b, c correspond to those in Fig. 14–2A) and their relationship to the parent arteries are well defined by this study. (C). The MCA and aneurysms are shown in relation to a simulated pterional opening, with the head positioned to approximate the intraoperative view of the aneurysms after exposure. (D). Intraoperative photo during exposure, demonstrating the surgical anatomy (labels a, b, and c correspond to the labels in Figs. 14–2A and 14–2B). Aneurysm is still hidden by a portion of the frontal cortex. Note that the anterior temporal artery (Ant Temp A.), which is approximately 900 microns in diameter, was not visualized on the preoperative CTA in Figure 14–2B or 14–2C. (E). Postoperative angiogram.

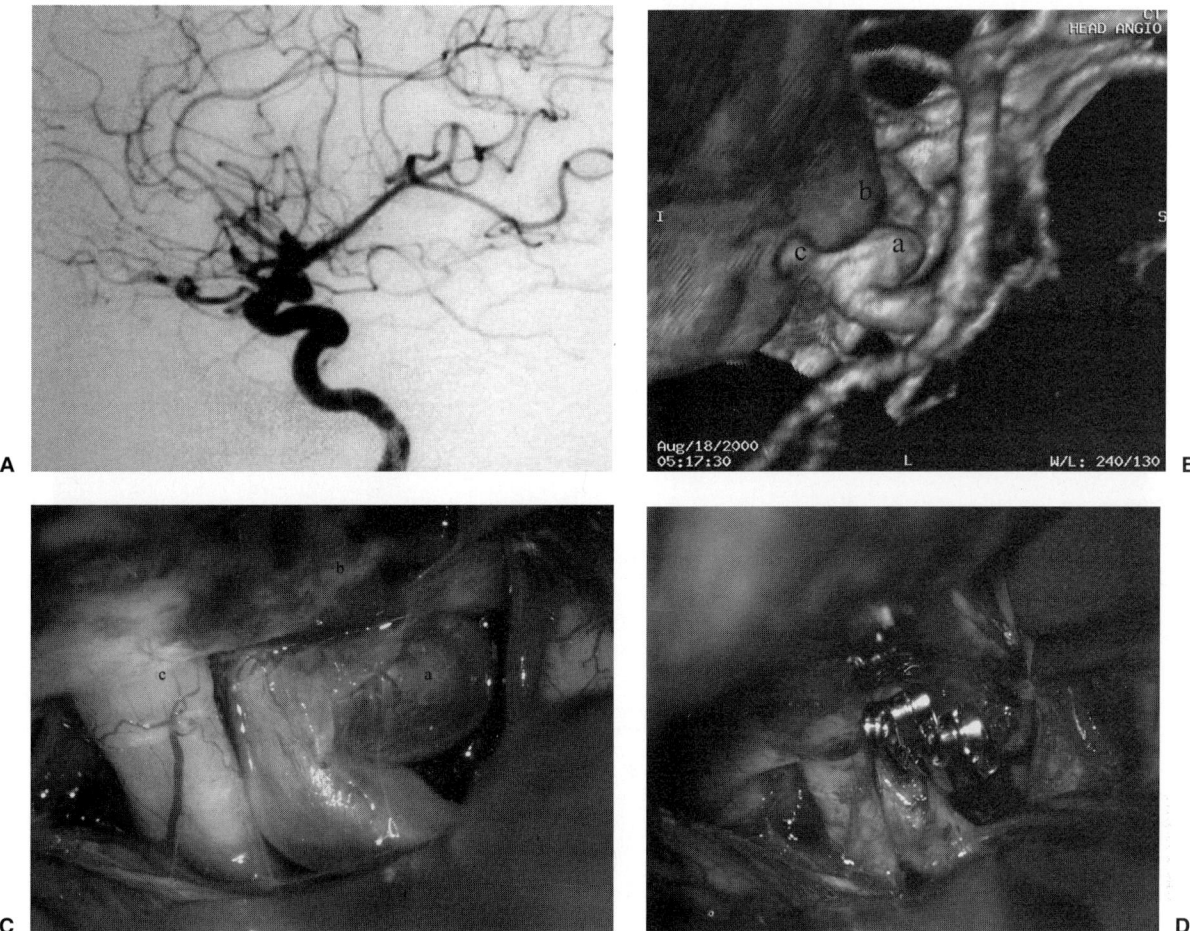

FIGURE 14–3. (A). Preoperative right carotid angiogram demonstrating a small, inferiorly projecting paraclinoid aneurysm. (B). Preoperative CTA with 3-D reconstruction and surface rendering. The anatomy of the aneurysm (a), in relation to the anterior clinoid process (b), is well visualized and suggests that only a small amount of drilling will be required. The optic canal (c) is seen, but not the optic nerve. (C). Intraoperative photo during initial exposure demonstrating the aneurysm (a). In contrast to the preoperative image the anterior clinoid process is hidden by dura (b), and the optic nerve fills the optic canal. (D). As predicted by the preoperative studies minimal drilling of the anterior clinoid process was required to secure the aneurysm.

reconstruction and surface rendering defined the relationship of the aneurysm to the distal internal carotid artery and the anterior clinoid process (Figs. 14–4B and 14–4C). In contrast to Case 3, these studies indicate that the aneurysm is surrounded by bone and will require extensive removal of the anterior clinoid process and medial sphenoid wing to obtain exposure. Although the internal carotid artery distal to the aneurysm is well defined by the CTA, the proximal artery and aneurysm neck are obscured by the surrounding bone. In addition the ophthalmic artery is not visualized. In this case preoperative simulation assists the surgeon in predicting how much drilling will be required before local proximal control can be obtained. The surgical anatomy (Fig. 14–4D) closely reflects what was visualized preoperatively, which facilitated uneventful clipping (Fig. 14–4E) and demonstrated angiography (Fig. 14–4F).

Discussion

Preoperative imaging studies provided critical information about the bony anatomy and lack of local proximal control, and facilitated surgical planning. Only the catheter angiogram demonstrated the ophthalmic artery, and no study fully defined the surgical anatomy.

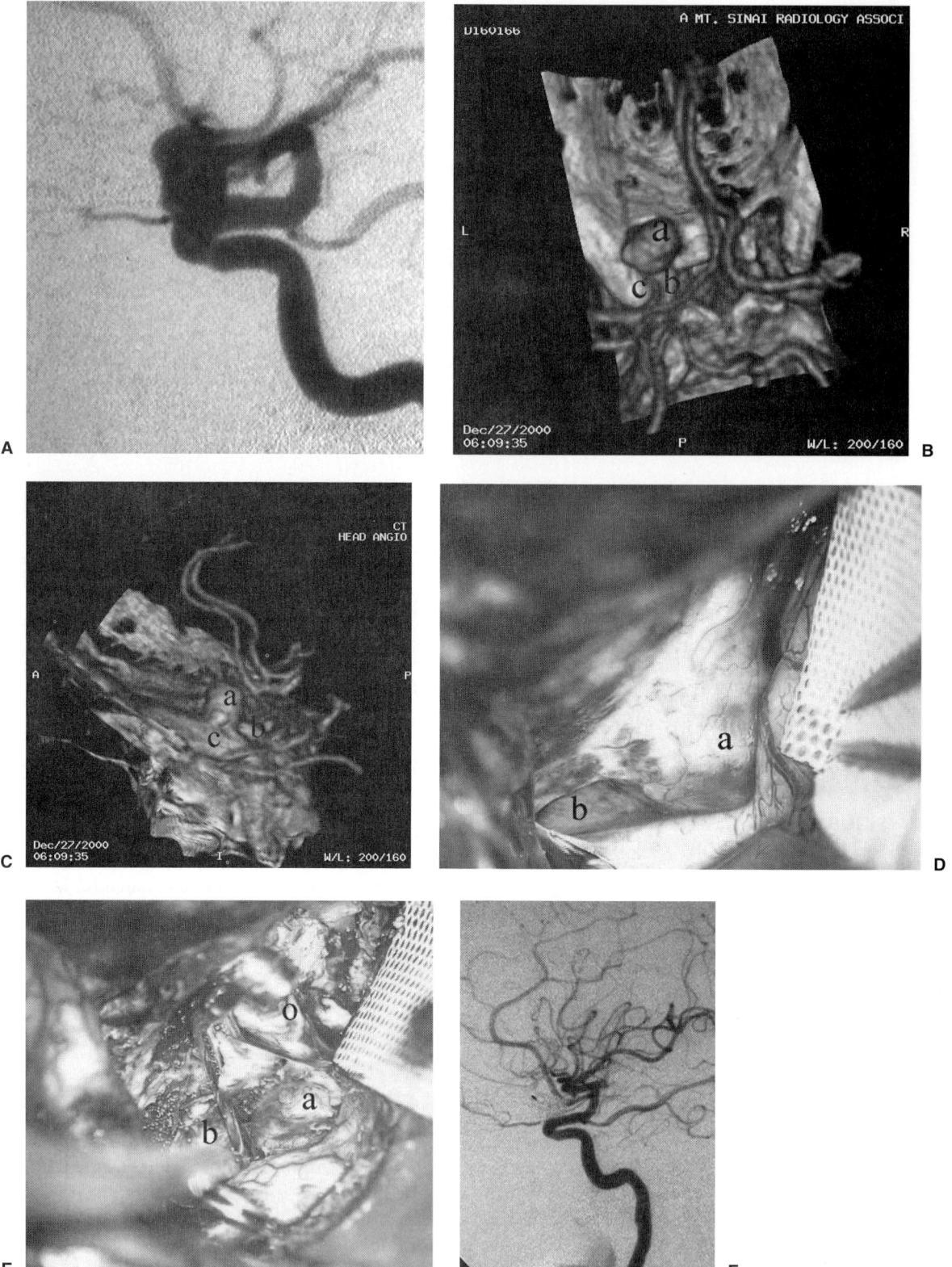

FIGURE 14–4. (A). Preoperative left carotid angiogram demonstrating a broad-based paraclinoid aneurysm. (B). Preoperative CTA with 3-D reconstruction and surface rendering. The anatomy of the aneurysm neck (a) is obscured by surrounding bone. The optic nerve and ophthalmic artery are not visualized. However, the aneurysm's relationship to the distal internal carotid artery (b) and the anterior clinoid process (c) is well defined. (C). Lateral view of the CTA, showing simulation of the operative approach. (D). Intraoperative photo during initial exposure demonstrating the dome of the aneurysm (a) projecting through the dura adjacent to the anterior clinoid process and its relation to the internal carotid artery (b), which is partially hidden by arachnoid. (E). Surgical view after clipping demonstrating the aneurysm (a), the internal carotid artery (b), and the optic nerve (o). Although removal of dura and mobilization of the optic nerve are critical to the success of the procedure, neither structure is visualized by the preoperative imaging studies. (F). Postoperative angiogram.

Case 5: Pretreatment evaluation of a paraclinoid aneurysm

Case description
A 45-year-old female was evaluated for an intracranial aneurysm discovered on MRI done to evaluate left nonspecific visual complaints and headache. Catheter angiography demonstrated right-sided carotid-ophthalmic aneurysm projecting superiorly (Fig. 14–5A). Preoperative CTA with 3-D reconstruction and surface rendering defined the relationship of the aneurysm to the distal internal carotid artery and the anterior clinoid process (Figs. 14–5B and 14–5C). As with Case 4, the internal carotid artery distal to the aneurysm is well defined by the CTA, but the proximal artery and aneurysm neck are obscured by surrounding bone. In addition the optic nerve, the ophthalmic artery, and the dura that encase the region are not visualized. In this case, although preoperative simulation assisted in uneventful clipping and in predicting how much drilling would be required, most of the critical structures exposed at surgery (Fig. 14–5D) were not visualized preoperatively.

Discussion
Preoperative imaging studies provided critical information about the bony anatomy and lack of local proximal control, and facilitated surgical planning. Only the catheter angiogram demonstrated the ophthalmic artery, and no study fully defined the surgical anatomy.

Case 6: Evaluation of postoperative patency of a carotid bypass vein graft

Case description
A 62-year-old male presented with panhypopituitarism from mass effect caused by an enlarging giant aneurysm of the left internal carotid artery (Fig. 14–6A). The aneurysm was treated with a saphenous vein bypass graft from the common carotid artery to the MCA and proximal occlusion of the internal carotid artery, as documented on the postoperative angiogram (Fig. 14–6B). The surgery and postoperative course were unremarkable, and the patient returned for radiological follow-up 14 months after surgery. The follow-up CTA demonstrated patency of the vein graft with no filling of the aneurysm (Fig. 14–6C and 14–6D).

Discussion
Noninvasive follow-up imaging confirmed patency of the graft, occlusion of the aneurysm, and additional detail about the postoperative anatomy. Noninvasive radiological imaging was useful in this patient because surgical clips and endovascular coils had not been used near the distal MCA anastomotic site. Had they been used, the anatomy would have been obscured by artifact.

Case 7: Intraoperative navigation for a cavernous malformation

Case description
A 47-year-old female presented with sudden headache and new seizures. Radiological evaluation led to the diagnosis of a right frontal cavernous malformation (Fig. 14–7A). Frameless stereotaxic navigation (Fig. 14–7B) was used to localize a small frontal craniotomy during exposure (Fig. 14–7C) and for highly accurate intraoperative navigation and lesion localization (Fig. 14–7D).

Discussion
Like its applications in neuro-oncology and diagnostic stereotaxy, frameless stereotaxy for intraoperative navigation and lesion localization is extremely useful. It permits smaller, less invasive openings, facilitates defining accurate trajectories, and aids considerably in lesion localization.

■ Summary

Noninvasive imaging with CTA and other modalities that permit 3-D reconstruction is a superb planning tool with great potential for future development. Current technologies provide excellent differentiation of major arteries to demonstrate aneurysm morphology. This information can be useful in making treatment decisions, in deciding about optimal treatment (e.g., coiling vs clipping), and in planning surgical approaches. Defining arterial structures in relation to the bony anatomy is also useful in many situations for preoperative surgical rehearsal. However, lack of true segmentation capabilities means that vascular structures that are surrounded by bone cannot be readily defined. CTA and other noninvasive imaging techniques are also useful for follow-up of known lesions that are treated conservatively. Postoperative evaluation when clipping or coiling has been performed usually requires catheter angiography because of artifact introduced by the clips and coils.

Currently, intraoperative lesion localization and navigation, although possible with existing technology, are not generally useful in the treatment of intracranial aneurysms. Preoperative noninvasive imaging is useful for lesion localization and navigation for cavernous malformations and for selected tumors of the cranial base. In these cases smaller craniotomies and less invasive procedures are facilitated by stereotaxic intraoperative navigation.

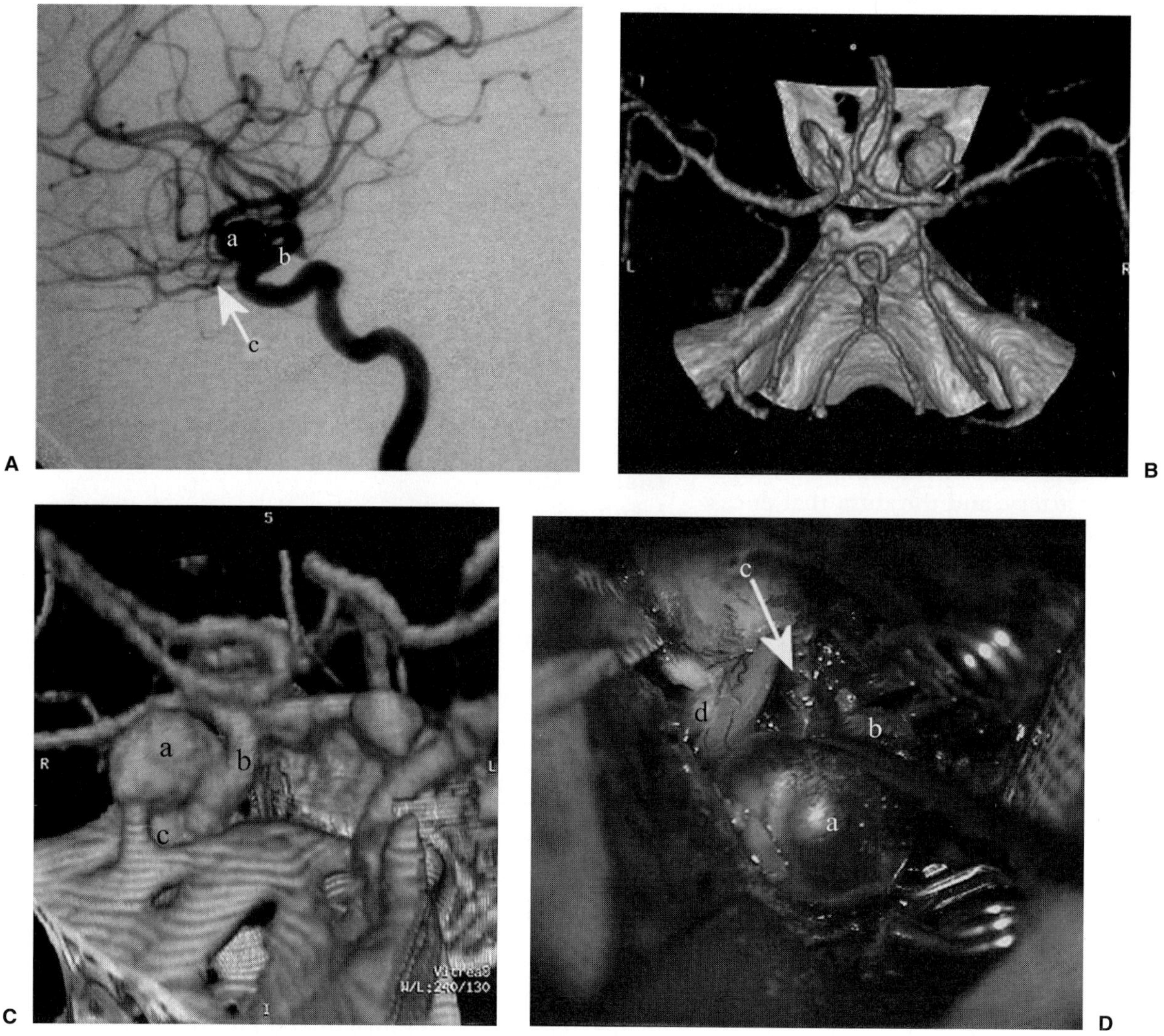

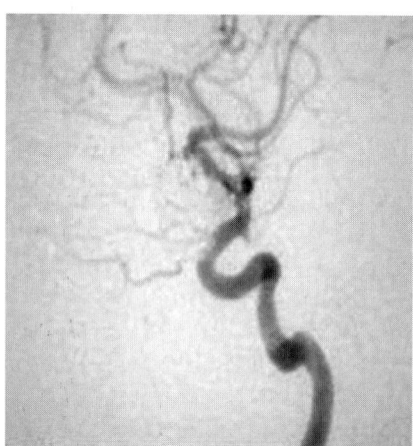

FIGURE 14–5. (A). Preoperative right carotid angiogram demonstrating a paraclinoid aneurysm (a) and its relation to the parent internal carotid artery (b) and the ophthalmic artery (c). (B). Preoperative CTA with 3-D reconstruction and surface rendering. The anatomy of the lateral aspect of the aneurysm neck is obscured by surrounding bone. Lateral view of the CTA showing simulation of the operative approach. (C). Anteromedial view of the preoperative CTA with 3-D reconstruction and surface rendering. The optic nerve and ophthalmic artery are not visualized though the optic canal is seen (c). However, because the lesion is not surrounded by bone, the aneurysm anatomy (a) and its relation to the internal carotid artery (b) are well visualized. (D). Intraoperative photo demonstrating the dome of the aneurysm (a), the internal carotid artery with temporary clips placed proximally and distally (b), the ophthalmic artery (c), and the optic nerve (d). As with the previous case, although removal of dura, mobilization of the optic nerve, and exposure of the ophthalmic artery are critical to the success of the procedure, these structures are not visualzed by the preoperative imaging studies. (E). Postoperative angiogram.

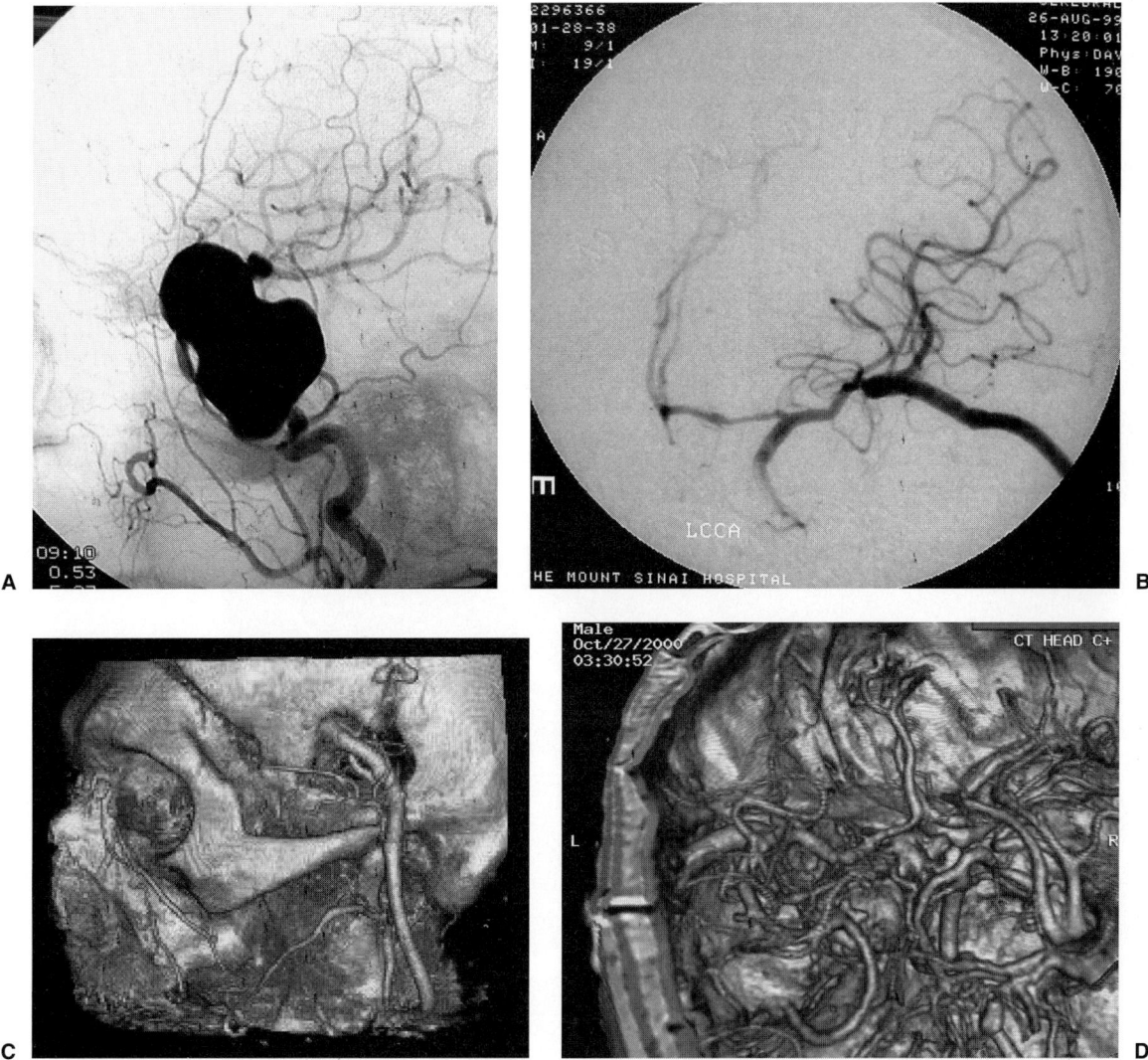

FIGURE 14–6. (A). Preoperative left carotid angiogram demonstrating the giant internal carotid artery aneurysm. (B). Postoperative angiogram demonstrating initial patency of the bypass graft and absent filling of the aneurysm. (C). Fourteen-month delayed follow-up CTA demonstrating patency of the vein graft. (D). Higher-magnification view of the delayed postoperative CTA, demonstrating the anatomy of the vein graft in relation to branches of the middle cerebral artery.

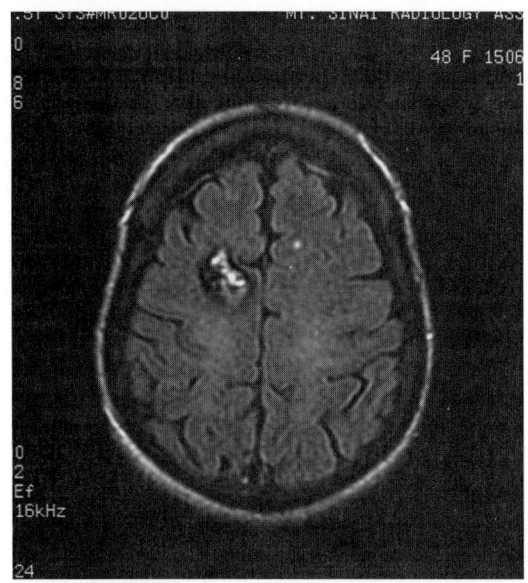

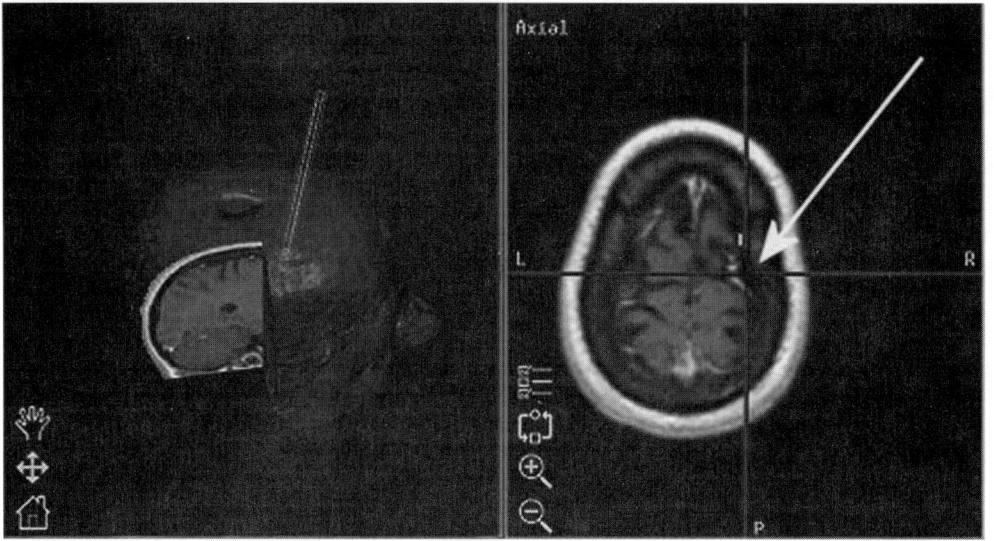

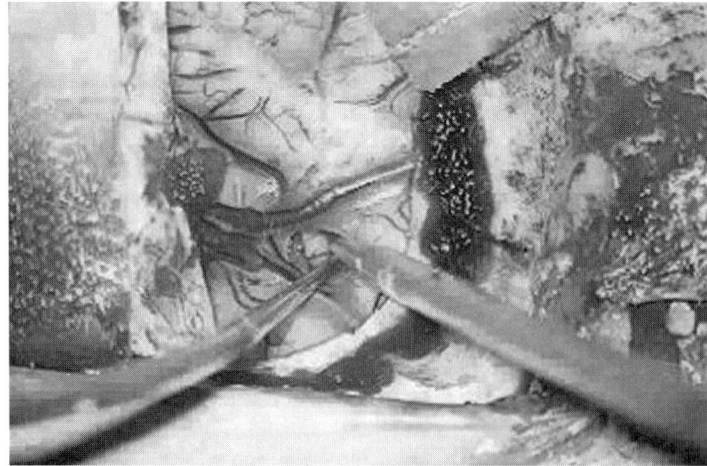

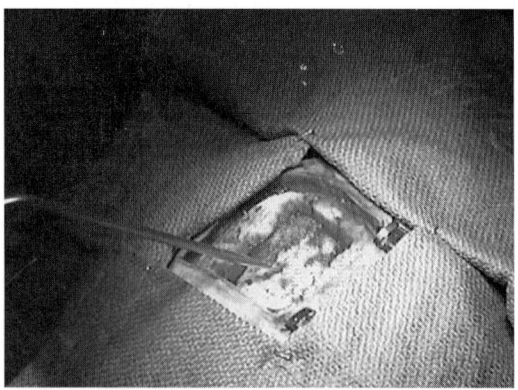

FIGURE 14–7. (A). Preoperative magnetic resonance imaging (MRI) demonstrating a right frontal cavernous malformation. (B) Intraoperative frameless MRI data set, demonstrating localization of the craniotomy and selection of surface landmarks and surgical trajectory. (E). Intraoperative photo demonstrating a small craniotomy chosen using image guidance. (D). Intraoperative photo during exposure demonstrating the high degree of correlation between the surgical surface anatomy and the preoperative images (Fig. 14–7B).

REFERENCES

1. Leffers AM, Wagner A. Neurologic complications of cerebral angiography: a retrospective study of complication rate and patient risk factors. *Acta Radiol* 2000;41(3):204–210.
2. Cloft HJ, Joseph GJ, Dion JE. Risk of cerebral angiography in patients with subarachnoid hemorrhage, cerebral aneurysm, and arteriovenous malformation: a meta-analysis. *Stroke* 1999;30(2):317–320.
3. Komiyama M, et al. Prospective analysis of complications of catheter cerebral angiography in the digital subtraction angiography and magnetic resonance era. *Neurol Med Chir* (Tokyo) 1998;38(9):534–539; discussion 539–540.
4. Gonzalez-Darder JM, Pesudo-Martinez JV, Feliu-Tatay RA. Microsurgical management of cerebral aneurysms based in CT angiography with three-dimensional reconstruction (3D-CTA) and without preoperative cerebral angiography. *Acta Neurochir* 2001;143(7):673–679.
5. Kato Y, et al. Application of three-dimensional CT angiography (3D-CTA) to cerebral aneurysms. *Surg Neurol* 1999;52(2):113–121; discussion 121–122.
6. Kato Y, et al. Can 3D-CTA surpass DSA in diagnosis of cerebral aneurysm? *Acta Neurochir* 2001;143(3):245–250.
7. Lee JY, et al. Brain surgery with image guidance: current recommendations based on a 20-year assessment. *Stereotact Funct Neurosurg* 2000;75(1):35–48.
8. Marro B, et al. Intracranial aneurysm on CTA: demonstration using a transparency volume-rendering technique. *J Comput Assist Tomogr* 2000;24(1):96–98.
9. Origitano TC, Anderson DE. CT angiographic-guided frameless stereotactic-assisted clipping of a distal posterior inferior cerebellar artery aneurysm: technical case report. *Surg Neurol* 1996;46(5):450–453; discussion 453–454.
10. Pedersen HK, et al. CTA in patients with acute subarachnoid haemorrhage: a comparative study with selective, digital angiography and blinded, independent review. *Acta Radiol* 2001;42(1):43–49.
11. Takizawa T, et al. Frameless isocentric stereotactic laser beam guide for image-directed microsurgery. *Acta Neurochir* 1993;125(1–4):177–180.
12. van der Weide R, et al. CTA-based angle selection for diagnostic and interventional angiography of saccular intracranial aneurysms. *IEEE Trans Med Imaging* 1998;17(5):831–841.
13. Villablanca JP, et al. Volume-rendered helical computerized tomography angiography in the detection and characterization of intracranial aneurysms. *J Neurosurg* 2000;93(2):254–264.
14. Harris A, et al. Infectious aneurysm clipping by an MRI/MRA wand-guided protocol: a case report and technical note. *Pediatr Neurosurg* 2001;35(2):90–93.
15. Isoda H, et al. MRA of intracranial aneurysm models: a comparison of contrast-enhanced three-dimensional MRA with time-of-flight MRA. *J Comput Assist Tomogr* 2000;24(2):308–315.
16. Jager HR, et al. MRA versus digital subtraction angiography in acute subarachnoid haemorrhage: a blinded multireader study of prospectively recruited patients. *Neuroradiology* 2000;42(5):313–326.
17. Kuzma BB, Goodman JM. Nonvisualization of known cerebral aneurysm on MRA. *Surg Neurol* 1999;51(1):110–112.
18. Zamani A. MRA of intracranial aneurysms. *Clin Neurosci* 1997;4(3):123–129.
19. Parenti G, Fiori L, Gasparotti R. Ruptured cerebral aneurysms operated on with only MRA: reports of two cases. *J Neurosurg Sci* 1995;39(1):21–25.
20. Patrux B, et al. Magnetic resonance angiography (MRA) of the circle of Willis: a prospective comparison with conventional angiography in 54 subjects. *Neuroradiology* 1994;36(3):193–197.
21. Houkin K, et al. Magnetic resonance angiography (MRA) of ruptured cerebral aneurysm. *Acta Neurochir* 1994;128(1–4):132–136.
22. Bradley WG Jr. MRA abets visualization of intracranial aneurysms. *Diagn Imaging* (San Francisco) 1992;14(11):122–128.
23. Matsumoto M, et al. Three-dimensional computerized tomography angiography-guided surgery of acutely ruptured cerebral aneurysms. *J Neurosurg* 2001;94(5):718–727.
24. Watanabe Z, et al. The usefulness of 3D MR angiography in surgery for ruptured cerebral aneurysms. *Surg Neurol* 2001;55(6):359–364.

15

Image-Guided Brain Tumor Resection

ISABELLE M. GERMANO AND SEIJI KONDO

Surgical treatment of primary brain tumors remains a considerable challenge for the neurosurgeon. Nonetheless, surgery is the mainstay of glioma therapy because it provides the means of obtaining absolute tissue diagnosis, mapping tumor margins, mechanical cytoreduction, and guidance of adjuvant therapy such as brachytherapy, gene therapy, or radiosurgery. Recent developments in computation technology have fundamentally enhanced the role of medical imaging, from diagnosis to computer-aided surgery. Today, computer-assisted methods provide real-time information for dynamic navigation, analysis, and inspection of three-dimensional (3-D) image structures for preoperative surgery, virtual surgery, and intraoperative localization.

Kelly's pioneering work to establish volumetric stereotactic resection techniques has provided a basis for assessing the benefits of surgical resection of deeply seated parenchymal tumors.[1] These techniques allow for proper diagnosis and definitive resection of benign and circumscribed gliomas as well as for radical cytoreduction of the bulk of high-grade tumors. Advances in image-guided technology greatly enhance a surgeon's ability to create a plan prior to surgery, to follow it during surgery, and to modify the surgical approach based on intraoperative information.

Although extent of resection of gliomas has not been analyzed as an influence on outcome in a prospective randomized trial, recent studies suggest improved length of survival after aggressive surgical resection.[2–7] Berger et al[8] have demonstrated that the degree of resection and amount of residual tumor are significantly related to the incidence of recurrence and to the tumor grade at recurrence. In the past, the task of correlating preoperative and intraoperative imaging studies was left to surgeons and depended on their knowledge of human anatomy. Stereotaxy enabled neurosurgeons to effectively correlate preoperative images with the patient's physical anatomy during the operation. Image-guidance technology allows the use of "frameless stereotaxy," offering accuracy similar to that of stereotactic neurosurgery while obviating some of the limitations.[9–10]

This chapter reviews the use, advantages, and limitations of frameless image guidance for neurosurgical treatment of brain tumors using the optical digitizer. Image guidance for biopsy and minimally invasive resection of brain tumors is reviewed as is the use of this technology for the administration of adjuvant treatment. Finally, the steps of these procedures as conducted at the authors' institution are described.

■ Needle Biopsy

Frameless, image-guided surgery can be successfully used for brain needle biopsy previously performed with frame-based stereotaxy. As part of the initial evaluation for an intracranial mass, patients may undergo stereotactic biopsy, given that numerous studies indicate that presumptive diagnoses based on preoperative clinical information and imaging studies alone are incorrect in as many as 25% of cases. With the use of image-guided techniques the surgical risk of biopsy has significantly declined. Therefore, empirically prescribed cytotoxic therapy with radiation or chemotherapy is usually no longer justified. Image-guided brain needle biopsy, because of its lesser risk, higher yield, and greater cost effectiveness, has superseded the former practice of performing an open craniotomy for biopsy.[11]

A hallmark of malignant gliomas is heterogeneity. Thus, careful planning is imperative to achieve satisfactory results. This includes tissue diagnosis and tissue sampling that are representative of the whole tumor. A typical example is that of a primary brain tumor nonenhancing after contrast on magnetic resonance (MR) images except in one or multiple small areas. Studies correlating imaging and histology have shown that the enhancing areas most likely contain tumor cells with anaplastic features and possibly of higher tumor grade.[12] Obtaining serial biopsies through the bulk of the tumor in a stepwise fashion increases the likelihood of accurate diagnosis. To that end, computer-assisted treatment planning programs are invaluable in selecting a safe and effective trajectory for biopsy. Frozen section analysis provides reassurance of a diagnostic biopsy prior to ending the procedure but should never be considered as sufficient to guide further therapy.

Fusion of positron emission tomography (PET) and MR spectroscopy (MRS) images has been reported to be useful in several areas of neurosurgery.[13] In most image-guided systems commercially available, these images can be fused to the routine preoperative MR images. This feature offers a promising role for MRS and especially for PET to enhance the intraoperative accuracy of image-guided stereotactic biopsy by intraoperatively guiding the biopsy to the regions of maximal metabolic rate and presumably highest tumor grade.

When planning a routine diagnostic biopsy a few technical aspects must be remembered. In particular, it is important to acknowledge that the radiographic appearance of glioblastomas and metastasis in some cases is characterized by a ring-enhancing appearance after contrast on preoperative images. The center of the lesion may consist of fluid or necrosis. In either case, when targeting the lesion, care should be taken to avoid the center of the lesion as the first or only target. If fluid is present within the lesion, drainage of it will cause brain shifting, and any additional biopsy at the same setting to obtain diagnostic tissue will most likely be unsuccessful. On the other hand, if necrotic tissue is obtained, it would not be diagnostic. Thus we advocate targeting the periphery first.

The senior author performs all diagnostic biopsies using the frameless equipment as previously reported.[11] Exceptions include brain stem biopsies when using a supratentorial approach and biopsy of lesions less than 1.5 cm in maximum longitudinal diameter.

■ Minimally Invasive Craniotomy and Open Resection

Intraoperative navigation allows the surgeon to locate a minimally invasive craniotomy flap, thereby reducing the size of the opening and optimizing the center of the craniotomy window. It is important to stress that endoscopy and ultrasound lack this important first step in preparing for resection of a brain tumor.

Although the benefit of aggressive resection of primary brain tumors, particularly high-grade malignancies, remains controversial, there is increasing clinical evidence that "complete" resections can prolong the patient's quality of life and extend survival.[2-8] It should be emphasized that when talking about volumetric resection or gross-total resection of a primary brain tumor, this is pertinent only to the "bulk" of the tumor. It is well known that gliomas have infiltrative cells beyond the limit of the resection that require adjuvant treatment in addition to surgery. Thus the image-guided navigator is helpful in allowing volumetric resection of the "ring-enhancing" lesion, typical of high-grade gliomas (Fig. 15–1), or the circumscribed area of "decreased signal intensity," typical of low-grade gliomas on MR images (Fig. 15–2).

Prior to beginning the operation, we perform "virtual surgery" on the computer screen. This step is usually conducted during the induction of anesthesia. When planning for resection of gliomas it is very important to have a precise understanding of the cortical eloquent areas surrounding the tumor (Fig. 15–3). In most cases, eloquent areas such as Broca's area and motor and sensory cortex can be visualized by the help of the reconstructed triplanar and 3-D images[14] (see Figs. 15–1B and 15–2B). Additionally, functional MRI can be fused to the anatomical views to increase the accuracy of functional localization. Although in our experience image guidance provides a very accurate identification of eloquent areas, we confirm our preoperative impression with intraoperative electrophysiological cortical mapping (see Fig. 15–3).

After the craniotomy flap is elevated and prior to beginning the corticotomy, it may be appropriate to perform cortical mapping with bipolar electrical stimulation. Intraoperative motor mapping may be used to minimize the risk of transversing the primary motor cortex. More importantly, functionally eloquent regions of the secondary motor associational cortex can be identified intraoperatively using mapping techniques. The phase reversal seen in somatosensory-evoked potential

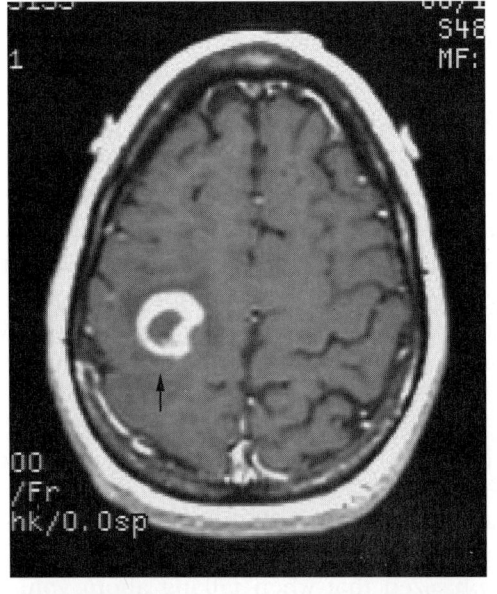
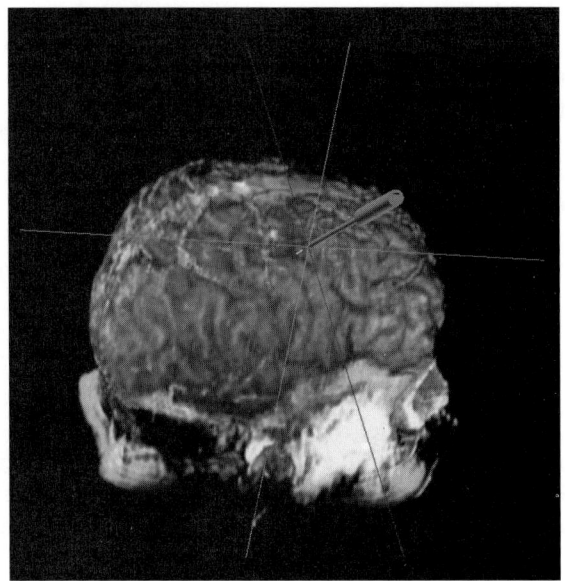
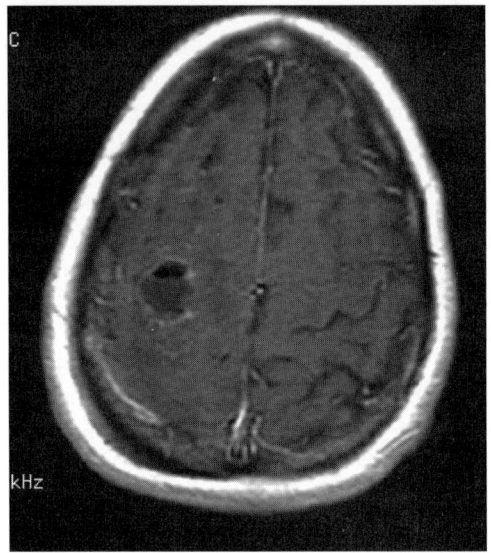

FIGURE 15–1. Brain magnetic resonance (MR) images after contrast of a 54-year-old woman presenting with left upper-extremity weakness. (A). Preoperative MRI shows the presence of a ring-enhancing lesion in the right frontal premotor cortex suggestive of a glioblastoma. (B). Three-dimensional reconstruction used for preoperative planning and intraoperative guidance, showing the cortical surface with the sulci, veins, and tumor (the arrow indicates the central sulcus determined preoperatively and confirmed intraoperatively) (CBYON system, Palo Alto, CA). (C). Postoperative MRI performed 24 hours after image-guided surgery showing volumetric resection of the tumor bulk. Histology confirmed the presence of glioblastoma. Postoperatively, the patient regained full strength of the left upper extremity.

recordings obtained from electrode arrays placed across the sensorimotor cortex is also very helpful in determining eloquent sensory-motor areas (see Fig. 15–3). Additionally, this technique does not require the patient's cooperation, and it is less time-consuming. Visual-evoked responses are occasionally employed to variable effect. Expressive language is tested using counting, alphabetical naming, and sentence-generation tests.

The use of the ultrasonic aspirator at low settings has been crucial to assure adequate resection of gliomas without overmanipulation of surrounding edematous and functionally compromised parenchyma. Image guidance benefits from the "inside-out" approach to debulk and to develop a pseudocapsular plan between the tumor bulk and the surrounding parenchyma.

At the conclusion of the resection procedure, the surgical work space is again sequentially sampled to confirm accomplishment of the planned surgical task (Fig. 15–4). On numerous occasions, a reappraisal is in order to reevaluate subjective intraoperative impressions regarding resectional volumetric estimates. The surgical judgment as to how to interpret these data is informed by numerous considerations not necessarily demonstrated on imaging studies.

Image-guided technology improves the extent of resection by better directing the approach to the lesion by clarifying the margins for resection when they are irregular or ill defined, by speeding resection and limiting surgeon fatigue, by identifying residual tumor after initial resection efforts, and by minimizing surgical

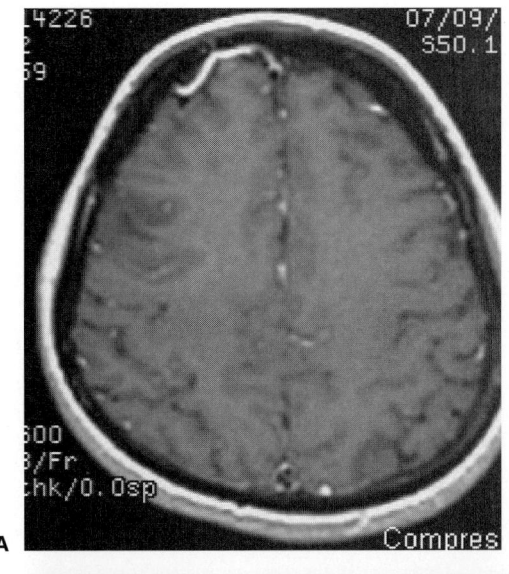
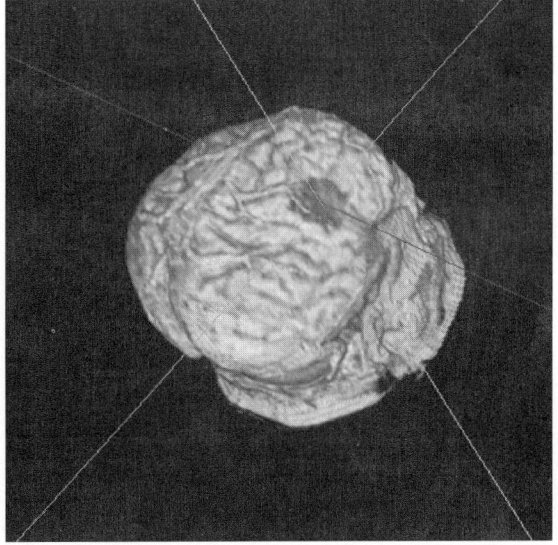
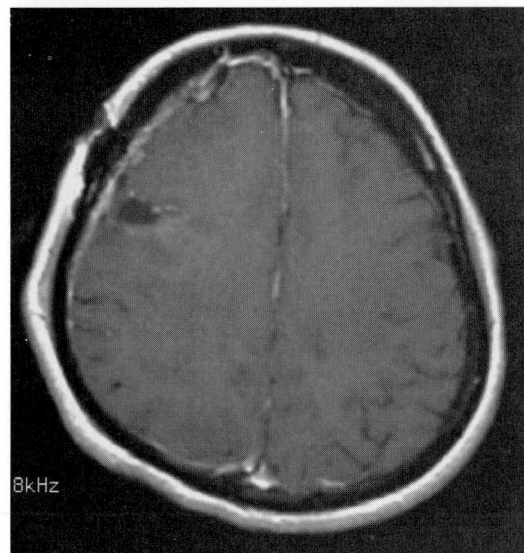

FIGURE 15–2. Brain magnetic resonance (MR) images after contrast of a 37-year-old woman presenting with new onset of seizure disorder. (A). Preoperative MRI shows the presence of an area of low-signal intensity in the right frontal area suggestive of a low-grade glioma. (B). Three-dimensional reconstruction used for preoperative planning and intraoperative guidance (CBYON system, Palo Alto, CA). (C). Postoperative MRI performed 24 hours after image-guided surgery showing volumetric resection of the tumor bulk. Histology confirmed the presence of an oligodendroglioma.

morbidity when related to navigational disorientation. This leads to fewer reoperations, better results from adjuvant therapies, and more predictable clinical outcomes.

■ Image-Guidance Caviats during Resection of Brain Tumor: Brain Shift and Images Updating

The surgeon should be familiar with the limitations and potential sources of error of the navigation system in use. Additionally, other sources of error, in particular brain shift and lack of real-time updating of images, should be kept in mind when using image guidance for tumor resection.

Intracranial shifts encountered during evacuation of cerebrospinal fluid from enlarged ventricles associated with centrally located tumors may prove to be a challenge to image guidance in terms of refining the surgical approach to the lesion. Shifts of intracranial soft tissue over the duration of the operation have been documented.[15] However, these have proven to be of remarkably less concern than initially feared. Nonetheless, different algorithms have been investigated to address these issues, including automated intraoperative, non-rigid body re-registration.

Brain shift has long being documented. This is most pronounced over the convexity and the poles, and it is minimal for the deep structures and structures in continuity with the dura, such as the corpus callosum and hippocampus.[16] Several strategies have been devised to

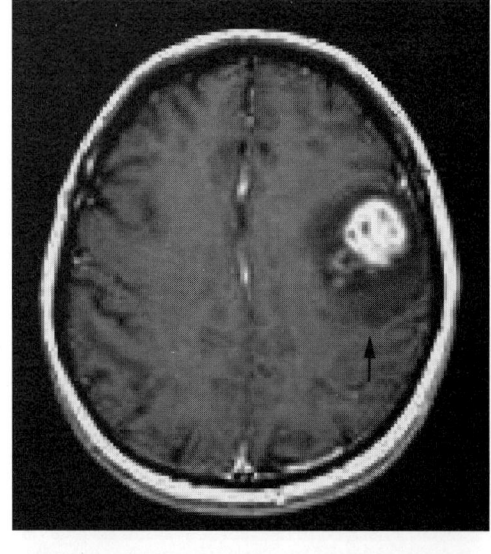
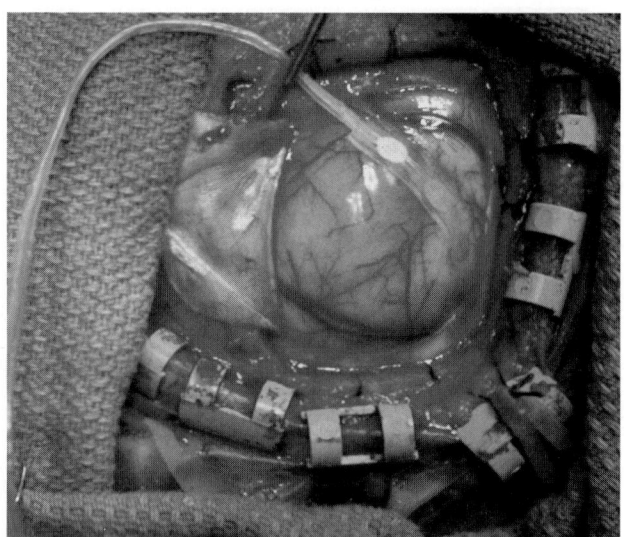
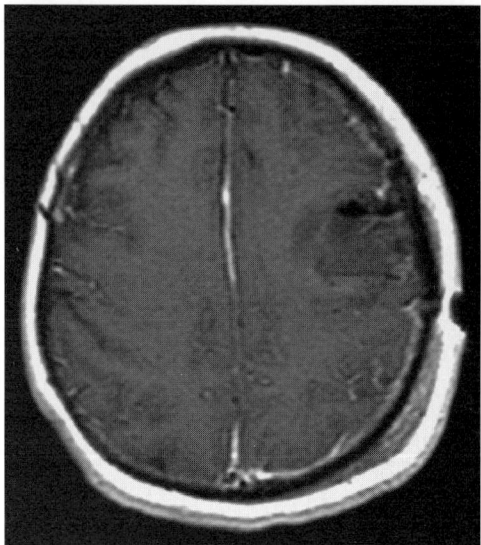

FIGURE 15–3. (A). Brain magnetic resonance (MR) images after contrast of a 51-year-old woman presenting with expressive dysphasia and dysarthria showing a left frontal enhancing lesion suggestive of high-grade glioma. Arrow indicates the central sulcus as determined preoperatively using the image-guided planning software (StealthStation, Medtronic SNT, Louisville, CO) and confirmed intraoperatively by cortical mapping. (B). Intraoperative photograph showing the craniotomy window, dural opening, and electrode strip used to perform cortical mapping to confirm the location of the central sulcus. Note the fullness of the brain (see text). (C). Postoperative MRI performed 24 hours after image-guided surgery showing volumetric resection of the tumor bulk. Histology confirmed the presence of glioblastoma. The patient's dysphasia improved significantly after surgery.

minimize shift.[1,17–19] In our practice, we follow the steps listed in Table 15–1 to minimize brain shift. When preparing to resect an intracranial tumor we avoid the use of mannitol and other diuretics. Hyperventilation is usually sufficient to significantly decrease the intracranial pressure and allow safe opening of the dura. The patient undergoes hyperventilation with a pCO_2 in the low twenties (20–25) torr. Typically, a greater "fullness" of the brain is tolerated when opening the dura to minimize "shift" secondary to massive diuresis (see Fig. 15–3). Naturally, the aggressive debulking of the tumor will decrease the intracranial pressure and render dural closure possible without any additional maneuver. In fact, in most cases, hyperventilation is reduced as soon as the bulk of the tumor is removed. We also carefully avoid the placement of lumbar or ventricular drains to avoid cerebrospinal fluid (CSF) diversion. Should postoperative CSF diversion be necessary, the drain is inserted prior to the surgery and kept clamped during the resection. When possible, surgery near the cyst is deferred until the end to avoid puncture of the cyst. En bloc resections are preferable to piecemeal resections for minimizing brain shift. Picket fencing techniques[19] are used prior to the resection to determine the depth of the tumor (see the section, Intraoperative Procedure).

Despite the registration of image space to physical space, digital scan information remains historical data and it is subject to becoming outdated during the course of surgical manipulation of the tissues. By digitizing the video output from intraoperative visualization techniques, such as ultrasonography, endoscopy, tomography, and electrophysiological recordings, these images can be treated as another source of spatially registered

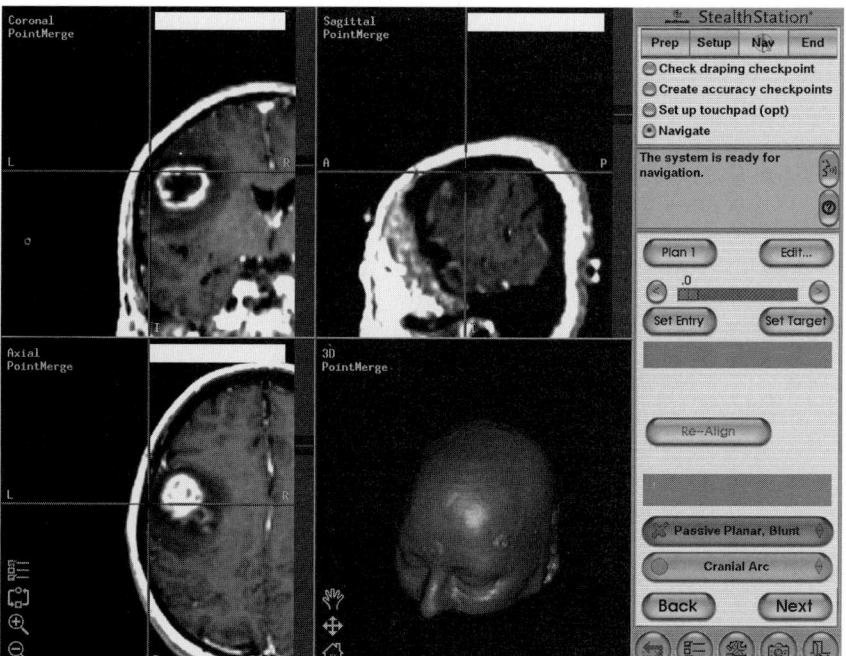
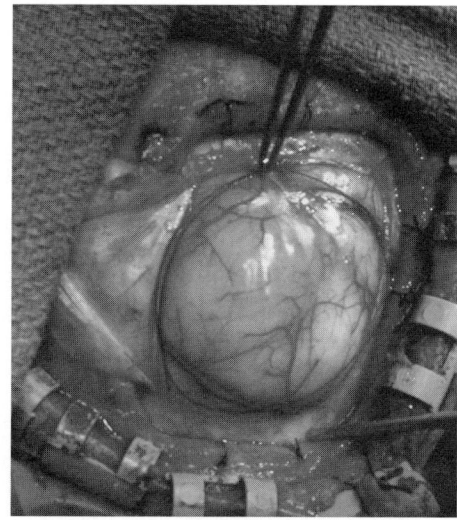

FIGURE 15–4. (A). Intraoperative computer screen photograph showing in clockwise fashion from the upper left panel coronal, sagittal, three-dimensional, and axial reformatted magnetic resonance (MR) images. The real-time location of the bipolar forceps used in (B) is indicated by the hairline crossing on the triplanar images. (B). Intraoperative photograph showing the bipolar forceps holding a silk suture while demarcating the periphery of the tumor with real-time feedback from the computer screen (see text). (C). Intraoperative computer screen photograph showing the real-time location of the bipolar forceps on the preoperative MR images at the end of the resection, checking for accuracy of extent of resection. From the upper left panel in clockwise fashion the following MR images are shown: coronal, sagittal, trajectory 1, axial, three-dimensional, and trajectory 2. Trajectory views are images reformatted in planes orthogonal to the bipolar forceps. (StealthStation, Medtronic SNT, Louisville, CO)

TABLE 15–1. Strategies to minimize brain shift during aggressive resection of brain tumor

Use hyperventilation
Avoid diuretics, including Mannitol
Avoid CSF diversion by spinal drain/ventricular tap/opening of ventricles
Mark tumor margins before resection
Remove tumor en bloc
Avoid puncture of tumor cyst(s)

medical information.[20–21] We have used the ultrasound (Aloka 5000, Wallington, CT) interfaced with the StealthStation (Medtronic SNT, Louisville, CO) to guide the resection of over 100 gliomas. This technique was deemed helpful in most instances (Fig. 15–5) to update the preoperative images. Additional details of our work on this topic will be published elsewhere. This topic also is covered in Chapter 16.

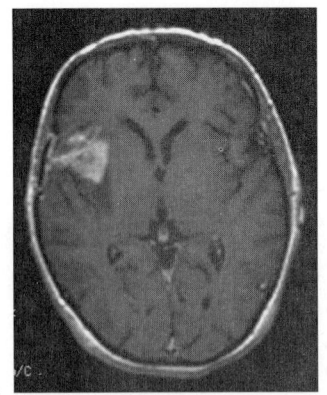
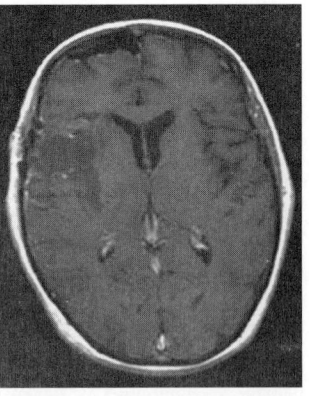
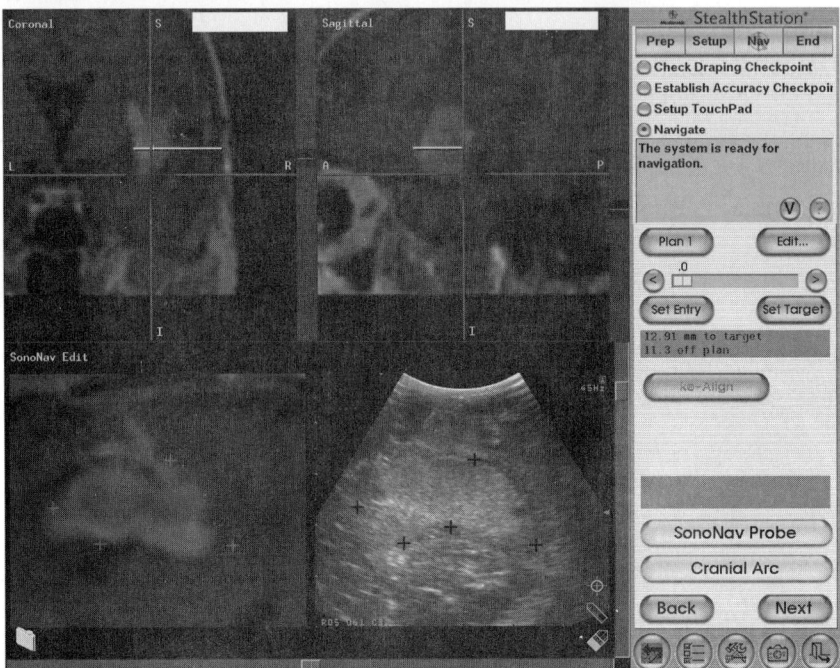
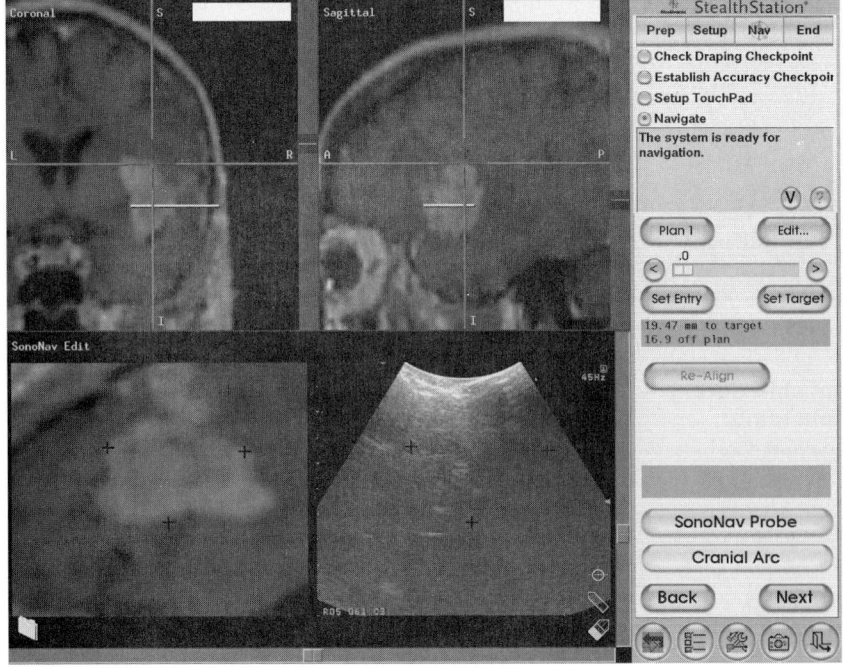

FIGURE 15–5. Brain magnetic resonance (MR) images after contrast of a 64-year-old woman with recurrent glioblastoma undergoing gene therapy (see text). (A). Preoperative MRI. (B). Postoperative MRI performed 24 hours after image-guided surgery showing volumetric resection of the tumor bulk. (C,D). Intraoperative computer screen photograph showing the preoperative MR images in the upper and left lower panels and the updated intraoperative ultrasound in the right lower panel (C) before tumor resection and (D) after tumor resection. The crosses on the ultrasound image correspond to the crosses delineating the tumor on the MR image reconstructed in the plane of the ultrasound probe (left lower panel). Note the lack of an echogenic mass in (D) on the ultrasound image, indicatating a gross total resection of the tumor bulk. (StealthStation, Medtronic SNT, Louisville, CO; Aloka 5000, Aloka, Wallingford, CT.)

Gene Therapy and Adjuvant Treatment

Adjuvant treatment after aggressive resection of primary brain tumor or without surgery in combination with conventional radiation has long been used for treatment of gliomas. Perhaps the first report of the use of stereotactic techniques for adjuvant treatment of brain tumors was by Murtagh et al in 1956.[22] These authors instilled ^{32}P into the cyst of a craniopharyngioma.

In the past decade, image-guided surgery became increasingly important in targeting administration of adjuvant treatment for brain tumors. Although there are several modalities that have been reported to be of value in the treatment of brain tumors, the combination of techniques seems to show the most promising results.[2-7,23-24] We recently presented our results on administration of gene therapy in 11 patients with recurrent glioblastoma (NIH-R03-CA-82804–01). Intraoperative image guidance was essential in this clinical study to ensure the accuracy of resection and treatment delivery. A detailed report will be published elsewhere.

Intraoperative Procedure

Intraoperative data display, planning, and virtual surgery

Details on image acquisition are described in Chapter 4. After the preoperative images are transferred to the computer, the software planning system allows the surgeon to create an intraoperative display semiautomatically to achieve optimal presentation of relevant surgical data. The surgeon selects those images deemed to be most beneficial for intraoperative viewing. Multiple images can be simultaneously displayed in separate display quadrants of the planning system. The display may include a 3-D rendering of the cranial contents as well as reformatted scan sets with triplanar and 3-D reconstruction (see Fig. 15–4A) or reconstruction based on an orthogonal approach view (see Fig. 15–4C). As the patient is being prepared for surgery and anesthesia is induced, we proceed with simulation of the procedure on the computer. This allows the neurosurgeon and the neurosurgeon-in-training to optimize the size and location of the craniotomy. Additionally, the location of eloquent areas can be visualized (see Fig. 15–3) and a surgical plan constructed to avoid them. Additional details on virtual surgery can be found in Chapter 4.

Registration and intraoperative navigation

After adequate anesthesia is achieved by general anesthesia or intravenous sedation, the patient's head is immobilized in a pinion head holder to maintain the registration relationship between the fiducial markers and the reference frame throughout the operation. When intravenous sedation is used, local anesthesia is used prior to placement of the head holder. After proper positioning of the patient and before registration of image space to physical space, a reference emitter is attached to the head holder. Registration of image space to physical space is then accomplished (see Chapter 4). At this point, the surgeon can use any surgical instrument with light emitting diodes (LEDs) to localize in real time on the preoperative images the location of the surgical instrument in relation to the patient's anatomy (see Fig. 15–4). Typically, we localize the tumor on the patient's scalp. This helps us to tailor a centered and minimally invasive bone flap. After the dura is opened, for tumors abutting the surface, tumor boundaries are established using the neuronavigator before starting the resection. Different techniques for marking the tumor perimeter have been described—we prefer the simple method of depositing a silk suture on the cortex while observing on the computer screen the location of the forceps holding the suture superimposed on the presurgical images (see Fig. 15–4). To establish the depth, picket fencing techniques are used.[19] The senior author uses the ultrasonic aspirator at low setting (25%) as a cutting knife to perform en bloc resections when feasible.

Conclusions

Current image-guided techniques provide the surgeon with new tools to plan and execute accurate and minimally invasive surgery for brain tumors. When coupled with good clinical judgment, they provide guidance in determining what is safely operable and may maximize the extent of the surgical resection. Intraoperative ultrasound may expand the utility of this technology by providing real-time updating of the images and allowing the surgeon to compensate for shift caused by positioning and resection. Cost-effectiveness evaluation of this technology has indicated that the use of this equipment is associated with a shorter hospital stay[10] and other potential financial benefits.[25] Because of these advantages, the authors have no doubt that image-guided resection of brain tumors will be considered standard-of-care in the near future.

REFERENCES

1. Kelly PJ. Computer-assisted stereotaxis: new approaches for the management of intracranial intra-axial tumors. *Neurology* 1986;36: 535–541.
2. Ammirati M, Vick N, Liao Y, et al. Effect of the extent of surgical resection on survival and quality of life in patients with supratento-

rial glioblastomas and anaplastic astrocytomas. *Neurosurg* 1987;21:201–206.
3. Devaux BC, O'Fallon JR, Kelly PJ. Resection, biopsy, and survival in malignant neoplasms. *J Neurosurg* 1993;78:767–775.
4. Warnick RE. The role of cytoreductive surgery in the treatment of intracranial gliomas. *Sem Rad Onc* 1991;1:10–16.
5. Black P. Management of malignant glioma: role for surgery in relation to multimodality therapy. *J Neurovirol* 1998;4:227–236.
6. Lipson AC, Gargollo PC, Black PM. Intraoperative magnetic resonance imaging: considerations for the operating room of the future. *J Clin Neurosci* 2001;8:305–310.
7. Azizi A, Black P, Miyamoto C, Croul SE. Treatment of malignant astrocytomas with repetitive resections: a longitudinal study. *Isr Med Assoc J* 2001;3:254–257.
8. Berger MS, Deliganis AV, Dobbins J, et al. The effect of extent of resection on recurrence in patients with low grade cerebral hemisphere low grade gliomas. *Cancer* 1994;74:1784–1791.
9. Germano IM. The NeuroStation System for image-guided, frameless stereotaxy. *Neurosurg* 1995;37:348–349.
10. Germano IM, Villalobos H, Silvers A, Post KP. Clinical use of the optical digitizer. *Neurosurgery* 1999;45:261–270.
11. Germano IM, Queenan JV. Clinical experience with intracranial brain needle biopsy using frameless surgical navigation. *Comp Aid Surgery* 1998;3:33–39.
12. Dumas-Duport C, Monsaingeon V, Szenthe L, et al. Serial stereotactic biopsies: a double histological code of gliomas according to malignancy and 3-D configuration, as an aid to therapeutic decision and assessment of results. *Appl Neurophysiol* 1982;45:431–437.
13. Pietrzyk U, Herholz K, Schuster A, et al. Clinical applications of registration and fusion of multimodality brain images from PET, SPECT, CT, and MRI. *Eur J Radiol* 1996;21:174–182.
14. Bucholz RD. The central sulcus and surgical planning. *Am J Neuroradiol* 1993;14:926–927.
15. Nabavi A, Black PM, Gering DT, et al. Serial intraoperative magnetic resonance imaging of brain shift. *Neurosurgery* 2001;48:787–797.
16. Olivier A, Germano IM, Cukiert A, Peters T. Frameless stereotaxy for surgery of the epilepsies: preliminary experience. *J Neurosurg* 1994;81:629–633.
17. Kelly PJ. Stereotactic resection: general principles. In: Kelly PJ, ed. *Tumor Stereotaxis*. Philadelphia: WB Saunders; 1991:268–295.
18. Moore MR, Black PM, Ellenbogen R, Gall CM, Eldredge E. Stereotactic craniotomy: methods and result using the Brown-Roberts-Wells stereotactic frame. *Neurosurgery* 1989;25:572–577.
19. Hassenbuch SJ, Anderson JS, Pillay PK. Brain tumor resection aided with markers placed using sterotaxis guided by magnetic resonance imaging and computed tomography. *Neurosurgery* 1991;28:801–806.
20. Hammound MA, Ligon BL, elSouki R, Shi WM, Schomer DF, Sawaya R. Use of intraoperative ultrasound for localizing tumors and determining the extent of resection: a comparative study with magnetic resonance imaging. *J Neurosurg* 1996;84:737–806.
21. Nimsky C, Ganslandt O, Kober H, Buchfelder M, Fahlbusch R. Intraoperative magnetic resonance imaging combined with neuronavigation: a new concept. *Neurosurgery* 2001;48:1082–1089.
22. Murtagh F, Wycis HT, Robbins R, Spiegel-Adolph M, Spiegel EA. Visualization and treatment of cystic brain tumors by stereoencephalotomy. *Acta Radiol* 1956;46:407–414.
23. Brem H, Piantadosi S, Burger PC, et al. Placebo-controlled trial of safety and efficacy of intraoperative controlled delivery by biodegradable polymers of chemotherapy for recurrent gliomas. *Lancet* 1995;345:1008–1012.
24. Black P. Management of malignant gliomas: role for surgery in relation to multimodality therapy. *J Neurovirol* 1998;4:227–236.
25. Paleologos TS, Wadley JP, Kitchen ND, Thomas DG. Clinical utility and cost-effectiveness of interactive image-guided craniotomy: clinical comparison between conventional and image-guided meningioma surgery. *Neurosurgery* 2000;47:40–47.

16

Intraoperative Image Update by Interface with Ultrasound

MITCHEL S. BERGER AND G. EVREN KELES

Despite advances in medical imaging techniques and their routine preoperative use, real-time intraoperative information regarding anatomy remains of significant importance to the neurosurgeon. Accurate localization of neurosurgical targets is essential to minimize surgical morbidity. To reach this goal, ultrasound was extensively used in neurosurgical procedures during the last quarter of the twentieth century, and the echogenic characteristics of various lesions were defined.[1] In addition, the quality of ultrasound images has improved significantly with newer technologies, and greater penetration at higher frequencies is achieved with new signal encoding techniques.

Ultrasound's most important advantage is its capability to depict in real time the anatomical characteristics of the surgical field. Furthermore, it does not require radiation, it is easy to use, and it is relatively inexpensive. Real-time information obtained from ultrasound images is helpful during both cranial and spinal procedures. Intraoperative ultrasound has been used to localize subcortical and deep lesions including tumors, abcesses, and hematomas; to define tumor margins; to evaluate the completeness of resection; and to determine the presence of surgical complications. During spinal procedures, a higher-frequency ultrasound probe may be used to verify that the bone removal is adequate to expose the entire solid component of a tumor. In addition, intramedullary lesions as well as pathologies located anterior to the spinal cord may be visualized by intraoperative ultrasonography.[2]

■ Neuronavigation

The development of neuronavigation systems was another major technical advance in neurosurgery. Neuronavigation methods help the neurosurgeon in planning surgery and approaching the tumor as well as during resection and in evaluating the extent of resection. Although conventional neurosurgery training and subsequent experience enable the surgeon to navigate safely within the brain parenchyma, additional intraoperative anatomical information is valuable, especially in situations where individual anatomical variations or prior treatment complicates the anatomy. Tumors, together with their surrounding edema, often distort normal anatomical relationships and thus pose a significant challenge to the neurosurgeon trying to navigate using conventional landmarks. Intraoperative image guidance may also provide critical information during resection of tumors with a consistency similar to normal brain tissue by delineating T2-weighted imaging margins.

The primary components of any contemporary navigational system include registration of the surgical target with respect to surrounding structures and physical space, interacting with a localization device, integration of real-time data, and interfacing with a computer.[3] Data from multiple images can be integrated using either natural landmarks or external fiducial markers. Frameless stereotactic navigation systems include ultrasonic digitizer systems, magnetic field digitizers, multijointed encoder arms, infrared flash systems, and robotic systems.

Multiple registration techniques are available to map images with respect to each other and to the surgical field. Regardless of the preferred registration method, frameless systems may provide an advantage over frame-based systems in defining precise localization because distortions of imagery are likely to be reflected in the landmarks as well as in the anatomy of interest. In addition, because frameless systems do not require fixation to an immobile frame, they may be used for craniotomies and spine surgeries. Several frameless stereotactic systems are now available for use in procedures together with ultrasound and light-emitting diode (LED)-based localization or with magnetic field-based tracking systems.[4–5]

Accuracy of a frameless stereotactic system using an instrument holder was assessed for images acquired using magnetic resonance (MR) or computed tomography (CT) scans.[6] In the first phase of the study, which consisted of 258 laboratory measurements on phantom frameless stereotactic procedures, a mean error of 1.1 ± 0.5 mm was found for CT-guided procedures, whereas the mean error rate was 1.4 ± 0.7 mm for MR-based stereotactic procedures. The clinical phase of the study, conducted on 21 procedures for intracranial mass lesions, revealed a mean linear error of 2.6 ± 1.9 mm and 2.5 ± 0.7 mm for MR and CT, respectively. In another study, the authors evaluated target-localizing accuracy of a neuronavigational system with passive optical tracking where reflection of infrared flashes from reflectors placed on surgical instruments was tracked by camera arrays.[7] In a study population of 125 patients with mostly tumor patients, a mean error rate of 4 ± 1.4 mm was detected.

■ Sononavigation

Alteration of the surgical anatomy of the lesion and surrounding structures may be the result of intraoperative displacement of the brain tissue due to surgical retraction or the resection cavity itself, as well as the shift caused by cerebrospinal fluid leakage. Roberts et al[8] reported their quantitative analysis of intraoperative cortical shift and deformation resulting in loss of spatial accuracy in the surgical field co-registered to preoperative imaging studies. Their results, based on 28 operative cases, showed a displacement of an average of 1 cm, with the dominant directional component being associated with gravity. The authors concluded that this loss of spatial registration with preoperative images, which did not correlate with the position, orientation, or size of the craniotomy, must be taken into account to achieve success during surgery.

The combination of neuronavigation systems with data obtained from intraoperative ultrasound has provided the opportunity to partially overcome errors due to tissue movement. Ultrasound has the unique distinction among other imaging modalities of producing real-time images. However, images are often difficult to interpret because echogenic structures cannot reliably discern normal from abnormal tissue. Additionally, blood products in the surgical field may cause misinterpretation of ultrasound images. Intraoperative ultrasound is controlled by a workstation that is attached to a transducer connected to a tracking attachment that tracks the position and orientation of the transducer and reports this information to the workstation. The position of the transducer is then recorded in coordinates with respect to both patient and physical space. These coordinates are then transformed onto maps created by MR or CT images.[4,9–10]

At our institution, for neuronavigation we use the StealthStation Image-Guided Surgery Platform (Surgical Navigation Technologies, Louisville, CO). Real-time intraoperative ultrasound data are provided by the SSD-2000 ultrasound machine (Aloka Company, Wallingford, CT) (Fig. 16–1). The 5 MHz ultrasound probe is attached to a frame with four LEDs (Fig. 16–2). As the probe is turned in any plane, the image corresponds directly to the same plane on MR. The registration accu-

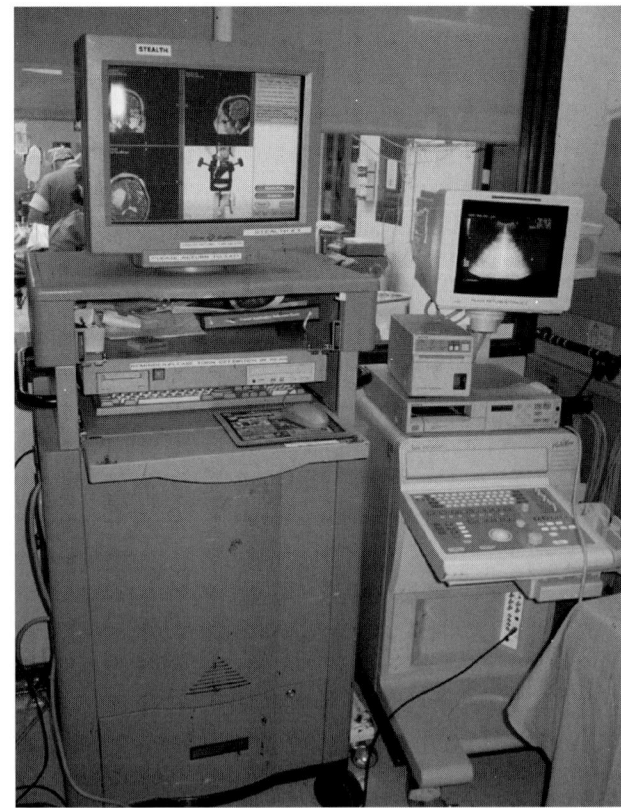

FIGURE 16–1. Operating room view with the Stealth navigation system (Medtronic SNT, Louisville, CO) (left) and the connected ultrasound setup (right).

16

Intraoperative Image Update by Interface with Ultrasound

MITCHEL S. BERGER AND G. EVREN KELES

Despite advances in medical imaging techniques and their routine preoperative use, real-time intraoperative information regarding anatomy remains of significant importance to the neurosurgeon. Accurate localization of neurosurgical targets is essential to minimize surgical morbidity. To reach this goal, ultrasound was extensively used in neurosurgical procedures during the last quarter of the twentieth century, and the echogenic characteristics of various lesions were defined.[1] In addition, the quality of ultrasound images has improved significantly with newer technologies, and greater penetration at higher frequencies is achieved with new signal encoding techniques.

Ultrasound's most important advantage is its capability to depict in real time the anatomical characteristics of the surgical field. Furthermore, it does not require radiation, it is easy to use, and it is relatively inexpensive. Real-time information obtained from ultrasound images is helpful during both cranial and spinal procedures. Intraoperative ultrasound has been used to localize subcortical and deep lesions including tumors, abcesses, and hematomas; to define tumor margins; to evaluate the completeness of resection; and to determine the presence of surgical complications. During spinal procedures, a higher-frequency ultrasound probe may be used to verify that the bone removal is adequate to expose the entire solid component of a tumor. In addition, intramedullary lesions as well as pathologies located anterior to the spinal cord may be visualized by intraoperative ultrasonography.[2]

■ Neuronavigation

The development of neuronavigation systems was another major technical advance in neurosurgery. Neuronavigation methods help the neurosurgeon in planning surgery and approaching the tumor as well as during resection and in evaluating the extent of resection. Although conventional neurosurgery training and subsequent experience enable the surgeon to navigate safely within the brain parenchyma, additional intraoperative anatomical information is valuable, especially in situations where individual anatomical variations or prior treatment complicates the anatomy. Tumors, together with their surrounding edema, often distort normal anatomical relationships and thus pose a significant challenge to the neurosurgeon trying to navigate using conventional landmarks. Intraoperative image guidance may also provide critical information during resection of tumors with a consistency similar to normal brain tissue by delineating T2-weighted imaging margins.

The primary components of any contemporary navigational system include registration of the surgical target with respect to surrounding structures and physical space, interacting with a localization device, integration of real-time data, and interfacing with a computer.[3] Data from multiple images can be integrated using either natural landmarks or external fiducial markers. Frameless stereotactic navigation systems include ultrasonic digitizer systems, magnetic field digitizers, multijointed encoder arms, infrared flash systems, and robotic systems.

Multiple registration techniques are available to map images with respect to each other and to the surgical field. Regardless of the preferred registration method, frameless systems may provide an advantage over frame-based systems in defining precise localization because distortions of imagery are likely to be reflected in the landmarks as well as in the anatomy of interest. In addition, because frameless systems do not require fixation to an immobile frame, they may be used for craniotomies and spine surgeries. Several frameless stereotactic systems are now available for use in procedures together with ultrasound and light-emitting diode (LED)-based localization or with magnetic field-based tracking systems.[4-5]

Accuracy of a frameless stereotactic system using an instrument holder was assessed for images acquired using magnetic resonance (MR) or computed tomography (CT) scans.[6] In the first phase of the study, which consisted of 258 laboratory measurements on phantom frameless stereotactic procedures, a mean error of 1.1 ± 0.5 mm was found for CT-guided procedures, whereas the mean error rate was 1.4 ± 0.7 mm for MR-based stereotactic procedures. The clinical phase of the study, conducted on 21 procedures for intracranial mass lesions, revealed a mean linear error of 2.6 ± 1.9 mm and 2.5 ± 0.7 mm for MR and CT, respectively. In another study, the authors evaluated target-localizing accuracy of a neuronavigational system with passive optical tracking where reflection of infrared flashes from reflectors placed on surgical instruments was tracked by camera arrays.[7] In a study population of 125 patients with mostly tumor patients, a mean error rate of 4 ± 1.4 mm was detected.

■ Sononavigation

Alteration of the surgical anatomy of the lesion and surrounding structures may be the result of intraoperative displacement of the brain tissue due to surgical retraction or the resection cavity itself, as well as the shift caused by cerebrospinal fluid leakage. Roberts et al[8] reported their quantitative analysis of intraoperative cortical shift and deformation resulting in loss of spatial accuracy in the surgical field co-registered to preoperative imaging studies. Their results, based on 28 operative cases, showed a displacement of an average of 1 cm, with the dominant directional component being associated with gravity. The authors concluded that this loss of spatial registration with preoperative images, which did not correlate with the position, orientation, or size of the craniotomy, must be taken into account to achieve success during surgery.

The combination of neuronavigation systems with data obtained from intraoperative ultrasound has provided the opportunity to partially overcome errors due to tissue movement. Ultrasound has the unique distinction among other imaging modalities of producing real-time images. However, images are often difficult to interpret because echogenic structures cannot reliably discern normal from abnormal tissue. Additionally, blood products in the surgical field may cause misinterpretation of ultrasound images. Intraoperative ultrasound is controlled by a workstation that is attached to a transducer connected to a tracking attachment that tracks the position and orientation of the transducer and reports this information to the workstation. The position of the transducer is then recorded in coordinates with respect to both patient and physical space. These coordinates are then transformed onto maps created by MR or CT images.[4,9-10]

At our institution, for neuronavigation we use the StealthStation Image-Guided Surgery Platform (Surgical Navigation Technologies, Louisville, CO). Real-time intraoperative ultrasound data are provided by the SSD-2000 ultrasound machine (Aloka Company, Wallingford, CT) (Fig. 16–1). The 5 MHz ultrasound probe is attached to a frame with four LEDs (Fig. 16–2). As the probe is turned in any plane, the image corresponds directly to the same plane on MR. The registration accu-

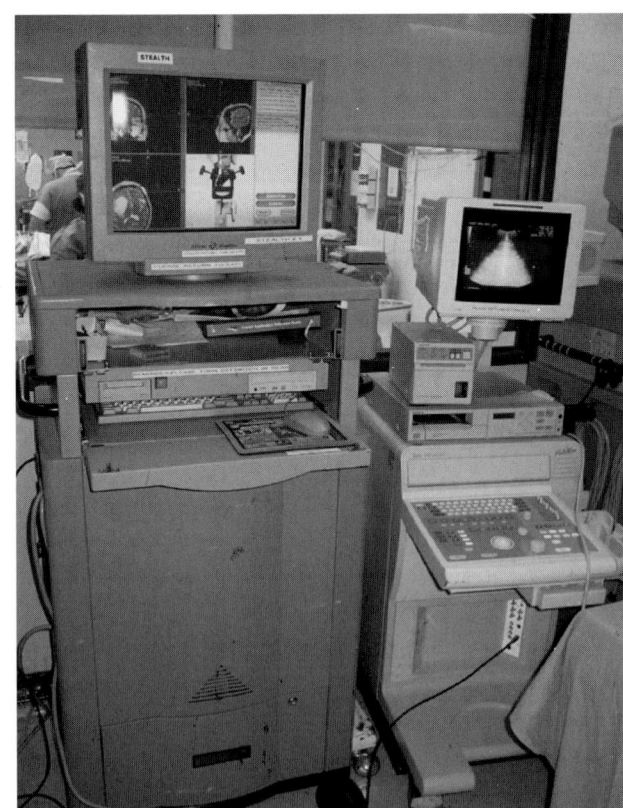

FIGURE 16–1. Operating room view with the Stealth navigation system (Medtronic SNT, Louisville, CO) (left) and the connected ultrasound setup (right).

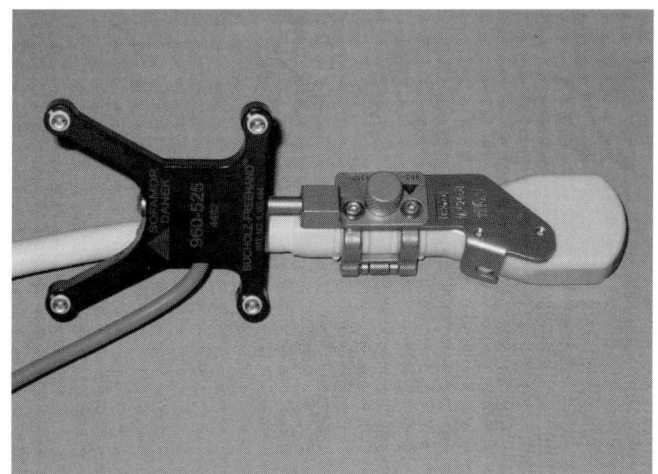

FIGURE 16–2. Image depicting the 5 MHz ultrasound probe with the attachment necessary for tracking by the Stealth neuronavigation system.

One of the earlier neuronavigation systems based on intraoperative ultrasonography for the verification of localization was developed at the University of Oulu, Finland.[11] The Oulu neuronavigator system enabled detection of brain shift and delineated contrast-enhancing tumor regions by overlaying the MR images onto the intraoperative ultrasound image.

Use of a hands-free stereotactic ultrasonic device effectively monitored volume changes and anatomical shifts in a study reported by Giorgi and Casolino.[4] In another study, ultrasonographic registration was utilized in conjunction with a frameless stereotactic neuronavigation system.[12] The authors used a computer system where CT or MR data were reconstructed in a new plane according to the location and orientation of the ultrasound probe. Subsequently, reformatted CT or MR data were superimposed with intraoperative information obtained by the ultrasound, allowing real-time adjustment of preoperatively acquired imaging data.

Comeau and colleagues[13] reported their experience with mapping intraoperative ultrasound information to preoperative MR and CT data. In a recent report by the same group, the authors showed that homologous points may be mapped from the intraoperative to the preoperative image space with an accuracy of better than 2 mm.[14] A similar accuracy of 1.36 mm was also reported by Pallatroni et al.[15] However, the greatest potential error is caused by intraoperative brain shift and not by reconstruction of the target. To eliminate this problem, Roberts et al[16] suggested the use of a computational method

racy between MR and ultrasound is between 1 and 2 mm. The first step is to align landmarks that typically do not shift (e.g., falx, choroid plexus) to make certain the ultrasound image corresponds to the same MR anatomy (Fig. 16–3). The boundaries of the lesion on ultrasound are marked and this also appears on the MR scan (Fig. 16–4). As the resection proceeds, the brain shift at different depths can be calculated, and this is configured when using the navigation probe to correct for the degree of shift (Fig. 16–5). Color Doppler may be used to visualize arteries (Fig. 16–6).

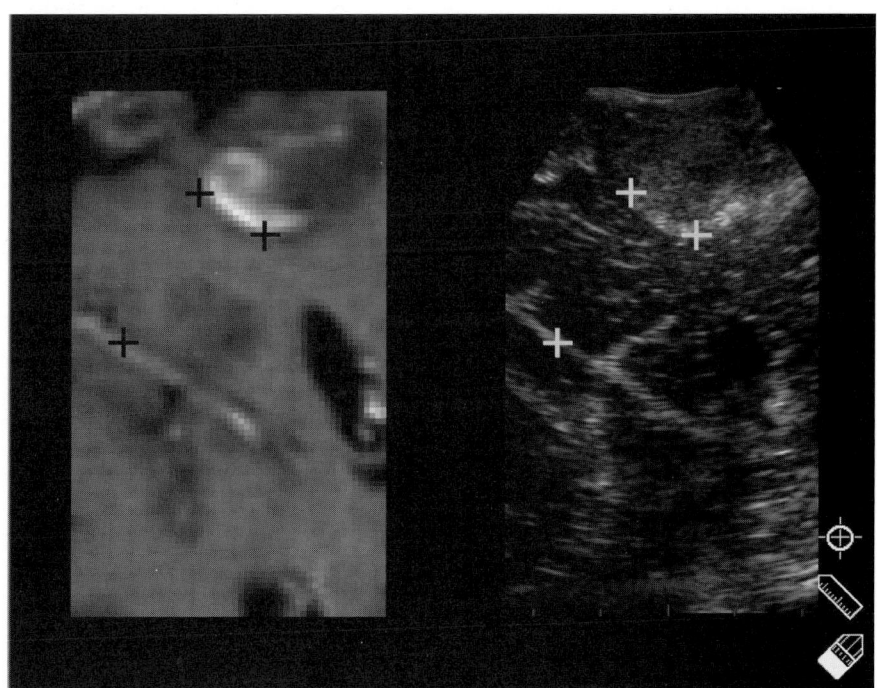

FIGURE 16–3. Preresection image demonstrating that the falx is in perfect alignment on both ultrasound and magnetic resonance, indicating excellent registration accuracy.

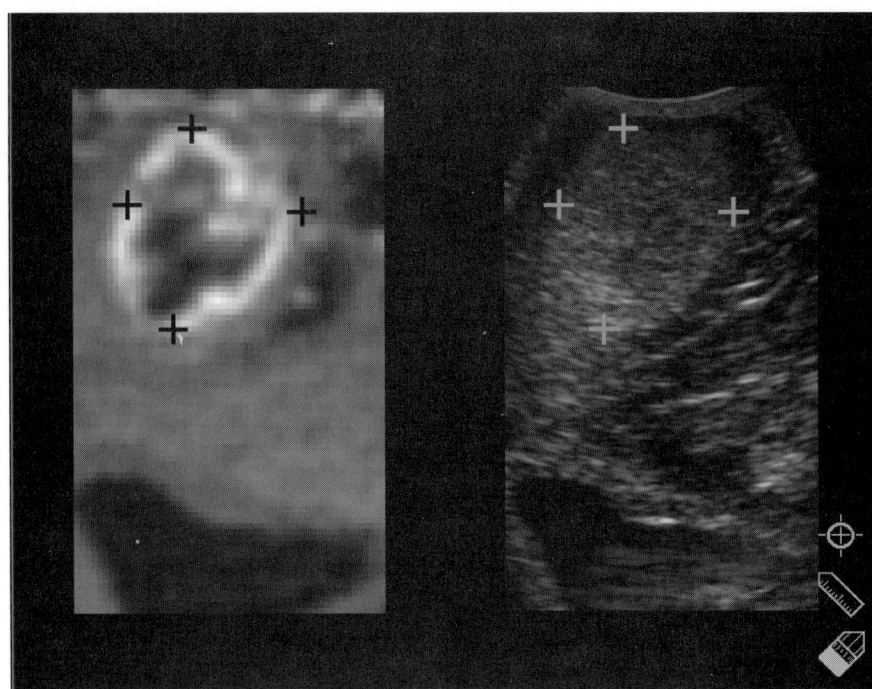

FIGURE 16–4. Preresection intraoperative ultrasound demonsrating the margins of the lesion.

based on data from intraoperative ultrasound and by tracking cortical displacement with digital images.

■ Conclusions

Despite extensive developments in image-guided surgery, it is still unclear whether patients harboring brain tumors benefit from the use of neuronavigation techniques in terms of lower morbidity, quality of life, and overall disease control. These issues, in addition to cost-effectiveness, have yet to be evaluated in prospective randomized studies. With their current use, intraoperative image-guidance techniques help the neurosurgeon in planning and performing surgery as well as in evaluating the extent of resection. In addition, the refinement

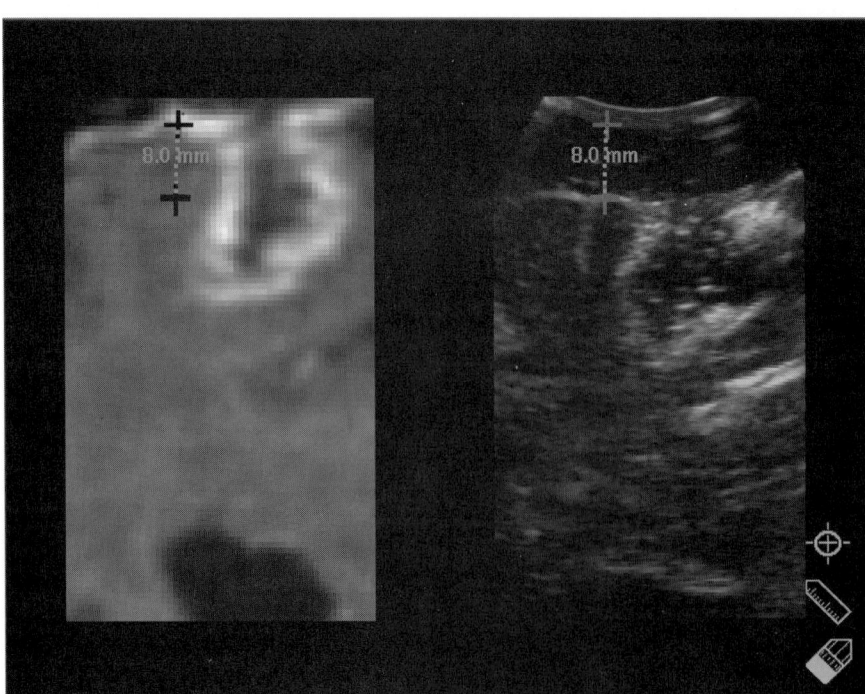

FIGURE 16–5. Following resection, the cortical surface has shifted.

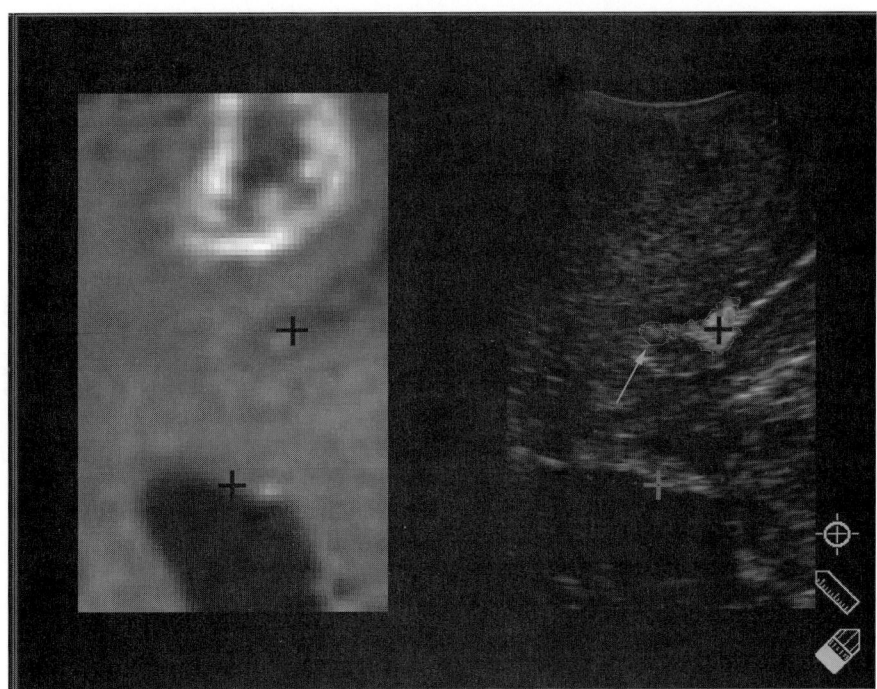

FIGURE 16–6. MR (left) and Doppler (right) demonstrating an artery in the subarachnoid space seen on the Doppler image (arrow).

of surgical navigation methods will enable the precise delivery of multimodal therapies including cell transplants, chemotherapeutics, and molecular tools for gene therapy.[17–19]

REFERENCES

1. Dohrmann GJ, Rubin JM. History of intraoperative ultrasound in neurosurgery. *Neurosurg Clin North Am* 2001;12(1):155–166.
2. Raghavendra BN, Epstein FJ, McCleary L. Intramedullary spinal cord tumors in children: localization by intraoperative sonography. *Am J Neuroradiol* 1884;5:395–397.
3. Zakhary R, Keles GE, Berger MS. Intraoperative imaging techniques in the treatment of brain tumors. *Current Opinion in Oncology* 1999;11(3):152–156.
4. Giorgi C, Casolino DS. Preliminary clinical experience with intraoperative stereotactic ultrasound imaging. *Stereotact Funct Neurosurg* 1997;68:54–58.
5. Roessler K, Ungersboeck K, Czech T, et al. Contour-guided brain tumor surgery using a stereotactic navigating microscope. *Stereotact Funct Neurosurg* 1997;68:33–38.
6. Dorward NL, Alberti O, Palmer JD, Kitchen ND, Thomas DGT. Accuracy of true frameless stereotaxy: in vivo measurement and laboratory phantom studies. *J Neurosurg* 1999;90:160–168.
7. Gumprecht HK, Widenka DC, Lumenta CB. BrainLab VectorVision neuronavigation system: technology and clinical experiences in 131 cases. *Neurosurgery* 1999;44:97–105.
8. Roberts DW, Hartov A, Kennedy FE, Miga MI, Paulsen KD. Intraoperative brain shift and deformation: a quantitative analysis of cortical displacement in 28 cases. *Neurosurgery* 1998;43:749–760.
9. Trobaugh J, Richard W, Smith K, Bucholz R. Frameless stereotactic ultrasonography. *Comput Med Imag Graph* 1994;18:235–246.
10. Zamorano LJ, Nolte L, Kadi AM, Jiang Z. Interactive intraoperative localization using an infrared-based system. *Neurol Res* 1993;15:290–298.
11. Oikarinen J, Alakuijala J, Louhisalmi Y, Sallinen S, Helminen H, Koivukangas J. The Oulu neuronavigator system: intraoperative ultrasonography in the verification and neurosurgical localization and visualization. In: Maciunas RJ, ed. *Interactive Image-Guided Neurosurgery*. Park Ridge, IL: American Association of Neurological Surgeons; 1993:233–246.
12. Hata N, Dohi T, Iseki H, Takakura K. Development of a frameless and armless stereotactic neuronavigation system with ultrasonographic registration. *Neurosurgery* 1997;41:608–614.
13. Comeau RM, Fenster A, Peters TM. Intraoperative US in interactive image-guided neurosurgery. *Radiographics* 1998;18:1019–1027.
14. Comeau RM, Sadikot AF, Fenster A, Peters TM. Intraoperative ultrasound for guidance and tissue shift correction in image-guided neurosurgery. *Med Phys* 2000;27(4):787–800.
15. Pallatroni H, Hartov A, McInerney J, et al. Co-registered ultrasound as a neurosurgical guide. *Stereotact Funct Neurosurg* 1999;73:143–147.
16. Roberts DW, Miga MI, Hartov A, et al. Intraoperatively updated neuroimaging using brain modeling and sparse data. *Neurosurgery* 1999;45:1199–1207.
17. Colombo F, Zanusso M, Casentini L, et al. Gene stereotactic neurosurgery for recurrent malignant gliomas. *Stereotact Funct Neurosurg* 1997;68:245–251.
18. Kelly P. Stereotactic procedures for molecular neurosurgery. *Exp Neurol* 1997;144:157–159.
19. Zlokovic B, Apuzzo M. Cellular and molecular neurosurgery: pathways from concept to reality, II: Vector systems and delivery methodologies for gene therapy of the central nervous system. *Neurosurgery* 1997;40:805–812.

17

Intraoperative Image Update by Magnetic Resonance Imaging

CHRISTOPHER NIMSKY, OLIVER GANSLANDT, AND RUDOLF FAHLBUSCH

Magnetic resonance imaging (MRI), in comparison to computed tomography (CT) and ultrasound, provides multiplanar imaging with a high soft-tissue resolution. It is generally accepted that MRI is the method of choice for the preoperative diagnostic evaluation of intracranial tumors. However, the closed-bore superconducting cylindrical design of MR scanners, with relatively long imaging times and difficult patient access, prevented their intraoperative application when MRI was introduced in clinical diagnostics. As a result, intraoperative imaging for evaluation of the resection completeness of a tumor was first investigated by ultrasound[1-3] and CT,[4-8] but the initial imaging quality and lesional resolution were not very satisfactory.

The development of MR systems with an open configuration has initiated the adaptation of these systems to the operating room (OR). Black and colleagues introduced a dedicated MRI system for intraoperative use in neurosurgery at Boston's Brigham and Women's Hospital.[9] Their MR scanner was developed in collaboration with the General Electric Company. The GE scanner (0.5 Tesla Signa SP) has solved the problem of patient access in a cylindrical MR system with the so-called double doughnut design. The central segment of the cylindrical system is removed, allowing patient access through this vertical gap. An alternative to the design of a dedicated MR system for intraoperative use was our adaptation of an open MR scanner that was originally designed for diagnostic use only. The 0.2 Tesla Magnetom Open scanner (Siemens AG, Erlangen, Germany) was adapted for intraoperative implementation in cooperation with the Siemens company and the departments of neurosurgery at the Universities of Heidelberg and Erlangen.[10-11] The unit has a biplanar magnet design that uses a resistive magnet. The C-shaped design with a horizontal gap allows wider access for patients.

The initial Erlangen concept,[12] developed in 1994, was based on the installation of the MR scanner in a twin-operating theater in combination with two neuronavigation systems, which allowed intraoperative imaging in combination with frameless stereotaxy, so-called neuronavigation. Subsequently the Magnetom Open was installed in our OR in 1995. Soon thereafterafter, we incorporated magnetoencephalography (MEG) and functional MRI (fMRI), which allowed intraoperative identification of eloquent brain areas, a method also known as functional neuronavigation.[13-16]

Rubino et al[17] were the first to report on the extension of this concept of surgery in the fringe field of the Magnetom Open scanner, which we had introduced for transsphenoidal procedures. They performed open cranium procedures directly on the MR table, with the head placed near the 5 Gauss line but without using additional neuronavigation guidance. In spring 1999, we began performing open cranium surgery in the fringe field of the MR scanner using the new NC4 navigation microscope (Carl Zeiss AG, Oberkochen, Germany), which could be operated in the low-magnetic field and rendered lengthy intraoperative patient transport unnecessary.[18]

To date, intraoperative MRI has been investigated in over 300 patients. Like other groups of investigators[9,11,17,19-23] we have not observed any negative effects of intraoperative MRI. In our experience, intraoperative

MRI is indicated in the surgical treatment of gliomas, especially low-grade gliomas, ventricular tumors, epilepsy,[24] and complicated pituitary tumors. Furthermore, intraoperative MRI could be used to compensate for the effects of brain shift, if in complicated cases tumor remnants were to be localized in the surgical field and ongoing neuronavigational guidance was needed.[25,26] Further indications, not yet investigated by our group, may be biopsy procedures with additional therapy control provided by the scanner (e.g., temperature monitoring in cryo- or laserablation).[19,21] This chapter focuses on our experiences using intraoperative MRI for resection control in transsphenoidal pituitary surgery and in glioma surgery.

■ Operating Room Setup for Intraoperative Magnetic Resonance Imaging

The initial setup of the twin-operating theater (Fig. 17–1) included a conventional OR allowing surgery with magnetically incompatible instruments and microscopes. Two neuronavigation systems could be used in this conventional OR: a pointer-based system (StealthStation, Medtronic SofamorDanek, Boulder, CO, USA), and a microscope-based system (MKM, Carl Zeiss AG, Oberkochen, Germany). The MR scanner (0.2 Tesla Magnetom Open, Siemens AG, Erlangen, Germany) was placed in an adjacent radio frequency-shielded OR that was specially designed for the requirements of intraoperative MRI. With this setup the patient could be placed in three basic positions for surgery: (1) directly inside the scanner, used in interventional procedures such as biopsies only; (2) on the extended table of the MR scanner in the fringe field, which was initially used in transsphenoidal surgery or for catheter placements only; and (3) in the adjacent conventional operating theater, necessitating intraoperative patient transport. A specially designed air-cushioned OR table allowed intraoperative movement (over a distance of 4 to 5 meters) of a patient with an open cranium from the conventional OR to the MR scanner for imaging. This separation of operating site and imaging site was necessary because in

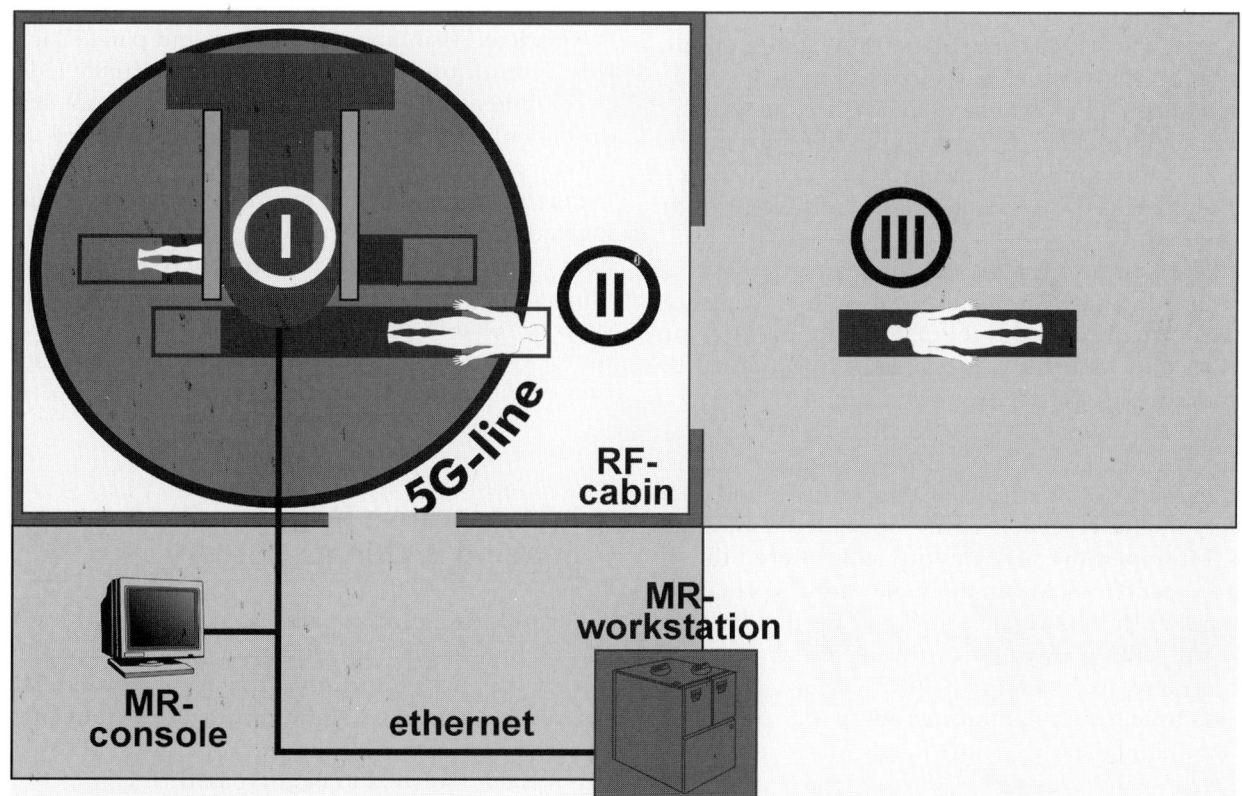

FIGURE 17–1. Operating theater setup with a 0.2 Tesla Magnetom Open MR scanner. There are three possible operating sites: (I) inside the scanner for interventional procedures, (II) at the 5 Gauss line for transsphenoidal surgery and craniotomy procedures using the NC4 navigation microscope, and (III) in the adjacent conventional operating room using the robotic MKM microscope (Zeiss, Oberkochen, Germany).

1995, microscope-based neuronavigation was available only in the form of the MR-incompatible MKM microscope. Since the introduction of the NC4 neuronavigation microscope, which can be used in the fringe field of the scanner, nearly all surgeries are performed in the radio frequency-shielded OR near the 5 Gauss line.[18] Rather than lengthy intraoperative patient transport for imaging, the MR table itself is moved into the center of the MR scanner in less than half a minute.

■ Intraoperative Magnetic Resonance Imaging in Transsphenoidal Surgery

Until now, only anecdotal reports on the use of intraoperative MRI in transsphenoidal pituitary surgery were published.[10,22,27–29] We investigated a series of 50 patients with large intra- and suprasellar, mainly hormonally inactive, pituitary tumors (44 adenomas, 6 craniopharyngiomas), which were operated using a transsphenoidal approach.[30] The patient was lying directly on the MR table of the scanner; a standard flexible coil was placed around the patient's head, which was embedded in a cushion. To obtain images in coronal and sagittal planes, T1-weighted spin echo sequences (slice thickness: 3 mm, TR: 340 ms, TE: 26 ms, FOV: 200 mm, matrix: 192×256) were measured. Optionally a T2-weighted turbo spin-echo sequence (slice thickness: 3 mm, TR: 5700 ms, TE: 117 ms, FOV: 230 mm, matrix: 224×256) was applied, allowing better delineation in cystic lesions and in cases where there was blood in the resection cavity.

In 72% of these 50 patients, intraoperative MRI allowed an ultra-early evaluation of tumor resection, which is normally only possible 2 to 3 months after surgery. A second look (i.e., a repeated inspection of the surgical field, $n = 24$) for suspected tumor remnants in the adenoma patients led to further resection in 15 patients (34%) (Fig. 17–2). However, image artifacts caused by metal debris from drilling or by blood accumulation in the resection cavity presented some challenges. Intraoperative MRI undoubtedly offered the option of a second look within the same surgical procedure if incomplete tumor resection was suspected. This improved the rate of procedures during which complete tumor removal was achieved. Furthermore, for those with incomplete tumor removal, additional treatments could be planned early—immediately following surgery. In contrast to intraoperative imaging, early postoperative MR studies performed a few days after surgery failed to show reliably the extent of the resection. In a significant proportion of cases, the extent of the mass lesion even exceeded its presurgery dimensions.[31] Therefore both early CT and early MR investigations are unsuitable means to assess the extent of tumor resections. Intraoperative imaging is advantageous in that it is comparable to delayed postoperative investigations, which are generally accepted as the standard diagnostic postoperative procedures.

Intraoperative MR in transsphenoidal surgery is most indicated for large tumors with a distinctive suprasellar extension. In the case of drilling artifacts, which may impede proper image interpretation, it is possible to evaluate the extent of the suprasellar resection, but intra- and parasellar structures may not be easily identified. Immediately following the resection of a pituitary tumor a swelling of the cavernous sinus may occur due to the movement of the compressed sinus into the resection cavity. This can impede proper interpretation of the extent of intrasellar resection. Small intrasellar lesions or lesions that invade the cavernous sinus are not ideal candidates for intraoperative MRI because it is very difficult to differentiate between remaining tumor, normal pituitary gland, structures of the cavernous sinus, and blood remaining in the resection cavity. Perhaps in these difficult cases intraoperative sonography will be of further help. Furthermore, intraoperative Doppler sonography offers the possibility to visualize the relation to vascular structures in real-time mode.[32–33]

Restricted visibility of the supra- and parasellar tumor extension in transsphenoidal surgery initially led to the development of mirrors to enhance the visual field. Endoscopes used in transsphenoidal surgery[34–35] further enhance the extent of the visual field and are a classic means of intraoperative imaging. But tumor remnants located in, for example, a suprasellar fold may not be visible, even with modern sophisticated endoscopic techniques. In these selected cases intraoperative MRI provides a reliable possibility to assess the extent of the tumor resection and may further improve the high efficacy of transsphenoidal microsurgery.

■ Intraoperative Magnetic Resonance Imaging in Glioma Surgery

All groups using intraoperative MR in recent years have shared the view that investigations in glioma patients are one of the main indications for intraoperative MR. Initial results published showed that the extent of tumor removal was increased by intraoperative MR[23,36]; even survival time seemed to be increased.[23]

For glioma surgery, our own group has combined intraoperative imaging with integrated functional neuronavigational support. On the one hand, MRI provides quality control to evaluate the extent of the resection; neuronavigation with integrated functional data, on the

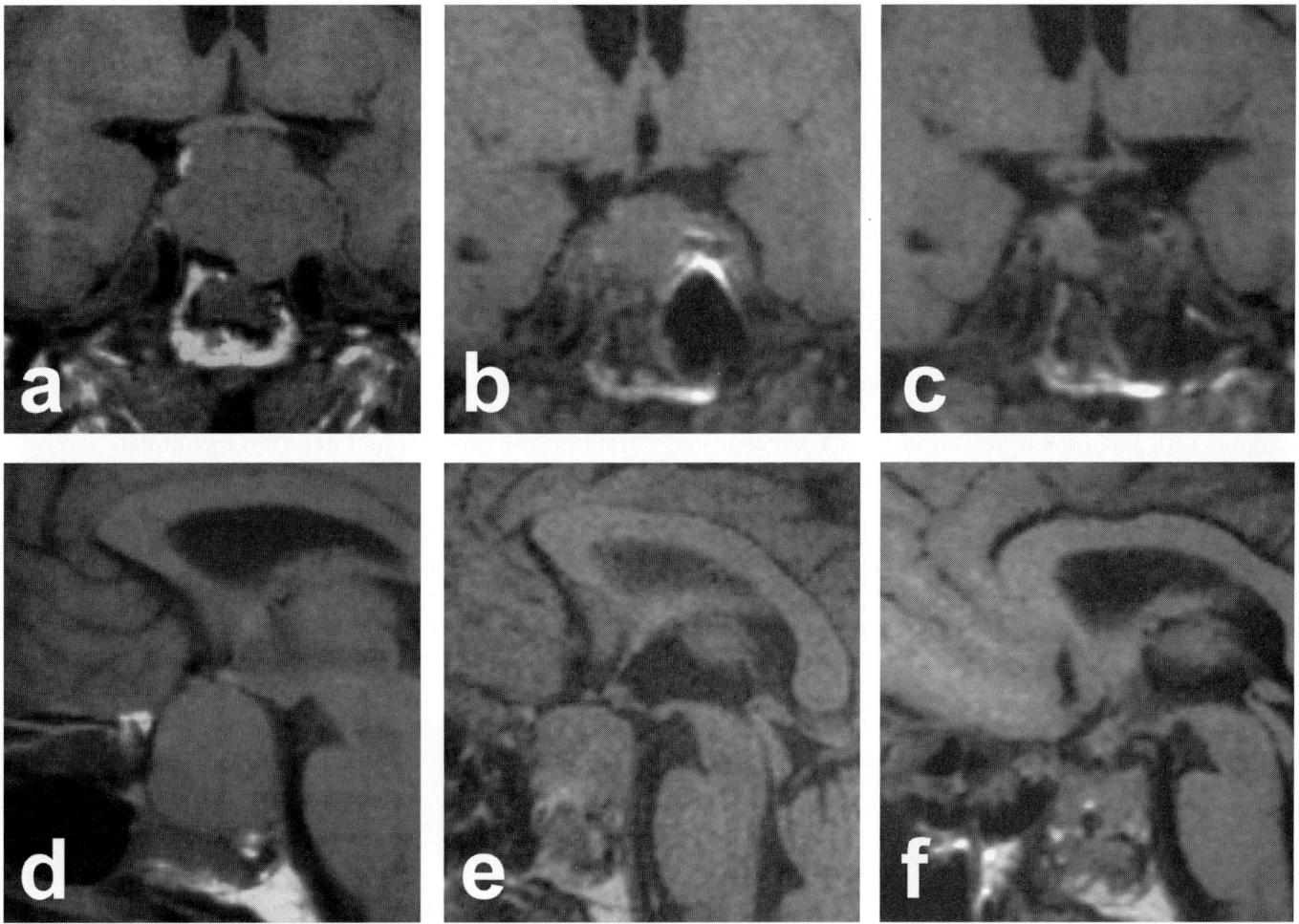

FIGURE 17–2. 51-year-old male with a large intra-, supra-, and parasellar, hormonally inactive pituitary adenoma. (A,D). Preoperative scans. (B,E). Intraoperative scans depict some remaining tumor. (C,F). After a second look and further tumor removal repeated imaging showed complete removal with preservation of the pituitary gland.

other hand, prevents too extensive resections, which would otherwise result in severe neurological deficits.[37]

The locations of eloquent brain areas such as the motor cortex, the sensory cortex, speech-related areas, and the visual cortex were displayed intraoperatively in the neurosurgeon's field of view using the heads-up display of the neuronavigation microscopes. To accomplish this "functional neuronavigation," the functional data, which were obtained by MEG[13–15] or fMRI,[16] were integrated into the anatomical MR data set that was normally used for neuronavigation. All the functional data were registered with the anatomical three-dimensional (3-D) data set using a contour fit algorithm.[38] The functional data were displayed in the anatomical dataset by markers inserted into the MR images. A pyramid or cube in the MR volume with white or black intensity accordingly represented a functional modality. The patient was registered with the navigation microscope (MKM or NC4-microscope with SMN-system, navigational software STP4.0; Zeiss, Oberkochen, Germany) at the beginning of surgery. The contours of the lesion, the predefined surgical approach, and the segmented markers for functional data were displayed using the heads-up display of the microscopes.

For imaging, the head was fixed in an MR-compatible ceramic head holder. A separable MR coil was used for imaging. The upper part of this coil, which can be sterilized, is applied just before the patient is moved into the center of the scanner for imaging. Routinely, a T1-weighted 3-D-FLASH (fast low-angle shot) gradient-echo sequence (TE: 7.0 ms, TR: 16.1 ms, flip angle: 30 degrees, slab 168 mm, 112 slices, FOV: 250 mm, matrix: 256×256) was used for imaging. This 3-D sequence allows free reformatting so that standard projections, independent from intraoperative head positioning, can be obtained. This facilitated comparison with the preoperative images to distinguish between remaining tumor and contrast media enhancements due to surgical manipulations at the resection border. Furthermore, in certain cases (especially in low-grade glioma) two-dimensional T2-weighted and inversion recovery sequences were applied. MR contrast agent (20 mL gadolinium-DTPA intravenously), which was given just prior to scanning, was administered if the tumor showed enhancement in the preoperative images. In the case of repeated imaging during one operation, contrast medium was not repeatedly given because otherwise severe interpretation artifacts occurred.

In our series of 96 glioma patients intraoperative MRI revealed incomplete tumor removal in 64%. In 29 of 61 patients with incomplete resection (48%), we repeated inspection of the surgical field. This reinspection led to further resection in 23 patients, in 14 of which we achieved total removal. This could increase the rate of gross total removal from 81 to 94% ($n = 16$) for World Health Organization (WHO) grade I gliomas. In grade II gliomas ($n = 32$) further tumor removal was performed in 16 patients. In 10 of these, we achieved complete removal. Thus the gross total removal rate in grade II gliomas increased from 25 to 56%. In the remaining 6 patients, despite further tumor removal, complete resection was not possible due to small tumor remnants infiltrating eloquent brain areas. In high-grade gliomas the extent of resection was enlarged in only 5 patients, resulting in an increased removal rate of 47 versus 42% in grade III gliomas and 24 versus 21% in grade IV patients (Fig. 17–3).

In nine of the low-grade gliomas (WHO grades I and II) the resection could not be extended primarily because eloquent brain areas were infiltrated. In the majority (29 out of 34) of the high-grade gliomas, where intraoperative imaging had depicted incomplete removal, it was the policy above all to avoid new neurological deficits.

Although it was sometimes difficult to depict the completeness of a resection in the T1-weighted 3-D images, especially in the grade II gliomas, in all of these cases the inversion recovery and dark fluid sequences were of sup-

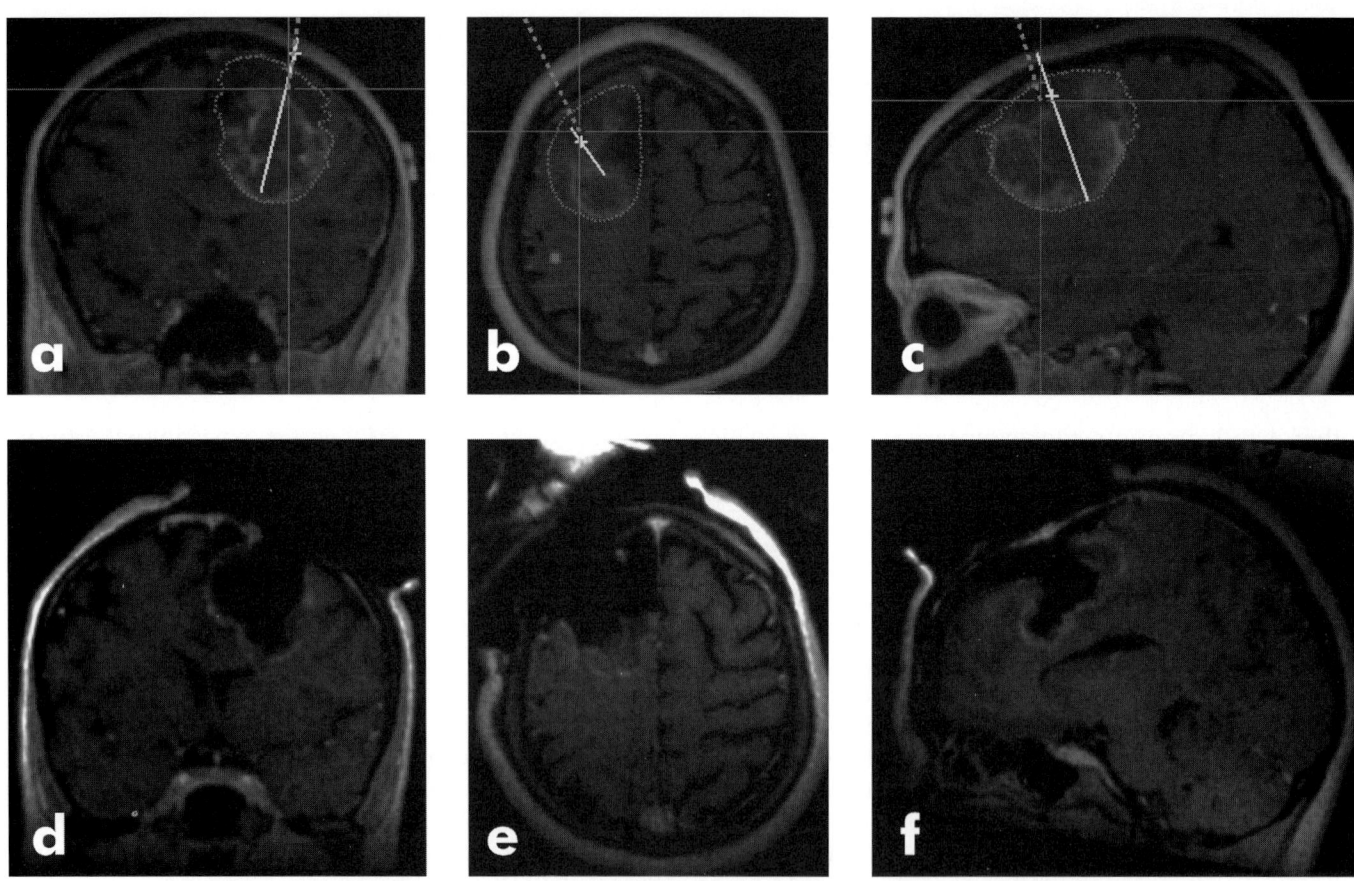

FIGURE 17–3. 31-year-old female with a right frontal glioblastoma. (A,B,C). Coronal/axial/sagittal display of the navigation screen. In (B) small black and white dots around the central region are markers from functional investigations, allowing functional neuronavigation. (D,E,F). Corresponding intraoperative images showing contrast enhancement at the resection border and some remaining tumor at the dorsal aspect and toward the corpus callosum.

plementary value in the evaluation of tumor resection. On the other hand application of contrast media in the high-grade gliomas often resulted in difficulties in image interpretation due to contrast media leakage and spreading into the borderline of the resection cavity (in 14 out of the 41). The comparison with preoperative scans, which were measured in the same fashion, and which after registration[39] could be displayed along the intraoperative images, provided valuable information for image interpretation. It was important to know, for example, whether special hemostyptic materials were applied or "contrast-media-loaded" blood could be detected at the resection border or in the resection cavity.[40] Perhaps new contrast media will prevent the surgically induced contrast enhancement in the future.[41]

Functional neuronavigation in cases where the tumor was located near eloquent areas allowed for preservation of neurological function.[13–16] We encountered an aggravation of the neurological deficit in only one patient of this subgroup with combined usage of intraoperative MRI and functional neuronavigation. In four other patients who did not receive functional neuronavigation support, neurological deterioration occurred.

Anatomical and functional neuronavigation were used as guidance to identify relevant structures. Intraoperative MRI allowed delineation of the extent of resection. The combination of both allowed the maximum possible resection with the least neurological deficits,[37] while taking into account incomplete tumor removal, when eloquent brain areas were infiltrated.

Based on our experience with intraoperative MR evaluation of glioma removal, we doubt the benefit of intraoperative MRI in high-grade glioma surgeries, although initial reports published on this topic claim a benefit even in such surgeries.[23,42] Controversial reports on life expectancy in high-grade gliomas emphasize that life expectancy is more dependent on low postoperative deficits than on macroscopic total tumor removal.[43] On the other hand, even though complete resection at a microscopic level is also not possible for low-grade gliomas, survival of these patients seems to be highly correlated with the extent of the tumor resection.[44–47] We believe that surgery of these tumors will benefit from intraoperative imaging. It is still too early to determine the effects on life expectancy in this subgroup, but it can be stated that more radical resections are possible with lower morbidity, especially when intraoperative imaging is supported by the use of functional neuronavigation.

■ Brain Shift and Image Updating

Tumor removal, brain swelling, the use of brain retractors, and cerebrospinal fluid drainage all result in an intraoperative brain deformation that is known as brain shift.[48–50] Thus the accuracy of neuronavigation systems relying on preoperative image data decreases during the surgical procedure. Intraoperative image data represent the real-time anatomical situation and therefore may allow surgeons to evaluate and visualize the extent of, and perhaps compensate for, the effects of, brain shift.[25–26]

In a case of suspected remaining tumor, five MR-visible bone fiducials (Howmedica-Leibinger, Freiburg, Germany) were placed around the craniotomy opening prior to intraoperative scanning. This allowed the intraoperative registration of the new image data to update neuronavigation. In selected cases, such as residual tumor and the possibility of further resection, the intraoperative images were used for an update of the neuronavigation system. The intraoperative 3-D MRI data were transferred via ethernet to the navigation system, and these images were registered with the help of the bone fiducials. If the tumor remnant was easily localized in the surgical field, a second inspection was performed without further neuronavigation to economize the procedure. The neuronavigation update added roughly 15 minutes to the operating time, including the time for image transfer, segmentation of suspected remaining tumor, defining the surgical approach, and re-referencing.

In a series of 16 glioma patients, we used intraoperative MRI to perform an intraoperative update of the neuronavigation system. In all of them the updating of the neuronavigation system with the intraoperative MR data was successful (Fig. 17–4). It led to reliable neuronavigation with high accuracy; the mean registration error of the update procedure was 1.1 mm. In all patients the area suspicious for remaining tumor was reached. Histopathological examination revealed tumor in 14 of these 16 patients. A final complete tumor removal could be achieved in 12 patients. In the remaining cases, an extension of the tumor into eloquent brain areas prevented a macroscopic complete excision. Updating a neuronavigation system with intraoperative MRI compensated reliably for the effects of brain shift.

Due to the intraoperative image update of the neuronavigation system the functional markers, which were integrated into the preoperative MR data set, are lost. To preserve the functional data for the updated navigation, pre- and intraoperative MR images have to be registered, and the new position of the functional markers has to be calculated. Initial attempts to establish an automatic algorithm for the transfer of functional markers into the intraoperative MR images have been successful.[51] Current work concentrates on an acceleration of this algorithm to allow intraoperative application without significant time delay. This integration of functional

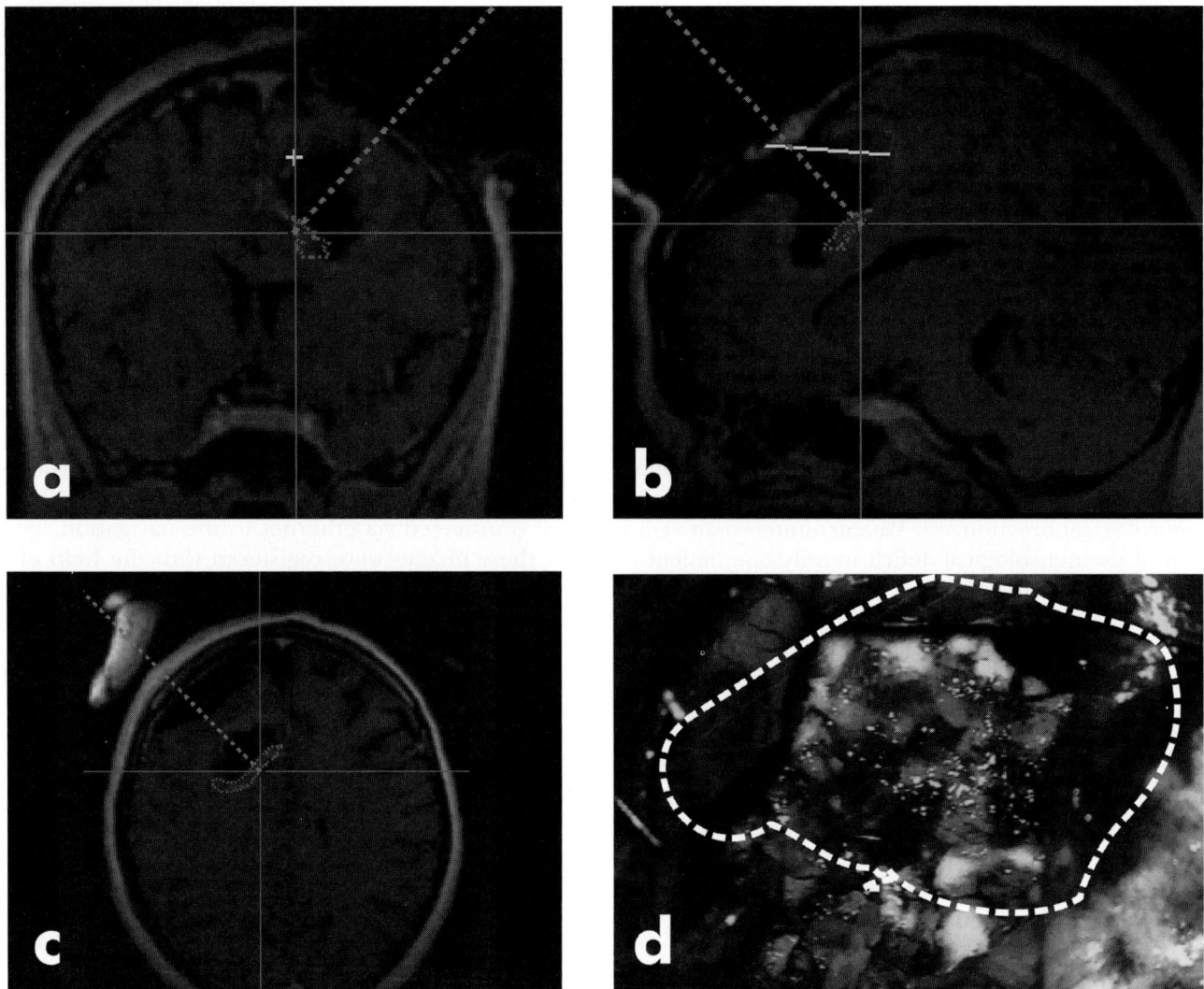

FIGURE 17–4. Intraoperative update of the neuronavigation with intraoperative image data (see Fig. 17–3). (A,B,C). Coronal, sagittal, and axial display of the updated navigation screen. (D). Intraoperative view with some of the remaining tumor segmented and displayed (the outline of the contour was enhanced for better reproduction).

data into intraoperative images is an important step for image updating in the future, when data about vascular structures and from white matter structure, measured by diffusion weighted imaging,[52–54] are integrated into the navigational setup and will therefore also have to be updated intraoperatively to compensate for brain shift.

Other attempts to compensate for the effects of brain shift rely on mathematical models that try to describe the behavior of the brain under surgery. They are primarily based on finite element techniques. Either so-called sparse data or data from intraoperative ultrasound images are input for the mathematical models to deform high-quality preoperative MRI data.[55–57] Comparing these deformed MR data with the real intraoperative MR images allows for evaluation and further refinement of the mathematical models.

■ Other Intraoperative Imaging Modalities

Regardless which MR system is compared with other imaging modalities, intraoperative MRI is without doubt the most advanced intraoperative imaging modality available. Ultrasound[1–3] provides real-time data at lower costs, but despite recent advances in image quality, soft-tissue contrast and signal-to-noise ratio in MRI are still superior to ultrasound.[58] The difficulties of 3-D orientation of ultrasound imaging may soon be resolved by integrating ultrasound with neuronavigation systems and by appliying 3-D ultrasound transducer abilities, which possibly can also compensate for the effects of brain shift.[59–60] High-end ultrasound systems are able to visualize not only tissue, but also vessels and flow in real time and therefore will be an important imaging modality addition in the OR setup of the future.[61]

Intraoperative CT, either with fixed systems as originally introduced[6–8,62] or on tracks,[5] or the recently presented system of mobile CT,[4,63–64] does not require special instruments except for radiation-compatible head fixation. However, low soft-tissue resolution as well as missing free-slice orientation and the need for x-ray protection requirements are major drawbacks compared with intraoperative MRI. Intraoperative CT has its advantages in the evaluation of bony structures, making it highly suitable for imaging in spine surgery.[65]

■ High-Field Magnetic Resonance

The next step in intraoperative MRI is the introduction of high-field MR systems into the operating theater. High-field MR scanners are the standard in neuroradiology diagnosis. They offer not only better image quality than the low-field systems, but also a wider range of sequences, including measurement modalities not available in a low-field system. This includes MR angiography, fMRI, diffusion-weighted imaging, and MR spectroscopy. With the rapid fall off of the static magnetic field achieved by actively shielded magnet design, it is possible to site a superconducting system in the near proximity of the surgical work space.[20]

Preliminary results demonstrated that the introduction of high-field MR scanners into the neurosurgical OR is feasible.[66–69] Whether the whole imaging armamentarium of a high-field scanner can be applied intraoperatively remains an open question. High-field MR scanners provide a possibility for an intraoperative image update in shorter times and perhaps with more information than just standard anatomical imaging. Intraoperative evaluation of pathways and function may be possible. We are planning the installation of a high-field MR scanner into our OR environment. With an OR table, which is adapted to a standard 1.5 Tesla MR scanner, surgery will be performed at the 5 Gauss line, allowing full neuronavigational support. An automatic registration of the patient with the intraoperative MR images, where the operating table may serve as a reference, should be possible. This should allow nearly instantaneous image updating, compensating for the effects of brain shift and providing anatomical and functional information about the current situation.

Although high-field MR seems to be the upcoming challenge for intraoperative imaging, major advancements in the future, besides integration of all manner of functional and anatomical data, including data from sophisticated brain atlases, may be new developments in MR technology. Extreme low-field MR technology with magnetic field strengths of 10 mT, via the so-called Overhauser effect,[70] may open new avenues for intraoperative imaging because small, "invisible" MR scanners that are below the operating table (and thus will not impair surgical maneuvers) will then become possible.

REFERENCES

1. Hammoud MA, Ligon BL, elSouki R, Shi WM, Schomer DF, Sawaya R. Use of intraoperative ultrasound for localizing tumors and determining the extent of resection: a comparative study with magnetic resonance imaging. *J Neurosurg* 1996;84(5):737–741.
2. LeRoux PD, Winter TC, Berger MS, Mack LA, Wang K, Elliott JP. A comparison between preoperative magnetic resonance and intraoperative ultrasound tumor volumes and margins. *J Clin Ultrasound* 1994;22(1):29–36.
3. Woydt M, Krone A, Becker G, Schmidt K, Roggendorf W, Roosen K. Correlation of intraoperative ultrasound with histopathologic findings after tumour resection in supratentorial gliomas: a method to improve gross total tumour resection. *Acta Neurochir* 1996;138(12):1391–1398.
4. Grunert P, Muller-Forell W, Darabi K, et al. Basic principles and clinical applications of neuronavigation and intraoperative computed tomography. *Comput Aided Surg* 1998;3(4):166–173.
5. Kabuto M, Kubota T, Kobayashi H, et al. Intraoperative CT imaging system using a mobile CT scanner gantry mounted on floor-embedded rails for neurosurgery. *No To Shinkei* 1998;50(11):1003–1008.
6. Lunsford LD, Parrish R, Albright L. Intraoperative imaging with a therapeutic computed tomographic scanner. *Neurosurgery* 1984;15(4):559–561.
7. Lunsford LD, Rosenbaum AE, Perry J. Stereotactic surgery using the "therapeutic" CT scanner. *Surg Neurol* 1982;18(2):116–122.
8. Okudera H, Kobayashi S, Kyoshima K, Gibo H, Takemae T, Sugita K. Development of the operating computerized tomographic scanner system for neurosurgery. *Acta Neurochir* 1991;111(1–2):61–63.
9. Black PM, Moriarty T, Alexander E III, et al. Development and implementation of intraoperative magnetic resonance imaging and its neurosurgical applications. *Neurosurgery* 1997;41(4):831–845.
10. Steinmeier R, Fahlbusch R, Ganslandt O, et al. Intraoperative magnetic resonance imaging with the Magnetom Open scanner: concepts, neurosurgical indications, and procedures: a preliminary report. *Neurosurgery* 1998;43(4):739–748.
11. Tronnier VM, Wirtz CR, Knauth M, et al. Intraoperative diagnostic and interventional magnetic resonance imaging in neurosurgery. *Neurosurgery* 1997;40(5):891–902.
12. Fahlbusch R, Nimsky C, Ganslandt O, Steinmeier R, Buchfelder M, Huk W. The erlangen concept of image-guided surgery. In: Lemke H, Vannier M, Inamura K, Farman A, eds. *CAR '98*. Amsterdam: Elsevier Science BV; 1998:583–588.
13. Ganslandt O, Fahlbusch R, Nimsky C, et al. Functional neuronavigation with magnetoencephalography: outcome in 50 patients with lesions around the motor cortex. *J Neurosurg* 1999;91(1):73–79.
14. Ganslandt O, Steinmeier R, Kober H, et al. Magnetic source imaging combined with image-guided frameless stereotaxy: a new

method in surgery around the motor strip. *Neurosurgery* 1997;41(3):621–628.
15. Möller M, Kober H, Ganslandt O, Nimsky C, Vieth J, Fahlbusch R. Functional mapping of speech evoked brain activity by magnetoencephalography and its clinical application. *Biomed Tech (Berlin)* 1999;44(suppl):159–161.
16. Nimsky C, Ganslandt O, Kober H, et al. Integration of functional magnetic resonance imaging supported by magnetoencephalography in functional neuronavigation. *Neurosurgery* 1999;44:1249–1256.
17. Rubino GJ, Farahani K, McGill D, Van De Wiele B, Villablanca JP, Wang-Mathieson A. Magnetic resonance imaging-guided neurosurgery in the magnetic fringe fields: the next step in neuronavigation. *Neurosurgery* 2000;46(3):643–654.
18. Nimsky C, Ganslandt O, Kober H, Buchfelder M, Fahlbusch R. Intraoperative magnetic resonance imaging combined with neuronavigation: a new concept. *Neurosurgery* 2001;48(5):1082–1091.
19. Lewin JS. Interventional MR imaging: concepts, systems, and applications in neuroradiology. *Am J Neuroradiol* 1999;20:735–748.
20. Lewin JS, Metzger A, Selman WR. Intraoperative magnetic resonance image guidance in neurosurgery. *J Magn Reson Imaging* 2000;12:512–524.
21. Schwartz RB, Hsu L, Wong TZ, et al. Intraoperative MR imaging guidance for intracranial neurosurgery: experience with the first 200 cases. *Radiology* 1999;211(2):477–488.
22. Seifert V, Zimmermann M, Trantakis C, et al. Open MRI-guided neurosurgery. *Acta Neurochir* 1999;141(5):455–464.
23. Wirtz CR, Knauth M, Staubert A, et al. Clinical evaluation and follow-up results for intraoperative magnetic resonance imaging in neurosurgery. *Neurosurgery* 2000;46(5):1112–1122.
24. Buchfelder M, Ganslandt O, Fahlbusch R, Nimsky C. Intraoperative magnetic resonance imaging in epilepsy surgery. *J Magn Reson Imaging* 2000;12:547–555.
25. Nimsky C, Ganslandt O, Cerny S, Hastreiter P, Greiner G, Fahlbusch R. Quantification of, visualization of, and compensation for brain shift using intraoperative magentic resonance imaging. *Neurosurgery* 2000;47:1070–1080.
26. Wirtz CR, Bonsanto MM, Knauth M, et al. Intraoperative magnetic resonance imaging to update interactive navigation in neurosurgery: method and preliminary experience. *Comput Aided Surg* 1997;2:172–179.
27. Bohinski RJ, Kokkino AK, Warnick RE, et al. Use of low field strength intraoperative MRI during transsphenoidal microsurgery for pituitary macroadenoma [abstract]. *Eur Radiol* 2000;10:C16.
28. Martin CH, Schwartz R, Jolesz F, Black PM. Transsphenoidal resection of pituitary adenomas in an intraoperative MRI unit. *Pituitary* 1999;2:155–162.
29. Pergolizzi R, Nabavi A, Schwartz BJ, et al. Intra-operative MR guidance during transsphenoidal pituitary resection: preliminary results. *J Magn Reson Imaging* 2001;13(1):136–141.
30. Fahlbusch R, Ganslandt O, Buchfelder M, Schott W, Nimsky C. Intraoperative magnetic resonance imaging in transsphenoidal surgery. *J Neurosurg* 2001;35(3):381–390.
31. Dina TS, Feaster SH, Laws ER, Davis DO. MR of the pituitary gland postsurgery: serial MR studies following transsphenoidal resection. *Am J Neuroradiol* 1993;14:763–769.
32. Atkinson JL, Kasperbauer JL, James EM, Lane JI, Nippoldt TB. Transcranial-transdural real-time ultrasonography during transsphenoidal resection of a large pituitary tumor: case report. *J Neurosurg* 2000;93(1):129–131.
33. Yamasaki T, Moritake K, Hatta J, Nagai H. Intraoperative monitoring with pulse Doppler ultrasonography in transsphenoidal surgery: technique application. *Neurosurgery* 1996;38(1):95–98.
34. Fahlbusch R, Heigl T, Huk W, Steinmeier R. The role of endoscopy and intraoperative MRI in transsphenoidal pituitary surgery. In: Werder v K, Fahlbusch R, eds. *Pituitary Adenomas from Basic Research to Diagnosis and Therapy*. Amsterdam: Elsevier; 1996:237–241.
35. Jho HD, Carrau RL. Endoscopic endonasal transsphenoidal surgery: experience with 50 patients. *J Neurosurg* 1997;87(1):44–51.
36. Black PM, Alexander E III, Martin C, et al. Craniotomy for tumor treatment in an intraoperative magnetic resonance imaging unit. *Neurosurgery* 1999;45(3):423–433.
37. Berger MS. Intraoperative MR imaging: making an impact on outcomes for patients with brain tumors. *Am J Neuroradiol* 2001;22(1):2.
38. Kober H, Grummich P, Vieth J. Fit of the digitized head surface with the surface reconstructed from MRI tomography. In: Baumgartner C, ed. *Biomagnetism: Fundamental Research and Clinical Applications*. Amsterdam: Elsevier Science, IOS Press; 1995:309–312.
39. Hastreiter P, Rezk-Salama C, Nimsky C, Lürig C, Greiner G, Ertl T. Registration techniques for the analysis of the brain shift in neurosurgery. *Computers and Graphics* 2000;24(3):385–389.
40. Knauth M, Aras N, Wirtz CR, Dorfler A, Engelhorn T, Sartor K. Surgically induced intracranial contrast enhancement: potential source of diagnostic error in intraoperative MR imaging. *Am J Neuroradiol* 1999;20(8):1547–1553.
41. Knauth M, Egelhof T, Roth SU, Wirtz CR, Sartor K. Monocrystalline iron oxide nanoparticles: possible solution to the problem of surgically induced intracranial contrast enhancement in intraoperative MR imaging. *Am J Neuroradiol* 2001;22(1):99–102.
42. Knauth M, Wirtz CR, Tronnier VM, Aras N, Kunze S, Sartor K. Intraoperative MR imaging increases the extent of tumor resection in patients with high-grade gliomas. *Am J Neuroradiol* 1999;20(9):1642–1646.
43. Kowalczuk A, Macdonald RL, Amidei C, et al. Quantitative imaging study of extent of surgical resection and prognosis of malignant astrocytomas. *Neurosurgery* 1997;41(5):1028–1038.
44. Berger MS, Deliganis AV, Dobbins J, Keles GE. The effect of extent of resection on recurrence in patients with low-grade cerebral hemispheric gliomas. *Cancer* 1994;74:1784–1791.
45. Karim AB, Maat B, Hatlevoll R, et al. A randomized trial on dose-response in radiation therapy of low-grade cerebral glioma: European Organization for Research and Treatment of Cancer (EORTC) study 22844. *Int J Radiat Oncol Biol Phys* 1996;36(3):549–556.
46. Nicolato A, Gerosa MA, Fina P, Iuzzolino P, Giorgiutti F, Bricolo A. Prognostic factors in low-grade supratentorial astrocytomas: a unimultivariate statistical analysis in 76 surgically treated adult patients. *Surg Neurol* 1995;44(3):208–223.
47. Piepmeier J, Christopher S, Spencer D, et al. Variations in the clinical history and survival of patients with supratentorial low-grade astrocytomas. *Neurosurgery* 1996;38(5):872–879.
48. Dorward NL, Alberti O, Velani B, et al. Postimaging brain distortion: magnitude, correlates, and impact on neuronavigation. *J Neurosurg* 1998;88(4):656–662.
49. Hill DLG, Maurer CR, Maciunas RJ, Barwise JA, Fitzpatrick JM, Wang MY. Measurement of intraoperative brain surface deformation under a craniotomy. *Neurosurgery* 1998;43(3):514–528.
50. Roberts DW, Hartov A, Kennedy FE, Miga MI, Paulsen KD. Intraoperative brain shift and deformation: a quantitative analysis of cortical displacement in 28 cases. *Neurosurgery* 1998;43(4):749–760.
51. Wolf M, Vogel T, Weierich P, Niemann H, Nimsky C. Automatic transfer of pre-operation fMRI markers into intra-operation MR-images for updating functional neuronavigation. In: Ikeuchi K, ed. *Proceedings of IAPR Workshop on Machine Vision Applications MVA2000*. Tokyo: University of Tokyo; 2000:405–408.
52. Inoue T, Shimizu H, Yoshimoto T. Imaging the pyramidal tract in patients with brain tumors. *Clin Neurol Neurosurg* 1999;101(1):4–10.
53. Karibe H, Shimizu H, Tominaga T, Koshu K, Yoshimoto T. Diffusion-weighted magnetic resonance imaging in the early evaluation

of corticospinal tract injury to predict functional motor outcome in patients with deep intracerebral hemorrhage. *J Neurosurg* 2000;92(1):58–63.
54. Virta A, Barnett A, Pierpaoli C. Visualizing and characterizing white matter fiber structure and architecture in the human pyramidal tract using diffusion tensor MRI. *Magn Reson Imaging* 1999; 17(8):1121–1133.
55. Ferrant M, Warfield SK, Nabavi A, Jolesz F, Kikinis R. Registration of 3D intraoperative MR images of the brain using a finite element biomechanical model. In: Delp SL, DiGioia AM, Jaramaz B, eds. *Medical Image Computing and Computer-Assisted Intervention—MICCAI 2000*. Berlin: Springer; 2000:19–28.
56. Miga MI, Staubert A, Paulsen KD, et al. Model-updated image-guided neurosurgery: preliminary analysis using intraoperative MR. In: Delp SL, DiGioia AM, Jaramaz B, eds. *Medical Image Computing and Computer-Assisted Intervention—MICCAI 2000*. Berlin: Springer; 2000:115–124.
57. Roberts DW, Miga MI, Hartov A, et al. Intraoperatively updated neuroimaging using brain modeling and sparse data. *Neurosurgery* 1999;45(5):1199–1207.
58. Tronnier VM, Bonsanto M, Staubert A, Knauth M, Kunze S, Wirtz CR. Comparison of intraoperative MR imaging and 3D-navigated ultrasonography in the detection and resection control of lesions. *Neurosurg Focus* 2001;10(2):Article 3.
59. Hata N, Dohi T, Iseki H, Takakura K. Development of a frameless and armless stereotactic neuronavigation system with ultrasonographic registration. *Neurosurgery* 1997;41(3):608–614.
60. Jödicke A, Deinsberger W, Erbe H, Kriete A, Böker DK. Intraoperative three-dimensional ultrasonography: an approach to register brain shift using multidimensional image processing. *Minim Invas Neurosurg* 1998;41(1):13–9.
61. Rubin JM, Quint DJ. Intraoperative US versus intraoperative MR imaging for guidance during intracranial neurosurgery. *Radiology* 2000;215(3):917–918.
62. Okudera H, Kyoshima K, Kobayashi S, Sugita K. Intraoperative CT scan findings during resection of glial tumours. *Neurol Res* 1994; 16(4):265–267.
63. Butler WE, Piaggio CM, Constantinou C, et al. A mobile computed tomographic scanner with intraoperative and intensive care unit applications. *Neurosurgery* 1998;42(6):1304–1311.
64. Matula C, Rossler K, Reddy M, Schindler E, Koos WT. Intraoperative computed tomography guided neuronavigation: concepts, efficiency, and work flow. *Comput Aided Surg* 1998;3(4):174–182.
65. Hum B, Feigenbaum F, Cleary K, Henderson F. Intraoperative computed tomography for complex craniocervical operations and spinal tumor resections. *Neurosurgery* 2000;47:374–381.
66. Hall WA, Liu H, Martin AJ, Pozza CH, Maxwell RE, Truwit CL. Safety, efficacy, and functionality of high-field strength interventional magnetic resonance imaging for neurosurgery. *Neurosurgery* 2000;46(3):632–642.
67. Hall WA, Martin AJ, Liu H, Nussbaum ES, Maxwell RE, Truwit CL. Brain biopsy using high-field strength interventional magnetic resonance imaging. *Neurosurgery* 1999;44(4):807–814.
68. Kaibara T, Saunders JK, Sutherland GR. Advances in mobile intraoperative magnetic resonance imaging. *Neurosurgery* 2000;47(1): 131–138.
69. Sutherland GR, Kaibara T, Louw D, Hoult DI, Tomanek B, Saunders J. A mobile high-field magnetic resonance system for neurosurgery. *J Neurosurg* 1999;91(5):804–813.
70. Katscher U, Petersson S. Kernspintomographie unter Nutzung des Overhauser-Effekts. *Phys Bl* 2000;56(2):51–54.

18

Image-Guided Epilepsy Surgery

ELDAD J. HADAR, ERIC L. LAPRESTO, AND WILLIAM E. BINGAMAN

Over the past several years, neurosurgery has witnessed a resurgence of interest in stereotactic and navigational techniques. There are several reasons for this renewed interest. The most important is the recent technical progress in brain imaging, specifically with regard to cross-sectional imaging such as computed tomography (CT) and high-resolution magnetic resonance imaging (MRI).[1] These imaging modalities have replaced the use of ventriculography and standardized brain atlases and allow direct, patient-specific anatomic targeting of brain structures. Along with advances in the development of compact, high-speed microprocessors, this has allowed for the commercial development of stereotactic navigation systems. Today, these systems are widely available and commonplace in most neurosurgical practices. The recent trend toward minimally invasive surgical procedures has also done its part to create interest in surgical stereotaxis. Stereotactic navigation allows for minimization of scalp incisions, craniotomies, and brain resections. This has the potential to make neurosurgical procedures more economical with shorter hospital stays and a more rapid return to preoperative lifestyle.[1–2]

Like other disciplines of neurosurgery, epilepsy surgery has benefited from the development and refinement of stereotactic navigation. Typical uses of intracranial stereotaxy in epilepsy surgery have included minimizing the invasiveness of diagnostic and resective procedures, defining trajectories to deep-seated cerebral structures, defining a navigational plan for the resection of small, subcortical lesions, and confirmation of resective boundaries in lesional resection. This chapter discusses some of these applications and describes a novel use of stereotaxy to assist in the perioperative evaluation of epilepsy surgery candidates.

■ Lesional Epilepsy Surgery

Stereotactic navigational techniques for lesional epilepsy surgery utilize the same principles already refined for image-guided resection of other radiographic lesions such as tumors and vascular malformations. In these cases, the navigational system can be used to plan the incision and craniotomy, localize the lesion, and confirm the extent of resective boundaries. Once again, navigational systems can be useful in localizing small, subcortical epileptogenic lesions such as cavernous malformations and low-grade tumors that may not produce grossly visible changes on the brain surface. This allows the surgeon to create a direct and minimally disruptive pathway to the lesion and surrounding epileptogenic zone. For more extensive resections, such as those performed in patients with cortical dysplasia, the primary utility is in defining the boundaries of lesional resection, which are often defined on fluid attenuated inversion recovery (FLAIR) and T1-weighted MRI. Such lesions often have a normal gross appearance, and intraoperative electrocorticography (ECoG) can yield variable results. This makes it difficult to assess the optimal extent of resection. Image guidance aids in defining the resection as long as the surgeon understands the relationship between radiographic changes and pathological substrate. The actual epileptogenic zone, which is defined as the area of cortex indispensable for the generation of clinical seizures, may be more or less extensive than those radiographic changes seen on MRI. The ability to define the "lesion" using stereotactic guidance is the first step toward a comprehensive operative plan that also includes metabolic, functional, and electrographic data. If ECoG is employed for research or clinical decision making, the navigation system can be used to demonstrate electrode position for the benefit of electroencephalographers and other ancillary staff in the operating room.[3]

■ Selective Amygdalohippocampectomy

Stereotactic techniques have been adapted to guide the selective resection of mesial temporal structures while sparing the temporal neocortex for the surgical treatment of mesial temporal lobe epilepsy. Such selective resection may confer protection to neuropsychological function, especially when surgery involves the dominant hemisphere.[4] Using image guidance, such a resection can be accomplished while minimizing neocortical disruption and the size of the skin incision and craniotomy. Without the benefit of image guidance, it would be necessary to employ a craniotomy large enough to expose recognized surgical landmarks such as the Sylvian fissure. Furthermore, it would be difficult to place the cortical incision in an optimal location for the most efficient resection of the mesial temporal structures. After patient positioning and registration, navigation systems allow the surgeon to determine the relationships of various intracranial structures with scalp position in order to optimize location of the skin incision. We utilize the navigation system both to place the skin incision in the same coronal plane as the junction of the amygdala and hippocampus and to guide the transection of the temporal stem white matter to the inferior (temporal) horn. By entering the ventricle at this location, we are able to minimize the size of the cortical opening and the extent of retraction needed to perform the amygdalar, hippocampal, and parahippocampal resections. Typically, a 1.5 to 2 cm cortical incision is large enough to allow resection of these structures. Other approaches to the mesotemporal structures have been described.[5] Navigational tools have been also used to assess the extent of hippocampal resection during selective amygdalohippocampectomy.[6]

■ Callosotomy

The use of navigational tools has also facilitated the safe and accurate performance of callosal disconnection. Although many procedures have evolved to replace callosotomy, this technique remains useful in a small subset of patients with severe, medically intractable epilepsy. The goal of surgery is typically disruption of the rostral two-thirds of the corpus callosum while sparing the more caudally located association fibers. Although this is a discrete, easily localized structure, the interhemispheric approach can be complicated by the presence of midline, cortical draining veins and their interference with retraction. In an attempt to limit such retraction, craniotomies and approaches that are located anterior to the coronal suture have been employed.[3] These approaches, however, make it difficult to accurately assess the extent of callosal disruption. Navigation systems allow for the determination of position along the corpus callosum while also allowing access from a safer approach. Furthermore, the midline location of the corpus callosum makes this structure less prone to intraoperative brain shift and, therefore, allows for accurate localization along its rostral-caudal extent.

■ Depth Electrode Placement

By the 1960s, Bancaud and Talairach had developed and popularized the use of depth electrodes in the workup of candidates for resective epilepsy surgery.[7] In many European epilepsy centers, evaluation with depth electrodes using their technique (or a slight modification of it) was required prior to resective intervention. Depth electrodes have also become a standard procedure in North American epilepsy centers for the localization and lateralization of focal epilepsies.[8,9] The most common application at our center is for the lateralization of seizure onset in cases of bitemporal or nonlateralizing mesial temporal lobe epilepsy. Electrodes can be inserted either parallel[8,10] or perpendicular[9] to the axis of the hippocampus. For the evaluation of deep, subcortical structures such as the amygdala, hippocampus, or ectopic gray matter, both frame-based and frameless image-guided depth electrode evaluations have been very helpful. Similar techniques are well established for performing needle biopsies and catheter placement, and the same principles are used to place depth electrodes into the areas of interest for chronic intracranial recordings. To accomplish this, the navigation system is employed in a trajectory mode that allows preoperative planning and manipulation of the electrode path to avoid injury to critical structures. This allows depth electrodes to be inserted in a safe, accurate, and minimally invasive procedure (Fig. 18–1).

■ Radiosurgery

No discussion of image-guided epilepsy surgery would be complete without some mention of radiosurgical procedures to treat chronic seizures. The majority of such

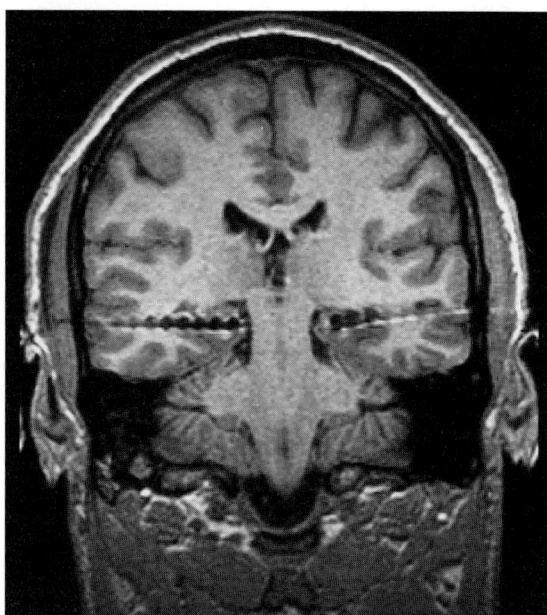

FIGURE 18–1. A postoperative coronal T1-weighted MR image demonstrates the bilateral placement of posterior hippocampal depth electrodes.

procedures have been used to treat lesional disorders such as tumors and vascular malformations that have secondarily resulted in chronic epilepsy. Typically, radiosurgical treatment of the primary lesion is undertaken with the thought that resolution of this lesion will lead to resolution of the patient's seizures. Recently, stereotactic radiosurgical techniques have also been used for the treatment of patients with mesial temporal lobe epilepsy (MTLE).[11,12] Regis et al have demonstrated a gamma knife technique that targets the head and anterior body of the hippocampus, the amygdala, and the entorhinal cortex.[11,12] Their results demonstrate a seizure-free rate of 81% in 16 patients with a follow-up interval of at least 24 months. The median latent interval from treatment to cessation of seizures was 10.5 months. Despite these promising results, the precise role and durability of radiosurgery in the treatment of focal epilepsy remains unclear. At the time of this publication, a prospective, multicenter study is under way to examine this technique and its utility in the treatment of patients with MTLE.

■ Multimodality Imaging

In the workup of seizure disorders, patients with nonlesional epilepsy and patients with lesional epilepsy that localizes to eloquent functional cortex are often candidates for the implantation of chronic subdural (SD) monitoring electrode grids. These are typically implanted with two purposes in mind; the first is to obtain accurate definition of the epileptogenic zone and the second is to allow for the extraoperative mapping of cerebral cortical functions such as speech and motor activity. The traditional method of localizing implanted electrodes required obtaining skull x-rays after implantation (Fig. 18–2). From this, an electrode map was hand drawn on a standard hard-copy template of the brain (Fig. 18–3). The main limitation of this method is the difficulty correlating the electrode positions to the sulcal and gyral cortical surface anatomy. This can be critically important information in developing a resective plan and prognosticating surgical risks.

To overcome this limitation, computer software has been developed that interactively displays the SD electrode positions as pseudocolored surface-rendered spheres on a three-dimensional, volume-rendered surface reconstruction of the brain, based on either pre- or postoperative MRI data (Fig. 18–4). Volume rendering,[13] as compared with surface rendering, is advantageous for the display of medical volume data for two reasons. Unlike surface rendering, volume rendering does not generate a polygonal wire-frame representation of the cortical surface. Instead, it models each three-dimensional volume element ("voxel") as having a variable, gray-level opacity value, which allows for a "fuzzier" identification of the cortical surface. Second, volume rendering retains the voxel signal data rather than eliminating all but the wire-framed surface data. This permits the user to visualize subsurface voxels by "pushing" into the volume deep to the cortical surface.

Intraoperatively, the software aids the surgeon in the placement of the SD grids. We obtain a standard preoperative stereotactic volume acquisition MRI with standard scalp fiducial markers in place then coregister the position of the fiducial markers on the scalp with their corresponding positions on the MRI. After craniotomy and exposure of the brain are completed, the electrodes are placed in their final position. The pointing tool is then used to register the positions of as many exposed electrodes as possible, such that a mathematical model of the SD grid can be calculated and displayed as pseudocolored plastic spheres in conjunction with the surface reconstruction. This effectively coregisters the position of each electrode to the MRI, allowing the surgeon to have immediate intraoperative feedback demonstrating the anatomic position of the SD grid.

Postoperatively, the software may again be used to detect and display the position of the SD grid electrodes. By obtaining a postoperative volume acquisition MRI, the electrodes can be identified and displayed on the surface reconstruction. Because the electrodes are composed of a nonferromagnetic platinum alloy, they appear as a low-signal artifact on the MRI images, which contrasts against the nearby higher-signal brain and parenchyma.[14] As with the intraoperative procedure, electrodes are identi-

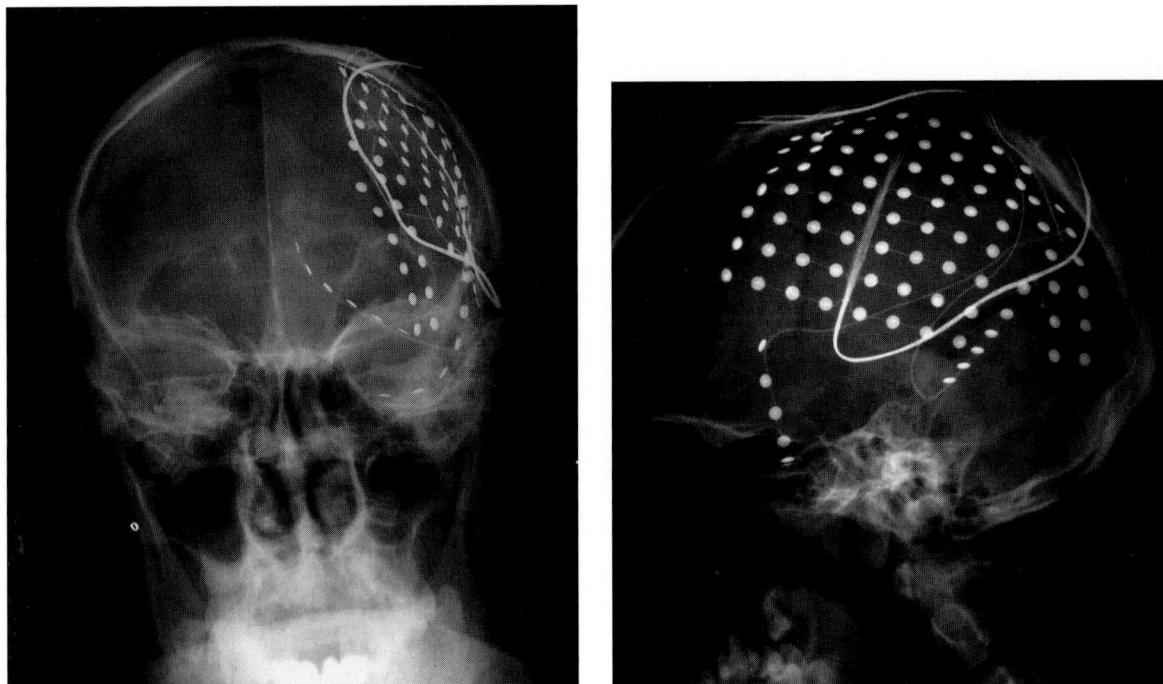

FIGURE 18–2. Anteroposterior and lateral postoperative skull x-rays demonstrate the position of subdural electrode grids. The relationships of electrode positions to defined bony landmarks are used to generate the electrode map seen in Figure 18–3.

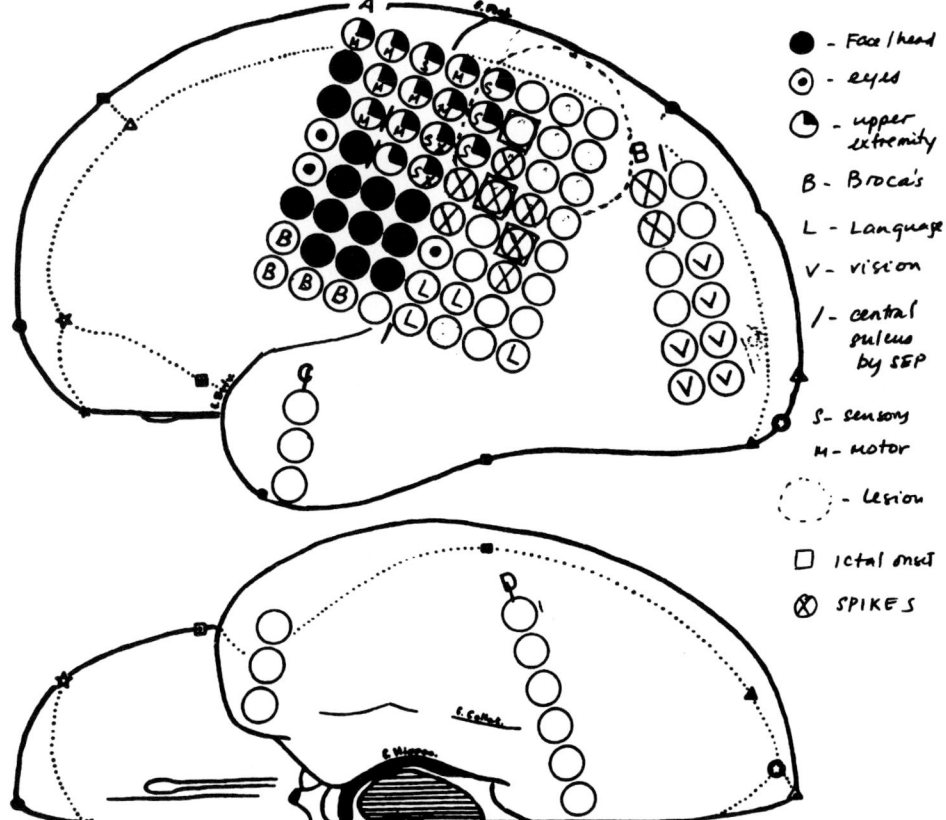

FIGURE 18–3. A hand-drawn electrode map was generated from the skull x-rays seen in Figure 18–2. This technique is limited by the difficulty of correlating electrode position with cortical anatomy.

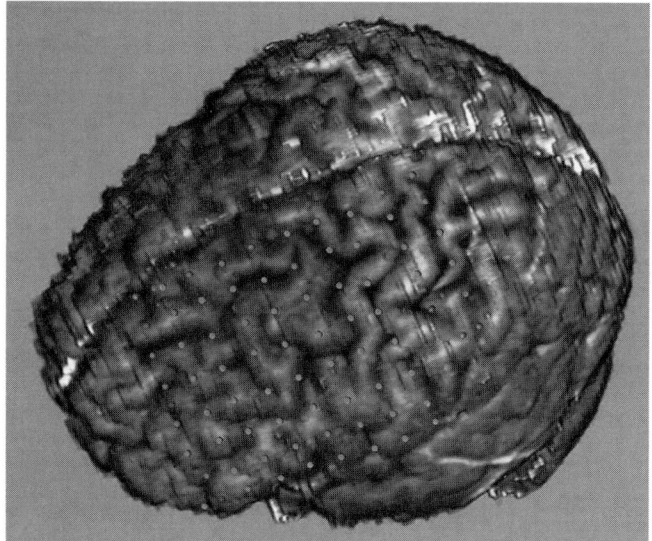

FIGURE 18–4. The positions of subdural electrodes in this patient are represented by spheres superimposed on a three-dimensional volume-rendered surface reconstruction of the brain generated from the preoperative magnetic resonance imaging data. This technique provides accurate correlation of electrode position with cortical anatomy.

fied until a suitably accurate model of the SD grid can be displayed.

Multimodality imaging allows the surgeon and epileptologist to coregister and fuse multiple preoperative imaging/metabolic tests during the initial consideration of surgical candidacy. Robust algorithms for coregistering intermodality and intramodality imaging studies now exist[15] that provide the means for visually fusing anatomic-based imaging (MRI, CT) to function-based imaging (positron emission tomography, single photon emission computed tomography, functional MRI). For the placement of SD grids, multimodality imaging guides the intraoperative placement and enables accurate postoperative anatomic localization of cortical structures to the electrical signature of the epilepsy (Fig. 18–5). This powerful technology allows more medically intractable seizure patients access to surgical treatment and aids in the execution of the surgical plan in the operating room.

■ Conclusions

Epilepsy surgery, like other neurosurgical subspecialty areas, has benefited from the development of stereotactic navigation. Today, new operative techniques make the surgical workup and treatment of seizures safer, less invasive, and highly accurate. As both anatomic and functional brain imaging become more refined and as computer microprocessors and detection systems gain speed and accuracy, we will likely see this trend continue with both epilepsy surgery and neurosurgery as a whole. As experience with this exciting technology grows, surgical outcomes for medically intractable epilepsy should continue to improve.

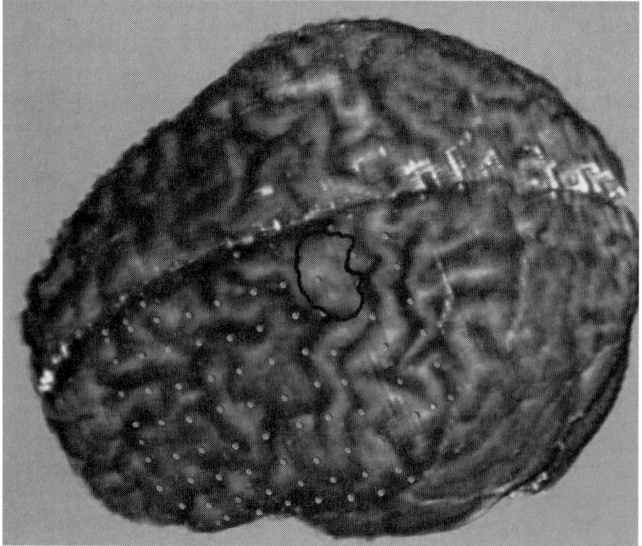

FIGURE 18–5. The same patient seen in Figure 18–4 underwent both baseline and ictal single photon emission computed tomography (SPECT) studies to generate a subtraction ictal SPECT profile. This data set has been coregistered to the magnetic resonance imaging data to provide correlation of the ictal onset zone (outlined in black) with anatomic and electrode positions.

REFERENCES

1. Parrent AG, Lozano AM. Stereotactic surgery for temporal lobe epilepsy. *Can J Neurol Sci* 2000;27(suppl 1):S79–S84.
2. Bingaman WE, Barnett GH. Social and economic impact of surgical navigation systems. In: Barnett GH, Roberts DW, Maciunas RJ, eds. *Image-Guided Neurosurgery: Clinical Applications of Surgical Navigation*. St. Louis: Quality Medical Publishing; 1998:231–250.
3. Olivier A, Germano IM, Cukiert A, Peters T. Frameless stereotaxy for surgery of the epilepsies: preliminary experience. *J Neurosurg* 1994;81:629.
4. Yasargil MG, Wieser HG, Valavanis A, von Ammon K, Roth P. Surgery and results of selective amygdala-hippocampectomy in one hundred patients with nonlesional limbic epilepsy. *Neurosurg Clin N Am* 1993;4(2):243–261.
5. Goncalves-Ferreira A, Miguens J, Farias JP, Melancia JL, Andrade M. Selective amygdalohippocampectomy: which route is the best? An experimental study in 80 human cerebral hemispheres. *Stereotact Funct Neurosurg* 1994;63(1–4):182–191.
6. Van Roost D, Schaller C, Meyer B, Schramm J. Can neuronavigation contribute to standardization of selective amygdalohippocampectomy? *Stereotact Funct Neurosurg* 1997;69(1–4 Pt 2):239–242.
7. Bancaud J, Talairach J, Bonis A, et al. *La stereo-electroencephalographie dans l'epilepsie: informations neurophysiopathologiques appotees par l'investigation functionelle stereotaxique*. Paris: Masson; 1965.
8. Blatt DR, Rober SN, Friedman WA. Invasive monitoring of limbic epilepsy using stereotactic depth and subdural strip electrodes: surgical technique. *Surg Neurol* 1997;48(1):74–79.

9. Wennberg R, Quesney F, Olivier A, Dubeau F. Mesial temporal versus lateral temporal interictal epileptiform activity: comparison of chronic and acute intracranial recordings. *Electroencephalogr Clin Neurophysiol* 1997;102(6):486–494.
10. Van Roost D, Solymosi L, Schramm J, van Oosterwyck B, Elger CE. Depth electrode implantation in the length axis of the hippocampus for the presurgical evaluation of medial temporal lobe epilepsy: a computed tomography-based stereotactic insertion technique and its accuracy. *Neurosurgery* 1998;43(4):819–826.
11. Regis J, Bartolomei F, Rey M, Hayashi M, Chauvel P, Peragut JC. Gamma knife surgery for mesial temporal lobe epilepsy. *J Neurosurg* 2000;93(suppl 3):141–146.
12. RegisJ, Bartolomei F, Rey M, et al. Gamma knife surgery for mesial temporal lobe epilepsy. *Epilepsia* 1999;40(11):1551–1556.
13. Fishman EK, Magid D, Ney DR, et al. Three-dimensional imaging. *Radiology* 1991;181(2):321–337.
14. Silberbusch MA, Rothman MI, Bergey GK, Zoarski GH, Zagardo MT. Subdural grid implantation for intracranial EEG recording: CT and MR appearance. *Am J Neuroradiol* 1998;19(6):1089–1093.
15. Maes F, Collignon A, Vandermeulen D, Marchal G, Suetens P. Multimodality image registration by maximization of mutual information. *IEEE Trans Med Imaging* 1997;16(2):187–198.

19

New Directions in Atlas-Assisted Stereotactic Functional Neurosurgery

WIESLAW L. NOWINSKI AND ALIM-LOUIS BENABID

The first stereotactic brain atlases in printed form, such as Talairach et al and Schaltenbrand and Bailey, [1,2] were constructed in the 1950s. Roughly two decades later, brain atlases in electronic formats were available in the clinical setting.[3] By the late 1990s, electronic brain atlases had become commonplace in stereotactic functional neurosurgery. The first author and his team have developed the Cerefy electronic brain atlas database, which has become the standard in stereotactic functional neurosurgery. Image-guided surgery companies including Medtronic/Sofamor-Danek, BrainLAB, Cedara/SNN, Elekta, and Integrated Surgical Systems have adopted the Cerefy atlas.

Beginning in the late 1990s, a new-generation brain atlas, referred to as a probabilistic functional atlas (PFA), has been under construction, and a novel way of using it has been proposed. The new atlas is built from electrophysiological and clinical brain mapping data acquired intraoperatively during the treatment of Parkinson's disease patients. This atlas will be used and its content expanded by the neurosurgical community via an Internet portal, which represents a paradigm shift from a manufacturer-centric to a community-centric atlas. The atlas will become a tool allowing intraoperative targeting based on the patient's internal landmarks and sufficiently precise to warrant its use for therapeutic purposes. The portal will facilitate data loading, parameter setting, PFA generation and display, and the combination of PFAs and data sets. The atlas and portal are described in greater detail in the section titled Internet Portal for Stereotactic Functional Neurosurgery.

■ Electronic Brain Atlas Database

The core of any atlas-assisted application is the brain atlas. Its construction may vary from a simple digitization of a printed atlas to a fully segmented, labeled, enhanced, extended, three-dimensionally expanded, and deformable atlas. We used the latter approach when developing our Cerefy electronic brain atlas database.[4,5] This database was derived from the brain atlases edited by Thieme Medical Publishers:

- *Atlas for Stereotaxy of the Human Brain* (Schaltenbrand and Wahren, 1977)[6]
- *Co-Planar Stereotactic Atlas of the Human Brain* (Talairach and Tournoux, 1988)[7]
- *Referentially Oriented Cerebral MRI Anatomy: Atlas of Stereotaxic Anatomical Correlations for Gray and White Matter* (Talairach and Tournoux, 1993)[8]
- *Atlas of the Cerebral Sulci* (Ono, Kubik, and Abernathey, 1990)[9]

We digitized these complementary atlases (with gross anatomy, brain connections, subcortical structures, and sulcal patterns) and then enhanced, extended, segmented (color-coded and/or contoured), labeled, aligned, and organized them into atlas volumes. Their three-dimensional extensions were constructed and all two-dimensional (2-D) and three-dimensional (3-D) atlases were mutually co-registered. The combined anatomical index has approximately 1000 structures per hemisphere and more than 400 sulcal patterns.

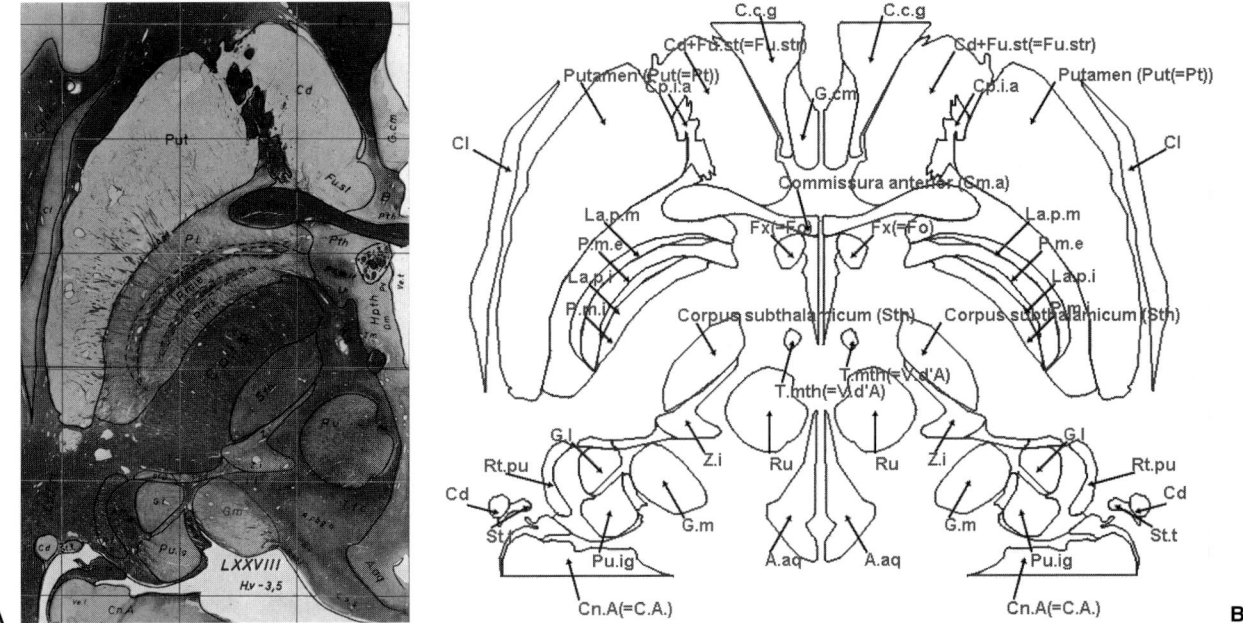

FIGURE 19–1. Schaltenbrand-Wahren brain atlas. (A). Digitized printed axial plate along with the overlay covering the right hemisphere only. (B). Corresponding derived electronic contour image covering both hemispheres with the structures labeled with full or abbreviated names.

The atlases most commonly used in stereotactic functional neurosurgery are the *Atlas for Stereotaxy of the Human Brain* by Schaltenbrand and Wahren (SW) and the *Co-Planar Stereotactic Atlas of the Human Brain* by Talairach and Tournoux (TT).

The SW atlas contains photographic plates of macroscopic and microscopic sections through the hemispheres and the brain stem. The microscopic myelin-stained sections show in great detail cerebral deep structures that usually are not well visible on computed tomographic (CT) and magnetic resonance imaging (MRI) scans. The original axial, coronal, and sagittal microseries were digitized with high resolution (Fig. 19–1A). The electronic contours were derived manually from the digitized atlas and labeled. The microseries images and contours were extended to cover both hemispheres. Three SW atlas volumes were constructed with about 600 segmented and labeled structures: coronal with 20 images, sagittal with 34 images, and axial with 20 images (Fig. 19–1B).

The TT atlas was constructed from a single, normal brain specimen (Fig. 19–2A). It had been sectioned and photographed sagittally, and the coronal and axial sections were subsequently interpolated manually. The printed plates were digitized with high resolution, and extensively processed, enhanced, and extended (Fig. 19–2B). The electronic TT atlas images were organized into five atlas volumes: sagittal with 35 images; coronal with 38 images; and three axial with 27 images each, first with standard images, second comprising parcellated cortex (as opposed to the annotated cortex in the original printed atlas) with color-coded Brodmann's areas on the left side and gyri on the right side, and third containing color-coded gyri on the left side and Brodmann's areas on the right side. In addition, a contour version of the TT atlas was constructed (Fig. 19–2C).

The 3-D versions of the SW and TT atlases were constructed and mutually co-registered, which enhances surgery planning by providing better insight into spatial relationships (Fig. 19–3).

The electronic atlas images were additionally pre-labeled to speed up structure labeling in atlas-based applications. In total, about 17,000 labels were placed manually for the entire electronic brain atlas database (see Figs. 19–1B and 19–2B). Atlas pre-labeling has been used in *The Electronic Clinical Brain Atlas*[10] and *Brain Atlas for Functional Imaging*.[11]

■ Atlas-Assisted Applications

Electronic brain atlases are commonplace in stereotactic functional neurosurgery. An atlas-assisted application may range from simple (*The Electronic Clinical Brain Atlas*[10]) to sophisticated (*NeuroPlanner*).[5,16] Brain atlases are used in various ways, based on several factors:

- Atlas type (2-D SW, 2-D TT, 3-D SW, 3-D TT, others)

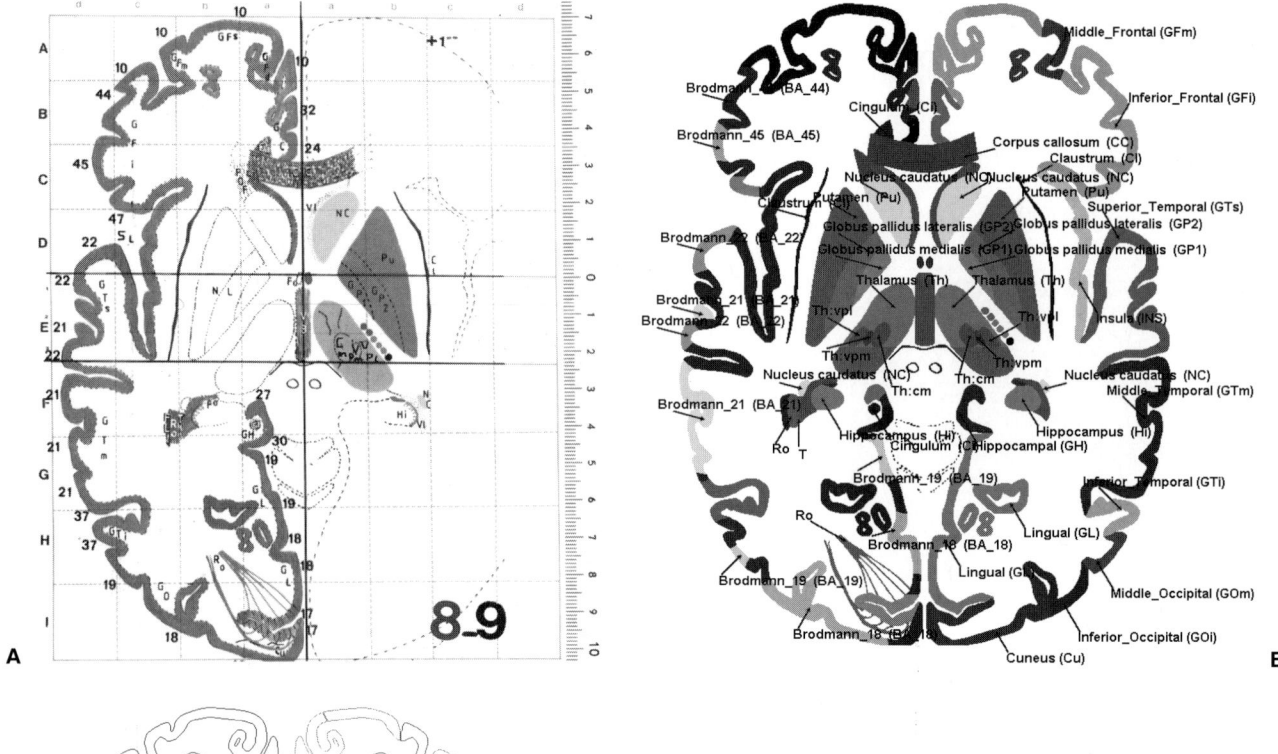

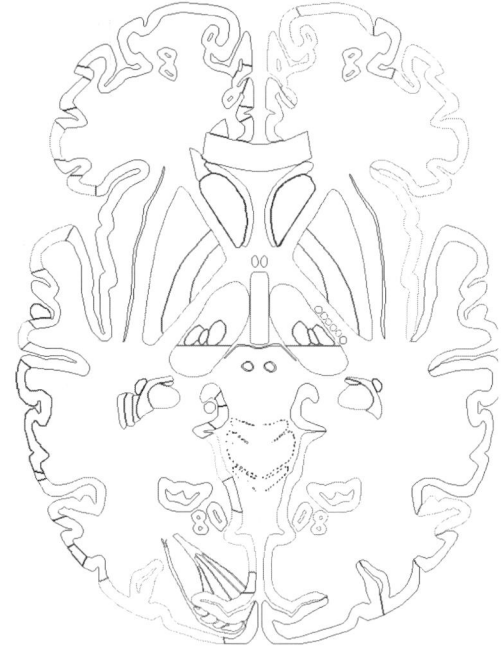

FIGURE 19–2. Talairach-Tournoux brain atlas. (A). Digitized printed axial plate; (B) corresponding electronic color-coded image labeled with subcortical structures, gyri, and Brodmann's areas (full or abbreviated names are used); (C) corresponding color-coded contours.

- Construction of the computerized atlas (direct digitization of printed plates versus an enhanced, extended, 3-D expanded, and deformable atlas)
- Atlas representation (image, contour, polygonal, volumetric)
- Availability and use of multiple atlases (single atlas, multiple independent atlases, multiple mutually co-registered atlases)
- Atlas-to-data registration method (fully automatic or based on user-specified features such as landmarks or scaling factors)
- Atlas-to-data warping transformation [linear scaling, 3-D piecewise linear scaling (Talairach transformation[7]) nonlinear warping]
- Availability of interactive atlas-to-data warping (nonavailable; available before planning; available at any

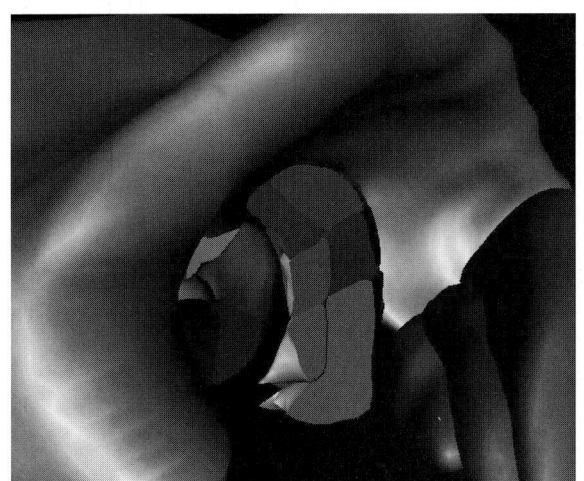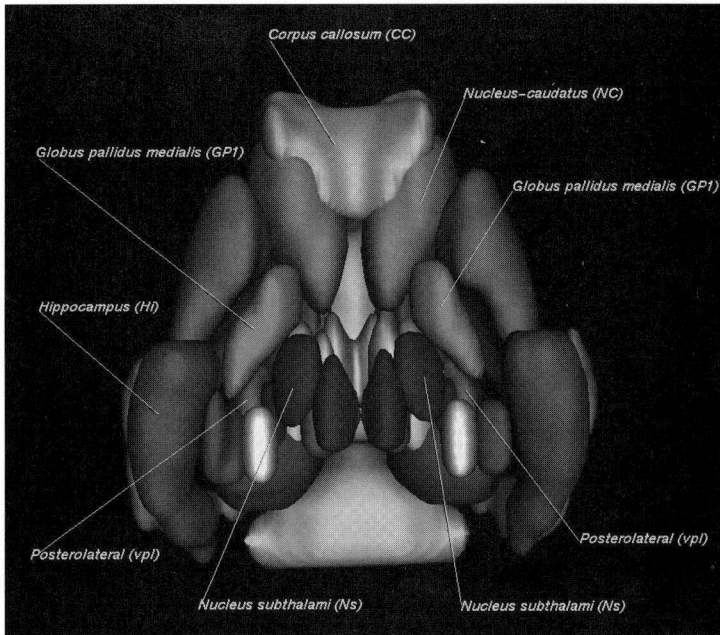

FIGURE 19–3. Three-dimensional atlases. (A). Talairach-Tournoux (TT) atlas co-registered with the Schaltenbrand-Wahren (SW) atlas: a view into the thalamic nuclei of the 3-D SW atlas combined with the basal ganglia and corpus callosum of the 3-D TT atlas. (B). Subcortical structures of the 3-D Talairach-Tournoux atlas with the stereotactic targets labeled on both sides.

time preoperatively, intraoperatively, and postoperatively)
- Atlas display (atlas alone, atlas next to data, atlas images overlaid on data, atlas images overlaid on data with user-controlled blending, atlas contours overlaid on data)
- Atlas-assisted operations (atlas labeling, data labeling, multiple orientation targeting, multiple atlas targeting, planning in 2-D and 3-D on the atlas-segmented anatomy)

Cerefy brain atlas applications

The *Electronic Clinical Brain Atlas* (ECBA)[10] on CD-ROM contains, among others, the SW and TT atlases. The ECBA provides features not available in the printed atlases such as: mutually co-registered atlases; fully pre-labeled 17,000 structures on 1500 atlas images; flexible display, manipulation, and printing of the atlas in multi-atlas and triplanar modes; and atlas warping. The ECBA generates individualized atlases without loading the patient-specific data, which is useful for targeting. The ECBA-based planning procedure for stereotactic functional neurosurgery has been described.[13] The atlas is conformed to the patient's scan by means of a 2-D local deformation done by matching the atlas rectangular region of interest to the corresponding data region of interest spanned on any landmarks. The deformation can be repeated in multiple orientations, if data are available, increasing the accuracy of targeting and the neurosurgeon's confidence level.

Two add-on brain atlas libraries are gaining increasing acceptance and use, the *Electronic Brain Atlas Library* and *Brain Atlas Geometrical Models*. The *Electronic Brain Atlas Library* (EBAL)[14] contains the brain atlas database with the SW and TT atlas images, and a browser. The browser provides means for exploring and understanding the atlas images and allows users to build their own atlas-assisted applications. It also allows the user to select atlas volume, display atlas images, find labels of structures, display atlas image location in 3-D space, display stereotactic grids, find stereotactic coordinates, and search for structure. These features also make the EBAL useful as a stand-alone atlas reference.

The *Brain Atlas Geometrical Models*[15] is a library with the atlases in contour and polygonal representations. The BAGM contains the brain atlas database and a viewer. The database comprises the SW atlas in contour representation and 3-D polygonal models of the SW and TT atlases. The viewer provides means for viewing and understanding the brain atlas database.

The detailed specifications of the EBAL content and the BAGM content along with file formats are available online at www.cerefy.com.

The *NeuroPlanner*[5,16] is a clinical prototype developed for preoperative planning and training, intraoperative procedures, and postoperative follow-up. It comprises all (mutually co-registered) atlases from the Cerefy brain atlas database, including their 3-D extensions. The atlases are available in image, contour, and polygonal representations as well as in multiple resolutions. The atlas-to-data registration is based on the Talairach landmarks specified in the data interactively; alternatively, the placement of the landmarks can be done automatically.[12] The *NeuroPlanner* is empowered with operations making atlas-to-data registration more accurate, efficient, and easy. They include global and local registrations, editing capabilities for the Talairach grid in 3-D, real-time interactive atlas warping feasible any time, targeting in multiple orientations, and targeting with multiple atlases. To warp the atlas against data, a two-step Talairach transformation, global and local, is used. The Talairach transformation scales the gross anatomy globally and does not compensate for the width of the third ventricle or internal capsule. Local warping (by using the same piecewise linear deformation mechanism) enhances the accuracy of registration in the region of interest for the previously globally selected atlas plates. When registering locally, any landmarks clearly visible in the data can be used to improve the delineation of the (usually not clearly visible) target structure. The use of the atlas in multiple orientations enhances the accuracy of targeting, gives more flexibility in choosing local landmarks, and provides an extra degree of confidence to the neurosurgeon. The global registration steps done simultaneously on all three orthogonal planes have been formulated, and the targeting steps and local registrations along with suitable landmarks for pallidotomy, thalamotomy, and subthalamotomy have been detailed by Nowinski.[17] Moreover, the use of multiple atlases provides complementary information and overcomes some limitations of the individual atlases, which additionally enhances targeting.[16] The Talairach transformation fits the Talairach grid to data, this operation is subject to several sources of errors including Talairach landmarks-grid inconsistency, inter-atlas co-registration, and global registration. Real-time interactive warping, applied to the atlas images, contours, and polygonal models, allows the neurosurgeon to fit any atlas to data and fine-tune the atlas-to-data match. This interactive warping can be done at any time—preoperatively, intraoperatively, or postoperatively.

In addition, the *NeuroPlanner* provides four groups of functions: data-related (data interpolation, reformatting, image processing), atlas-related (2-D and 3-D interactive labeling), atlas-data exploration-related (interaction in one 3-D and three orthogonal views, continuous data-atlas exploration), neurosurgery-related (targeting, path planning, mensuration, simulating the insertion of a microelectrode, simulating therapeutic lesioning) (Fig. 19–4).

The *NeuroPlanner* has been licensed for trial to several commercial, clinical, and research sites. It has been playing an important educative role as well as influencing the design of the commercial systems that use the EBAL and BAGM libraries.

One of the major advantages of atlas-assisted surgery planning using a tool such as the *NeuroPlanner* is a potential saving in terms of cost, time, and invasiveness. The initial validation suggests that the functional target can be confirmed electrophysiologically with the first microelectrode used.[16] Because the number of tracts is typically from three to seven, this number can potentially be reduced to a single tract, resulting in an average saving of four tracts per surgery (Fig. 19–5). This has the potential to reduce the cost and invasiveness of the procedure and save time for the neurosurgeon and personnel in the operating room (OR). The precise criteria have not been arrived at for determining the optimal (single) track, which is what the multitrack approach is aimed at.

Brain atlases in commercial systems

Electronic brain atlases are commonplace in stereotactic functional neurosurgery systems. The *Electronic Brain Atlas Library* and *Brain Atlas Geometrical Models* are becoming the standard in stereotactic functional surgery, available in the StealthStation (Medtronic SNT, Louisville, CO), Target (BrainLAB, Redwood City, CA), SNN 3 Image-Guided Surgery System (Cedara/SNN, Mississauga, Ontario, Canada), and SurgiPlan (Elekta, Stockholm, Sweden), and in the neurosurgical robot NeuroMate (Integrated Surgical Systems, Davis, CA). Other companies have developed their own digital versions of printed atlases, such as Tyco/Radionics (Burlington, MA) or Stryker/Leibinger (Kalamazoo, MI) described in the following text. Electronic atlases are also available in the COMPASS System of Stereotactic Medical Systems[18] and in the CASS system of MIDCO.[19]

The StealthStation uses the *Electronic Brain Atlas Library*. The atlases are registered with the patient-specific data by means of the Talairach transformation. The images of atlas contours are overlaid on the data and are available on axial, coronal, and sagittal planes, allowing the neurosurgeon to do planning on atlas-segmented anatomy (Fig. 19–6).

Stryker Navigation System Neuro includes the following features:

- Schaltenbrand-Wahren and Talairach-Tournoux brain atlases are supported.
- The atlases are available as slice images in three orientations: axial, coronal, and sagittal.
- The different atlas series are correlated together (one correlation with the patient is sufficient for any atlas series; in addition, the differences in the usage of the commissures are taken into account by the system).
- Two methods for atlas-to-data correlation are available: (1) with the Talairach grid (12 independent re-

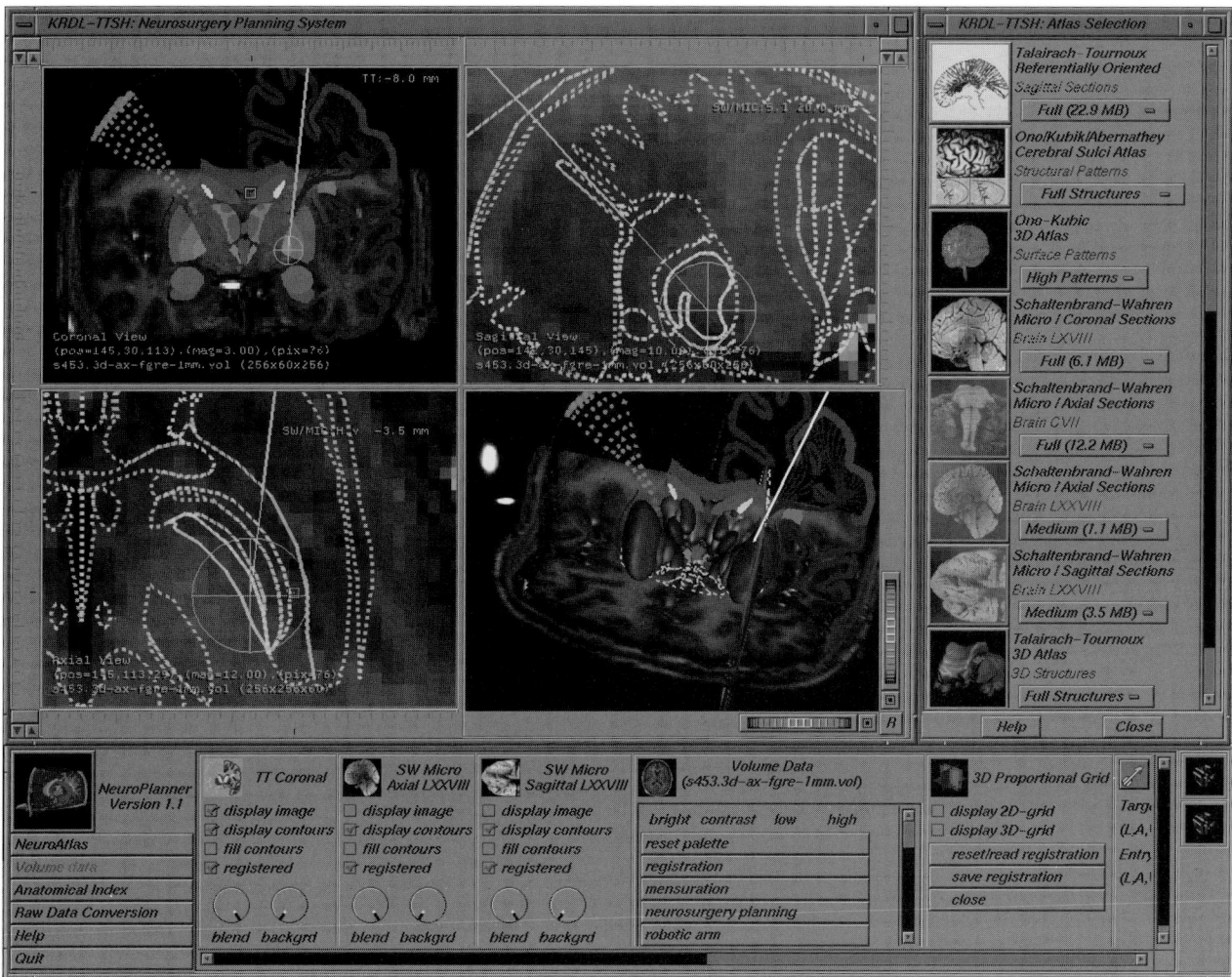

FIGURE 19–4. User interface of the *NeuroPlanner*. Pallidotomy planning using multiple atlases in multiple orientations. (Center). Main window with four smoothly and continuously resizable views, allowing the neurosurgeon to balance between the 2-D and 3-D presentations. The views show the orthogonal data sections registered with the 2-D SW (in contour representation) and 2-D TT atlases, and data-atlas triplanar registered with the 3-D TT atlas. The stereotactic trajectory (the thin line) along with the current position of the microelectrode (the thick line) are displayed in all views. (Right). Atlas selection panel with multiple atlases in multiple resolutions. (Bottom). Control panel with the surgery planning modules and atlas controls.

gions individually matched to patient's anatomy), and (2) a simple match with one linear distortion factor determined by the anterior commissure-posterior commissure (AC-PC) distance.

- The overlay contours of the Schaltenbrand-Wahren atlas are available.
- The system establishes coordinates and orientations on patient data as in the atlas.
- The system allows assessment of trajectories in terms relative to the commissures (e.g., direct input of functional targets).
- The system displays reference planes (intercommissural plane, midsagittal plane, and coronal planes passing through the AC and PC landmarks) in patient images.
- The system integrates the atlases as if they were images of the patient. For instance, it is possible in the atlases to define and display trajectories, determine coordinates, measure distances, fuse (overlay) with images of the patient (available for both atlas-to-data correlation methods) (Fig. 19–7).

The StereoPlan 2.1 of Tyco/Radionics contains the AtlasPlan module, which provides access to the SW atlas. The SW printed axial, coronal, and sagittal microseries were digitized and labeled. The electronic SW atlas is available in image representation for a single hemisphere. The AtlasPlan module allows neurosurgeons to perform the following tasks:

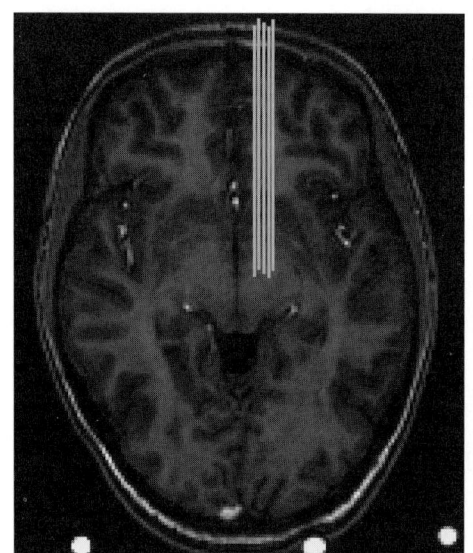 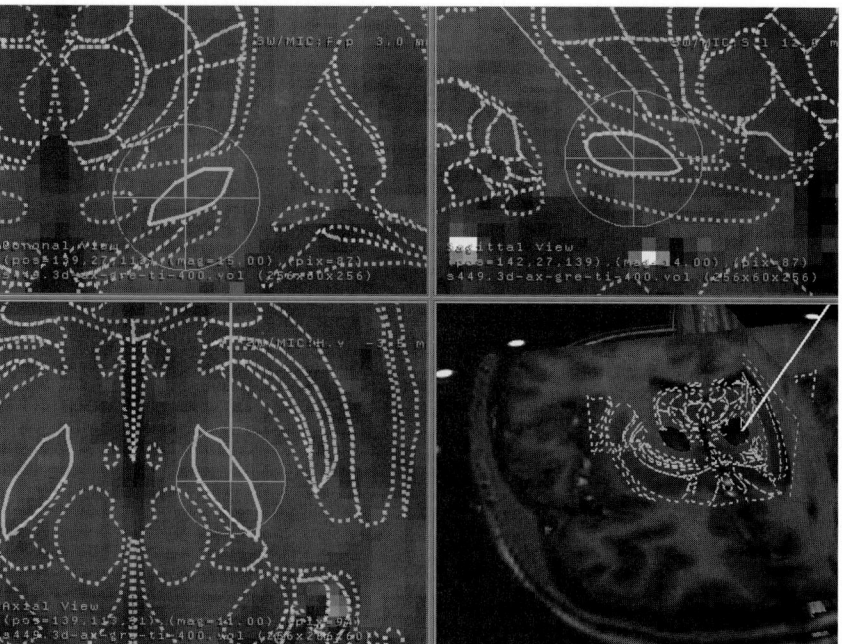

FIGURE 19–5. Illustration of potential of atlas-enhanced targeting. (A). Non-atlas targeting requires using five electrodes on average to cope with the individual variability and brain movements during surgery induced by the introduction of electrodes. (B). On the other hand, atlas-assisted targeting done in multiple orientations may suffice using a single electrode resulting in an average saving of four electrodes per hemisphere, provided that the statistical high coherence of the atlas structures with the real anatomical structures has been proven.

- Register the Schaltenbrand-Wahren atlas to the patient anatomy in 3-D. The atlas is translated and scaled to match the AC and PC landmarks. Lateral and vertical scales are set to account for variations in ventricular widths, and so forth.
- Select and project target points from the atlas to the patient slices or from the patient slices to the atlas while viewing the atlas plates and patient slices simultaneously. Because the atlas is not superimposed on the data, this approach provides a one-to-one correlation between the atlas and the data.
- View the outlines and names of the nuclei on the atlas plates.
- Flip automatically the atlas orientation for the target chosen.
- View the atlas plates in conjunction with the patient scans and 3-D view to analyze and confirm probe approaches (Fig. 19–8).

■ Probabilistic Functional Atlas

The current electronic stereotactic atlases have two major limitations. First, the original printed atlas plates are sparse and constructed from only a few brain specimens: the TT atlas from a single brain and the SW atlas microseries from two different brains (three various hemispheres) despite using 111 brains as the initial material. Second, these atlases are anatomical, whereas the stereotactic targets are functional. The probabilistic functional atlas, the preliminary version of which has been constructed for the Vim (ventrointermedius nucleus), STN (subthalamic nucleus), and GPi (globus pallidus internus), overcomes both limitations.

To build the PFA, we use electrophysiological and clinical brain mapping data acquired intraoperatively during the treatment of Parkinson's disease patients. The high-quality brain mapping data have been collected for several years by the second author and are available for hundreds of patients, most of them operated bilaterally. The OR environment for data collection has been described by Benabid et al.[20] The data containing the positions of the chronically implanted electrodes and their best (most clinically active) contacts are represented as a four-level data tree. The first level is the list of cerebral structures. At the second level, for each structure the list of patients is given. For each patient, the intercommissural distance and the height of the thalamus are available. At the third level, for each patient the list of electrodes is provided along with their type and status (i.e., active or passive). The type of electrode uniquely identifies its geometry, including diameter, number of contacts, contact height, and gap between contacts. At the fourth level, the list of contacts for each electrode is

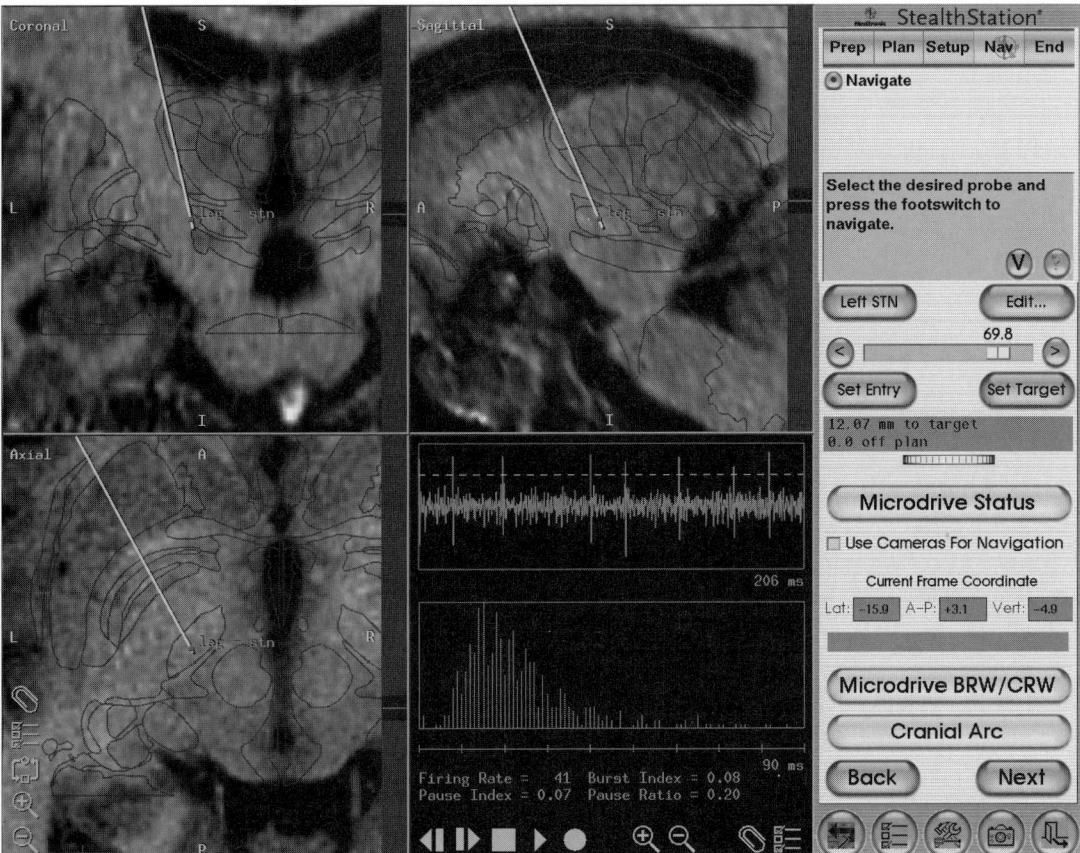

FIGURE 19–6. The user interface of the StealthStation of Medtronic SNT (Louisville, CO). Subthalamotomy planning simultaneously on axial, coronal, and sagittal planes assisted by the Schaltenbrand-Wahren contours from the *Electronic Brain Atlas Library*. (Image courtesy of Dr. J. Henderson, St. Louis University Health Sciences Center.)

given. Each contact has its identifier, coordinates, and status (best, not best). Either the complete data tree or any subtree containing the data of interest can be selected for the calculation of the PFA.

Based on electrode geometry, its 3-D model is constructed. For every treated patient, the corresponding electrode model is placed in the patient space according to its coordinates. To build a PFA across the whole population, the patient-specific data have to be normalized and placed in a common atlas space where different brains can be compared. The 3-D electrode models, originally located in the patient spaces, are normalized and placed in the atlas space (Fig. 19–9A). The operation used for electrode model normalization is linear scaling along the intercommissural distance and the height of the thalamus. The best contacts are then selected from the considered set of the electrodes and used for the calculation of the PFA (Fig. 19–9B).

The atlas is calculated for all best contacts available across all patients. For a calculated atlas structure, the best atlas target is the subset of this structure having the maximum atlas value. Two approaches are used to calculate the atlas probability: intuitive—easy to understand and use by the clinicians; and formal—defined in a mathematical sense. The atlas continuous function has to be converted into discrete representation suitable for processing, storing, and displaying. The discrete atlas is composed of voxels, elementary uniform parallelepipeds; the value of each determines the density of contacts within the voxel. Atlas discretization requires the normalized cylinders to be voxelized. Mathematically, the problem of locating a point relative to a normalized cylinder is simple. Computationally, this problem is more demanding because all best cylindrical contacts and all voxels in the atlas space relative to the processed cylindrical contact have to be tested. At the same time, the atlas calculation must be rapid, particularly for remote operations. Once the discrete volumetric atlas has been constructed, the structures can additionally be smoothed, if necessary, by using three-dimensional antialiasing.

This method calculates the atlas function for the entire atlas space, provided that the number of the best contacts available is sufficient. For instance, if the distri-

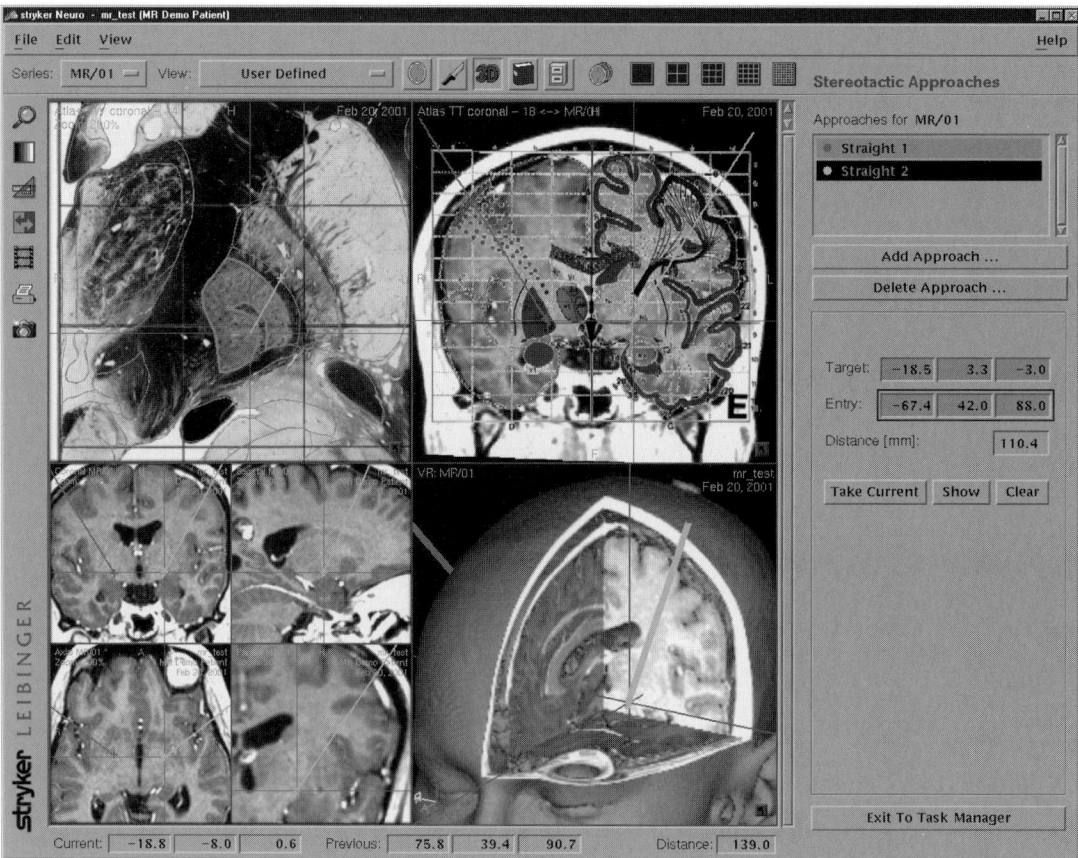

FIGURE 19–7. Stryker (Kalamazoo, MI) Navigation System Neuro: screenshot of planning situation. From upper left to lower right: a Schaltenbrand-Wahren atlas plate with an overlay and trajectory; image fusion with the Talairach-Tournoux atlas including trajectories; four reconstructed sectional patient images; and 3-D volume-rendered image. (Image courtesy of H. Schoepp, Stryker/Leibinger.)

bution of the best contacts would be uniform, then their number should be higher than the volume of structure to the volume of contact ratio. When the number of the best contacts available is not high enough, the originally calculated atlas may not be determined in some regions or it may have abrupt changes in value. Then, by treating the original atlas as a set of samples, the atlas can be smoothly reconstructed from these samples based on the theory of probability (Fig. 19–10).

■ Internet Portal for Stereotactic Functional Neurosurgery

As previously mentioned, the current surgical practice is manufacturer-centric. Surgeons are dependent and rely on the equipment and tools provided by manufacturers. We have been working on a community-centric solution that will represent a paradigm shift, at least for stereotactic functional neurosurgeons. The earlier described Internet portal has been developed to provide user services for stereotactic functional neurosurgeons. The portal contains the PFA and the tools for its calculation, presentation, and use. Neurosurgeons themselves will be able to expand the content of this PFA.

The core PFA built from the available data along with the developed algorithm for PFA calculation can be useful both for experienced functional neurosurgeons who have gathered numerous cases, and for neurosurgeons who are just starting their first cases. We envisage four scenarios of atlas use. First, the core PFA is used to enhance targeting, a scenario most likely useful for beginners. Second, the neurosurgeon generates an individualized PFA. This application will be beneficial for experienced neurosurgeons having gathered numerous cases. Third, the neurosurgeon calculates a combined PFA from the data of other neurosurgeons available in the PFA database. And finally, the neurosurgeon generates an individualized combined PFA by combining his or her own data with the selected data of others. This increases the neurosurgeons' confidence level. The PFA

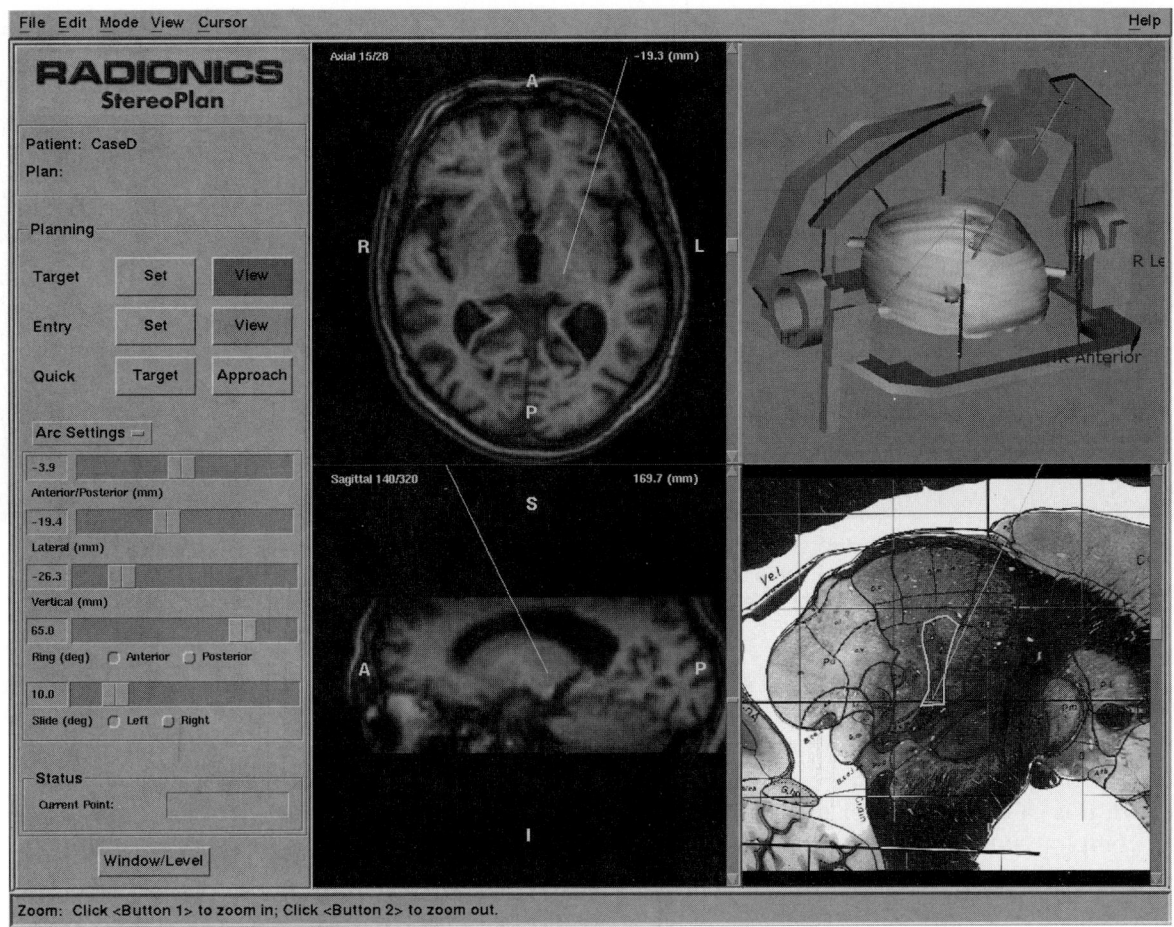

FIGURE 19–8. User interface of the Stereoplan, Tyco/Radionics (Burlington, MA). Thalamotomy planning: the stereotactic trajectory is displayed with respect to the patient-specific data, the Schaltenbrand-Wahren atlas, and the stereotactic frame. (Image courtesy of A. Csavoy, Tyco/Radionics.)

portal supports all four scenarios. It will also allow users to edit, complete, or replace the data sets they have already placed in the PFA database.

The core PFA and the tools for PFA generation have to be available to the neurosurgeon as well as the neurosurgical community in an efficient and user-friendly manner. We have developed a Web-enabled, multiple-window application for this purpose. This initial version of the PFA portal provides the following key functions: (1) data loading and editing, (2) parameter setting, (3) PFA generation, (4) PFA display, and (5) combination of PFAs and/or data sets. The portal is available at www.cerefy.com.

Data loading and editing

The data-related functions allow neurosurgeons to load and explore their data. They are able to add, delete, and edit the structure, patient, electrode, and contact data.

Parameter setting

Numerous options enable the neurosurgeon to set parameters, such as selecting the atlas type (original or reconstructed) and the type of probability, setting the atlas threshold and separating its visible from hidden parts, selecting a group of voxels, setting voxel size (i.e., the resolution of the calculated atlas can be set by the neurosurgeon), and controlling atlas display. After parameters are set, the atlas can be recalculated.

Probabilistic functional atlas display

The neurosurgeon is able to display the PFA as 3-D objects (see Fig. 19–10A) or as a 2-D slice in axial, coronal, or sagittal orientation (see Fig. 19–10B). Functions for atlas exploration are provided, such as scaling, rotation, translation, showing/hiding structures. Voxels to be displayed can be selected by using numerous criteria. In particular, two major operations facilitating targeting

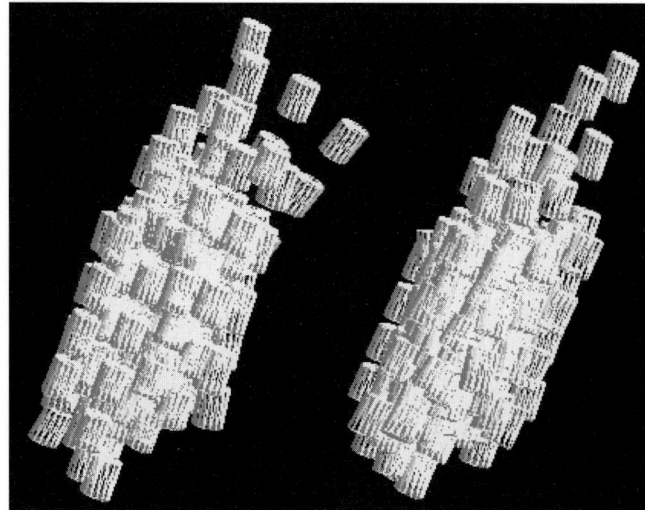
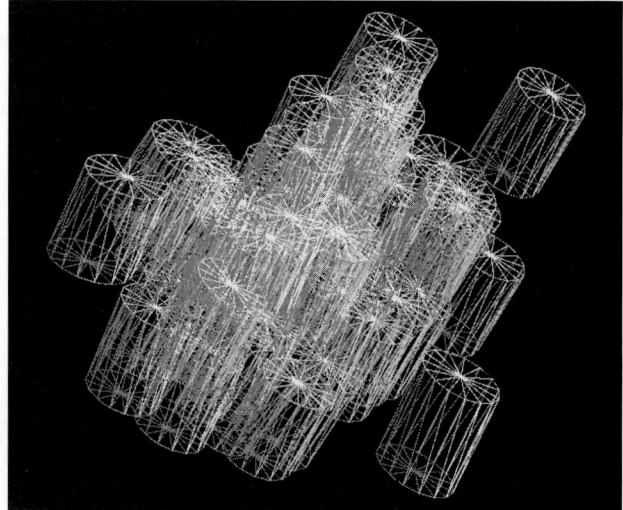

FIGURE 19–9. Calculation of the probabilistic functional atlas for the subthalamic nucleus. The normalized (placed in the atlas space) wire-frame models of (A) electrodes for both hemispheres, (B) best contacts for one hemisphere.

are provided: (1) the probability for a given region defined in the atlas by the neurosurgeon can be calculated; and (2) for a given probability determined by the neurosurgeon, the corresponding atlas region or the number of contacts in it is calculated. Other operations include displaying complete information about a selected voxel (probability, number of respective contacts and their characteristics); mensuration (distances between selected voxels, area of intersection by a plane, and volume of a selected region); displaying the mean value and standard deviation of the atlas; displaying the atlas with variable transparency such that voxel opacity is proportional to its probability. In addition, the PFA can be displayed in registration with the Cerefy anatomical atlases (see Fig. 19–10B).

Combination of probabilistic functional atlases and/or data sets

The PFA portal allows the neurosurgeon to combine atlases and data sets from multiple sources. Two PFAs are easily combined by adding their atlas functions. When a

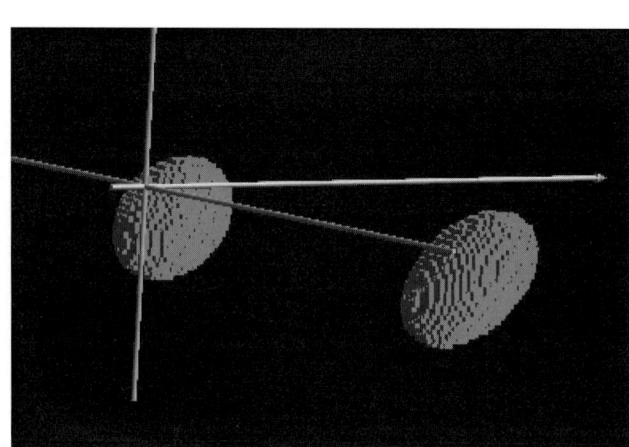
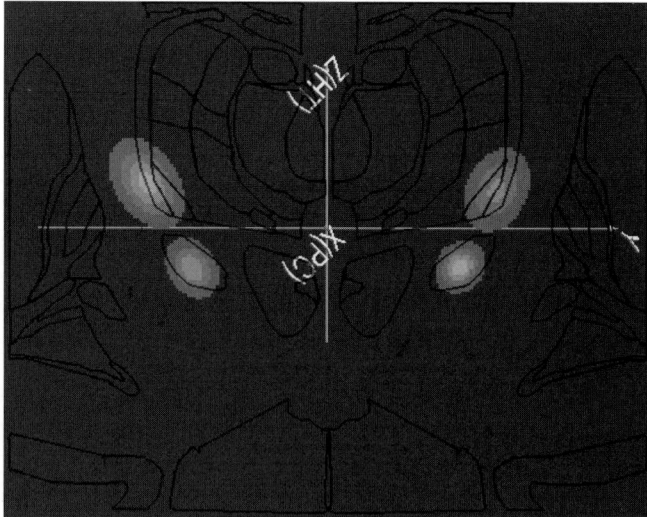

FIGURE 19–10. Reconstructed probabilistic functional atlas. (A). Three-dimensional volumetric model of the subthalamic nucleus calculated with the step of 0.25 mm from a set of the most active contacts of patients operated bilaterally. (B). Schaltenbrand-Wahren Fp 4.0 atlas plate blended with the corresponding slice from the probabilistic functional atlas. The ventrointermedius nucleus and subthalamic nucleus structures are shown such that the atlas value is proportional to image intensity.

PFA is combined with a new data set, the atlas function for the new data set is calculated first and both atlas functions are added. Similarly, if two data sets are combined, their atlas functions are calculated and then added. This combination mechanism can be done recursively, allowing neurosurgeons to combine their data, create the combined probabilistic functional atlas, and use it for more accurate targeting. When a new data set is combined with several PFAs available in the PFA database, the combined PFA is created by adding its component atlas functions; then the PFA for the new data set is calculated and added to the combined atlas function. Optionally, the new PFA can be incorporated into the PFA database and made available to the community. The best target from multiple PFAs and user's data is calculated as the best target of the combined atlas.

In addition, probabilities can also be combined. Their atlas functions have to be determined first by inversing the calculation of probability.

■ Summary

Brain atlases have become commonplace in stereotactic functional neurosurgery. The most commonly used are electronic versions of the Schaltenbrand and Wahren, and Talairach and Tournoux atlases. The Cerefy electronic brain atlas database, containing these two and other atlases, is the widely accepted standard in stereotactic functional neurosurgery. Despite their growing use, the Cerefy atlases have two major limitations. First, the original printed material is sparse and based on a few brain specimens only. And second, these atlases are anatomical, whereas the stereotactic targets are functional. The stereotactic PFA, constructed from intraoperative electrophysiological and clinical brain mapping data collected for hundreds of patients, overcomes both limitations. The use and expansion of the PFA content by means of an Internet portal represent a paradigm shift from manufacturer- to community-centric atlases. The PFA portal, supporting four scenarios of atlas use, will be useful for both experienced and novice functional neurosurgeons.

■ Acknowledgments

The authors are very grateful to the following persons for providing additional technical information: Ms. Deirdre Butler of Medtronic Surgical Navigation Technologies, Mr. Hans Schoepp of Stryker/Leibinger, and Dr. Zachary Leber of Radionics, a division of Tyco, Healthcare Group LP.

The key contributors to the construction of the electronic brain atlas database and development of the atlas-assisted applications include A. Thirunavuukarasuu, D. Belov, G. L. Yang, A. Fang, and B. T. Nguyen, among others. The *NeuroPlanner* was developed within a joint project with Dr. T. T. Yeo of Tan Tock Seng Hospital/National Neuroscience Institute, Singapore. *The Electronic Clinical Brain Atlas* was developed jointly with Prof. R. N. Bryan of Johns Hopkins Hospital, USA.

REFERENCES

1. Talairach J, David M, Tournoux P, Corredor H, Kvasina T. *Atlas d'Anatomie Stereotaxique des Noyaux Gris Centraux*. Paris: Masson; 1957.
2. Schaltenbrand G, Bailey W. *Introduction to Stereotaxis with an Atlas of the Human Brain*. Stuttgart: Georg Thieme Verlag; 1959.
3. Bertrand G, Olivier A, Thompson CJ. Computer display of stereotaxic brain maps and probe tracts. *Acta Neurochir* 1974;(suppl 21): 235–243.
4. Nowinski WL, Fang A, Nguyen BT, et al. Multiple brain atlas database and atlas-based neuroimaging system. *Computer Aided Surgery* 1997;2(1):42–66.
5. Nowinski WL. Computerized brain atlases for surgery of movement disorders. *Seminars in Neurosurgery* 2001;12(2):183–194.
6. Schaltenbrand G, Wahren W. *Atlas for Stereotaxy of the Human Brain*. Stuttgart: Georg Thieme Verlag; 1977.
7. Talairach J, Tournoux P. *Co-Planar Stereotactic Atlas of the Human Brain*. Stuttgart: Georg Thieme Verlag; 1988.
8. Talairach J, Tournoux P. *Referentially Oriented Cerebral MRI Anatomy: Atlas of Stereotaxic Anatomical Correlations for Gray and White Matter*. Stuttgart: Georg Thieme Verlag; 1993.
9. Ono M, Kubik S, Abernathey CD. *Atlas of the Cerebral Sulci*. Stuttgart: Georg Thieme Verlag; 1990.
10. Nowinski WL, Bryan RN, Raghavan R. *The Electronic Clinical Brain Atlas: Multiplanar Navigation of the Human Brain*. New York: Thieme Medical Publishers; 1997.
11. Nowinski WL, Thirunavuukarasuu A, Kennedy DN. *Brain Atlas for Functional Imaging: Clinical and Research Applications*. New York: Thieme Medical Publishers; 2000.
12. Nowinski WL, Thirunavuukarasuu A. *Methods and Apparatus for Processing Medical Images*. Patent application PCT/SG00/00185; 2000.
13. Nowinski WL, Yeo TT, Thirunavuukarasuu A. Microelectrode-guided functional neurosurgery assisted by Electronic Clinical Brain Atlas CD-ROM. *Computer Aided Surgery* 1998;3(3):115–122.
14. Nowinski WL, Thirunavuukarasuu A. *Electronic Brain Atlas Library*. New York: Thieme; Singapore: KRDL; 1998. [EBAL specification is available at www.cerefy.com].
15. Nowinski WL. *Brain Atlas Geometrical Models*. New York: Thieme Medical Publisers; Singapore: KRDL; 1998. [BAGM specification is available at www.cerefy.com].
16. Nowinski WL, Yang GL, Yeo TT. Computer-aided stereotactic functional neurosurgery enhanced by the use of the multiple brain atlas database. *IEEE Transactions on Medical Imaging* 2000;19(1): 62–69.
17. Nowinski WL. Anatomical targeting in functional neurosurgery by the simultaneous use of multiple Schaltenbrand-Wahren brain atlas microseries. *Stereotactic and Functional Neurosurgery* 1998;71: 103–116.
18. Kall BA. Computer-assisted stereotactic functional neurosurgery. In: Kelly PJ, Kall BA, eds. *Computers in Stereotactic Neurosurgery*. Boston: Blackwell; 1992:134–142.
19. Hardy TL, Deming LR, Harris-Collazo R. Computerized stereotactic atlases. In: Alexander E III, Maciunas RJ, eds. *Advanced Neurosurgical Navigation*. New York: Thieme; 1999:115–124.
20. Benabid AL, Lavallee S, Hoffmann, D, Cinquin P, Le Bas JF, Demongeot J. Computer support for the Talairach system. In: Kelly PJ, Kall BA, eds. *Computers in Stereotactic Neurosurgery*. Boston: Blackwell; 1992:230–245.

PART IIB

Spinal Applications

20

Image-Guided Cervical Instrumentation

GORDON D. C. DANDIE AND MICHAEL G. FEHLINGS

The surgical treatment of cervical spine disorders is a demanding art. This is particularly so when decompression and stabilization of the craniocervical junction, upper cervical spine, or thoracocervical junction is required. Frequently the operative field provides only a limited interface between the surgeon and complex regional anatomy. The degree of difficulty is often compounded by congenital anomalies or destructive pathological processes causing distortion of the anatomic relationships.[1]

Traditionally surgeons have had to rely on the ability to assimilate information gained from preoperative imaging with their anatomic knowledge and surgical experience, supplemented with intraoperative fluoroscopy, to determine the extent of decompression and placement of instrumentation in the cervical spine. Operative techniques developed to guide the insertion of instrumentation into cervical vertebrae are often based on cadaveric anatomic studies with limited numbers[2] and may not be appropriate for each individual case. This applies particularly to C1–C2 anatomy, which varies so significantly between patients that it precludes establishing absolute parameters for transarticular screw placement.[3] The incidence of vertebral artery injury from this procedure is greater than 4%.[4]

Frameless stereotaxy was initially applied to intracranial surgery,[5] and the technology has been adapted to assist spinal surgery.[6] As an adjunct to cervical spine surgery, use of image guidance has now been reported in transoral odontoid resection,[7] atlantoaxial fusion with C1–C2 transarticular screws,[8] occipitocervical fusion,[9] posterior cervical fusion with lateral mass plates,[9] anterior cervical decompression,[10] and cervical pedicle screw insertion.[11]

Due to the factors already discussed (limited surgical exposure, complex regional anatomy, and distortion of relational anatomy) image-guidance technology lends itself extremely well as an adjunct to cervical spine instrumentation. The surgeon is provided with a three-dimensional (3-D) anatomical correlation between the operative field and imaging data to guide surgical maneuvers, producing greater accuracy and consistency when placing instrumentation.[8] The inherent inaccuracies with the intracranial application of frameless stereotaxy due to "brain shift" and surface fiducial markers do not apply in spinal surgery.[12] The bony anatomy of the vertebrae remains consistent from preoperative imaging to intraoperative registration and is distinctive enough to provide recognizable landmarks that can be used as fiducial points. Any "intersegmental shift" is overcome by sequential registration of each vertebra to be instrumented,[12] with fluoroscopy used for cross checking alignment if required. Furthermore, the ability to universally calibrate a wide range of surgical instruments used in cervical spine surgery has expanded the benefits of image guidance beyond simply pointing with a probe to estimate trajectories.[13] Decompression can be undertaken with calibrated upcutting rongeurs,[14] or screwholes drilled through calibrated guide tubes with real-time image guidance.[12]

Some of the disadvantages of image-guided cervical surgery include the initial cost of the equipment,[8] the time added to the overall length of the procedure by registration,[15] increased imaging and therefore increased radiation dose to the patient,[16] and potential inaccuracies associated with relying on preoperative imaging of a mobile structure.[17] We believe that when image guidance is applied appropriately to cervical instrumentation procedures (see following text), most of these limitations can be answered. After the initial learning curve, intraoperative registration is a step that usually only takes 1 to 2 minutes per vertebra, time that is often recouped due to the surgeon's increased confidence in the accurate placement of the instrumentation when using the system.[9] For most of the cervical procedures in which we use the image-guidance system, patients require preoperative assessment with a fine-cut computed tomographic (CT) scan of the bony anatomy (and 3-D reconstructions) in addition to the imaging they presented with anyway, and therefore usually do not receive an increased radiation dose over and above that which our usual practice would entail.

A number of techniques are employed to overcome "motion inaccuracies." Intraoperative motion between segments due to respiration is compensated for by "dynamic referencing,"[12] a process whereby movement of the reference arc is tracked by the electro-optical camera at a frequency of 30 to 60 Hz, and the images on the workstation are constantly updated to compensate for the movement. As previously mentioned, "intersegmental shift" is overcome by sequential referencing of each vertebra as required. Instability at the site of the pathology can be negated by imaging the patient in a halo vest, which can be worn intraoperatively to maintain the same alignment. Alternatively intraoperative fluoroscopy can be employed to check alignment and confirm the relationship of two adjacent vertebrae (e.g., C1 and C2).

■ Indications

Despite the reported use of image guidance as an adjunct to all major types of cervical instrumentation,[7–11] we believe its main indications in cervical surgery are assisting the placement of C1–C2 transarticular screws, assisting the placement of pedicle screws, and guiding transoral decompression of the ventral cervicomedullary junction. If the image-guidance system is being employed to assist insertion of transarticular or pedicle screws, and the construct also requires lateral mass screws, we find it helpful in assisting their placement also, but we do not routinely use image guidance for lateral mass screws alone. Nor do we routinely use image guidance for anterior cervical decompression (discectomy, foraminotomy, corporectomy) and instrumentation (Table 20–1).

TABLE 20–1. Indications for Image Guidance in Complex Cervical Spine Surgery

Definite indications	C1–C2 transarticular screw insertion (occipitocervical fusion, atlantoaxial fusion)
	Transoral decompression ventral craniocervical junction
	Cervicle pedicle screws
Helpful	Lateral mass screws (including C1 lateral mass screws)
	C2 pars screws
	Tumor resections
Occasionally of assistance	Anterior cervical discectomy and fusion
	Anterior cervical corporectomy and fusion

Insertion of C1–C2 transarticular screws, whether associated with atlantoaxial fusion, occipitocervical fusion, or axial-subaxial fusion, is the indication par excellence for image-guided cervical instrumentation. As already mentioned, the high degree of anatomical variability in the C1–C2 region prevents a formulaic approach to transarticular screw insertion.[3] Individual features to be considered when planning screw placement include the size of the C2 pars, the degree to which the C1–C2 articulation is aligned, and whether the patient has a "high riding" transverse foramen. Standard operative techniques still result in inadequate screw positioning in over 5% of cases.[18] In addition, lateral fluoroscopy has been shown to be unreliable in determining optimal transarticular C1–C2 screw length, with a risk of anterior cortical perforation and the potential for hypoglossal nerve injury.[19] To illustrate how we employ image guidance as an adjunct to cervical instrumentation, we will describe its application to C1–C2 transarticular screw insertion.

■ Technique

Preoperative imaging for all of our patients undergoing C1–C2 transarticular instrumentation includes plain cervical spine radiographs, including dynamic flexion and extension views if feasible, magnetic resonance imaging (MRI) of the craniocervical junction (Figs. 20–1A and 20–1B), and 1 mm fine-slice CT scanning. We have found that 1 mm slices (as opposed to 1.5 mm and 3 mm) provide the most accurate reconstructions for image guidance applied to the cervical spine, where finer tolerances are required than for the lower spine. Patients requiring reduction or immobilization preoperatively are placed in a halo vest prior to imaging. The data from the CT study are transferred via ethernet to the image-guidance workstation (Surgical Navigation Specialists Inc., Mississauga, Ontario) and reconstructed to provide images in three planes and a 3-D model of the

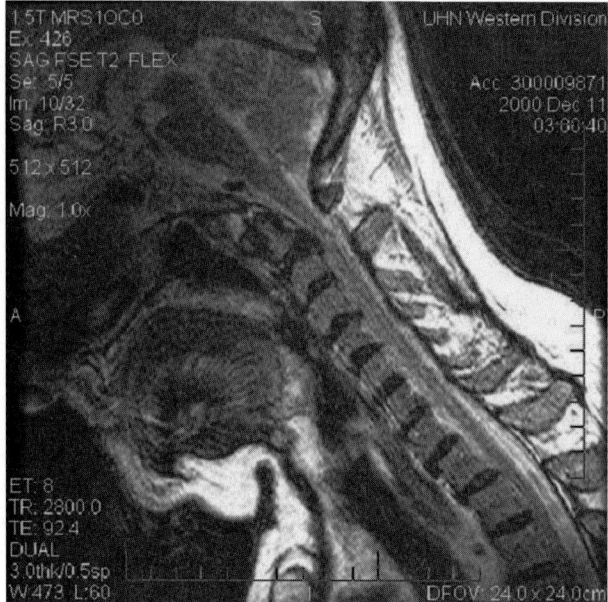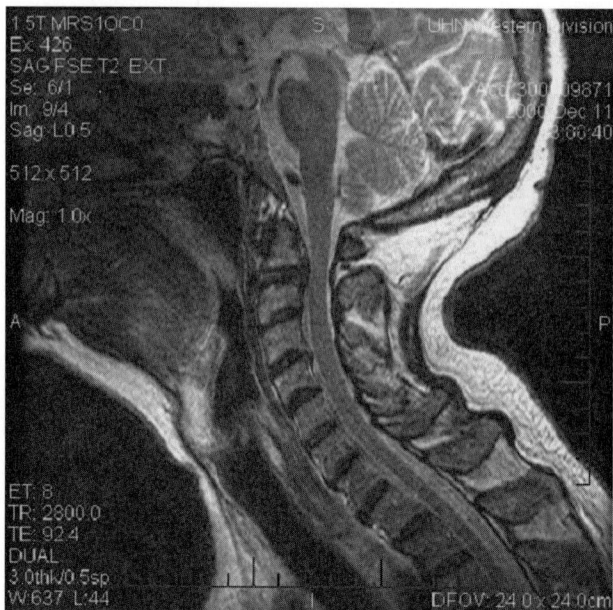

FIGURE 20–1. (A). T2-weighted magnetic resonance image (MRI) showing dynamic compression at C2 due to pseudoarthrosis (flexion). (B). T2-weighted MRI showing dynamic compression at C2 due to pseudoarthrosis (extension).

bony anatomy. If the procedure involves resection of tumor, CT/MRI fusion is also utilized.

The patient is transferred to the operating suite and undergoes awake fiber-optic intubation and general anesthesia. Somatosensory-evoked potentials are monitored and prophylactic antibiotics are administered. While anesthesia is being induced the surgeons undertake final preoperative planning and selection of anatomical fiducial points on the workstation images that will be used for registration. The two main modalities of registration are the paired-point and surface-fit methods.[20] Paired-point registration involves defining corresponding points on the images and the patient and thereby linking the two coordinate systems. Extrinsic points (skin markers) are usually used for cranial image guidance, whereas intrinsic points (anatomic features) can be more readily utilized in spinal surgery. Surface-fit registration matches a large set of points derived from the surface contour of the patient's anatomy with the best fit of the imaged contour. Surface-fit registration tends to be more time-consuming and less accurate than paired-point registration.[20]

The principles for paired-point fiducial selection have been described elsewhere,[21] the main criteria being to avoid linear fiducial configurations, center the fiducial configuration on the operative target, keep the fiducials as far away from each other as possible, and use as many fiducials as possible. Accordingly, we use a system of six paired points per vertebra, selecting the midpoint of the medial border of the lateral mass, the midpoint of the inferior articular process, and the midpoint of the lateral border of the lateral mass (Fig. 20–2). After the patient is positioned on the operating table, a C-arm image-intensifier is positioned to enable lateral fluoroscopy during the procedure (Fig. 20–3).

Following surgical exposure of the occiput and upper cervical spine, the stereotactic reference arc is then attached to the spinous process of C2 via a thin articulated arm (Fig. 20–4) and positioned away from the operative field, in direct view of the electro-optical camera system. Registration of the C2 vertebra is then per-

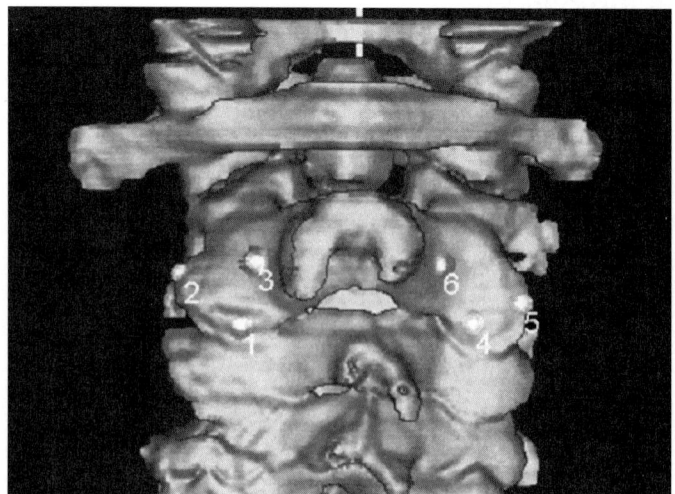

FIGURE 20–2. Three-dimensional reconstruction showing selected positions of paired-point anatomical fiducials.

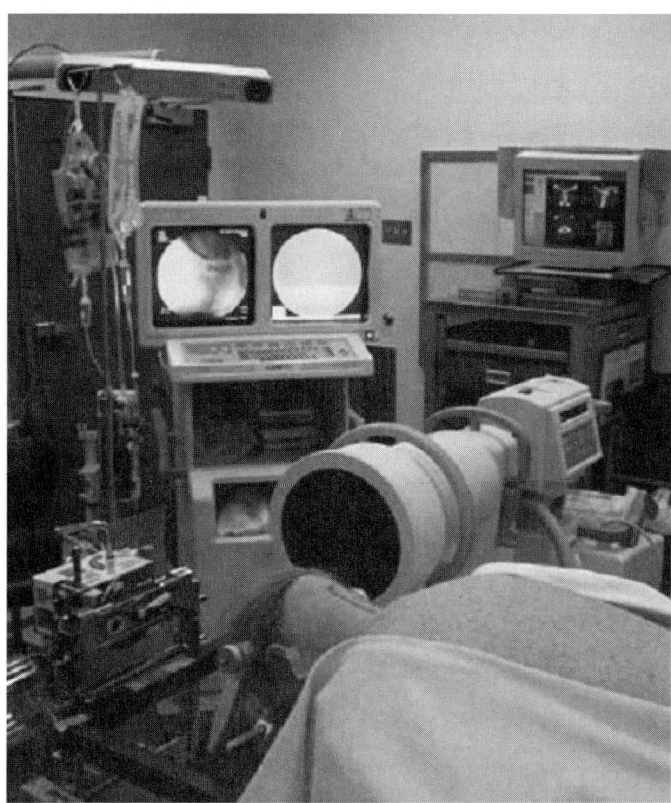

FIGURE 20–3. Operative setup. Note position of fluoroscope, optical tracking camera (small arrow), and computer workstation screen (large arrow).

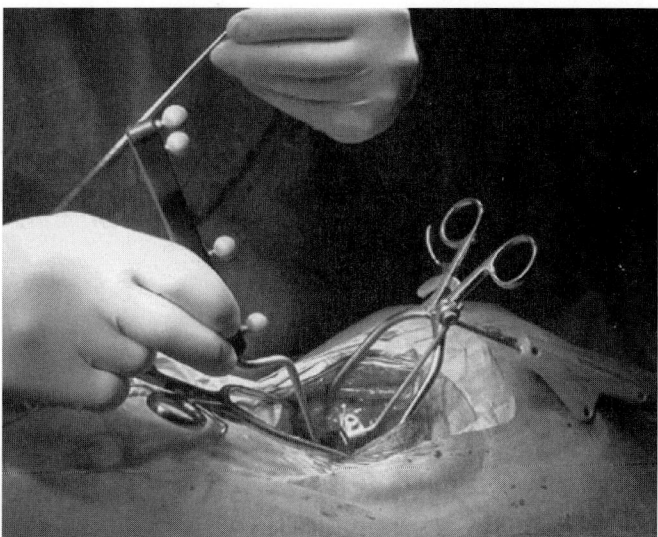

FIGURE 20–4. Articulated arm with reference arc in position (arrow).

formed using the preselected six paired points and accuracy checked by positioning the probe on well-defined anatomical landmarks, such as the tips of the spinous process, and viewing the corresponding position indicated on the workstation monitor. It is important for the surgeon to use familiar image configurations to ensure ease of application. We find a combination of axial, sagittal, coronal, and 3-D reconstructions most useful. Occasionally, other views, including a trajectory view when placing screws, can be helpful.

When testing accuracy after registration, the surgeon's perception of the accuracy of the correlation of the surgical anatomy with the image anatomy is as important as the "margin of error" figures generated by the system software. As already discussed, it is critical to validate the accuracy of registration by referring to fixed anatomic points. Image-guidance systems remain an adjunct to assist surgical maneuvers; they do not replace the surgeon's intuitive skills and knowledge of the intraoperative anatomy.

The stereotactic probe is then used to select the entry points for the C1–C2 transarticular screws to enable a safe passage through the C2 pars (Fig. 20–5), and the sites are decorticated with a high-speed drill (2 mm round diamond burr). A variable-depth stereotactic probe may also be used to guide incision sites for the percutaneous drill guide tubes. With the guide tubes inserted the fluoroscopy C-arm is positioned and drill trajectory confirmed with both the stereotactic probe and the fluoroscope. A 2.7 mm drill bit is then directed across the midportion of the C1–C2 articulation and toward the C1 anterior tubercle under intermittent fluoroscopic guidance. Fluoroscopy can be misleading if used to determine screw length[19] so we use the image-guidance system to help measure accurate screw dimensions. The hole is then further prepared with a 3.5 mm tap and an appropriate 3.5 mm diameter screw inserted under intermittent fluoroscopic guidance. The procedure is repeated on the opposite side, and autologous bone graft is laid over the C1–C2 facet after decortication with a high-speed dill. The rest of the construct is then applied as required (e.g., occipitocervical plate, interspinous graft, or lateral mass screws and plates). We routinely check the construct postoperatively with plain radiographs. We currently use 3-D CT to assess C1–C2 transarticular screw position postoperatively (Fig. 20–6).

■ Clinical Experience

At the University Health Network Spinal Program, University of Toronto, we recently assessed 35 complex cervical spine instrumentation procedures performed by the senior author in which image guidance was utilized. The 35 patients had an age range of 14 to 84 years (mean 55 years) and comprised 21 females and 14 males. The pathologies treated included rheumatoid arthritis, trauma, congenital anomalies, pseudotumor, osteoarthritis, tumor, and ossification of the posterior

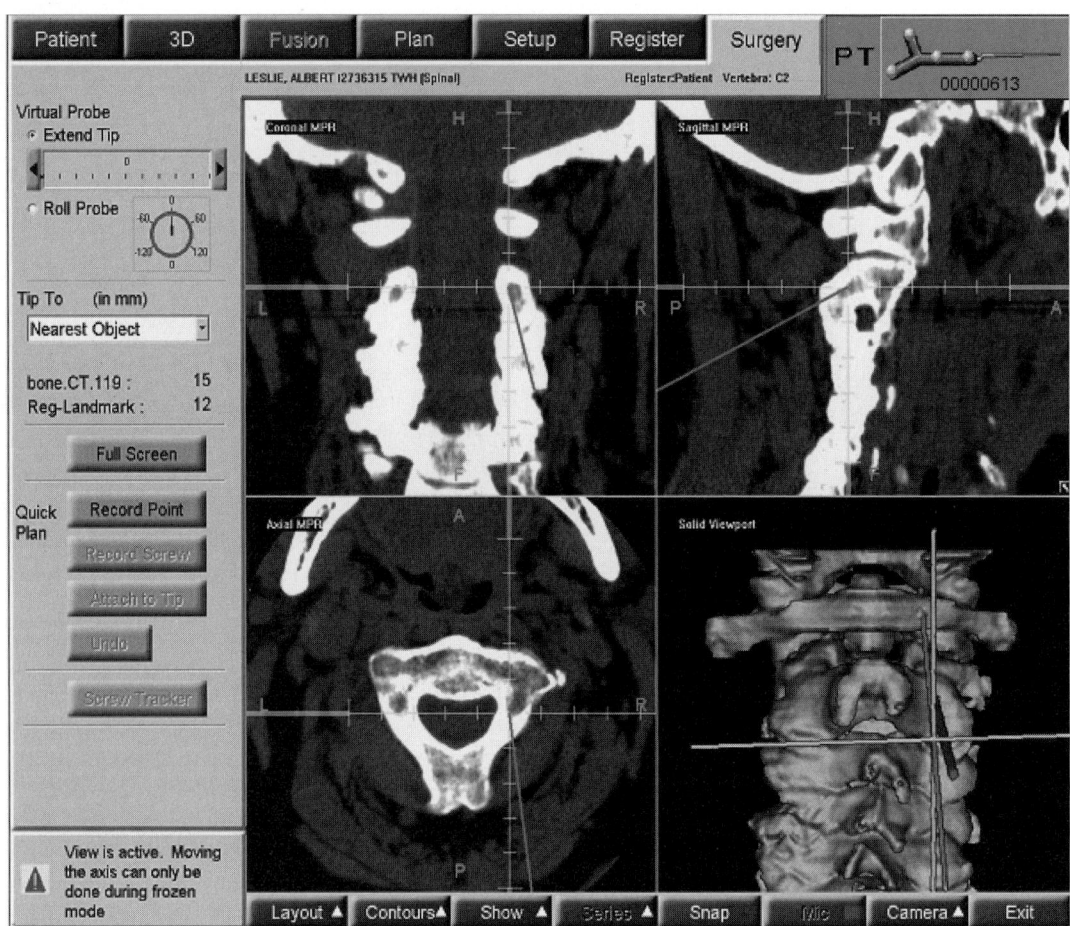

FIGURE 20–5. Workstation screen showing selection of entry point and proposed trajectory of C1–C2 transarticular screw (Surgical Navigation Specialists, Mississauga, Ontario, Canada).

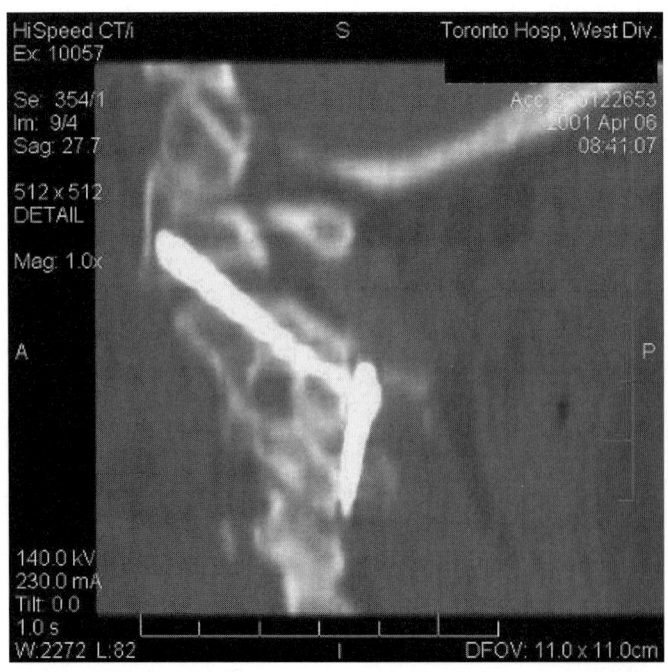

FIGURE 20–6. Postoperative computed tomography showing C1–C2 transarticular screw position.

longitudinal ligament. Image guidance was found useful for transoral decompression, occipitocervical fusion (transarticular screws), atlantoaxial fusion (transarticular screws), complex axial-subaxial fusion, and cervicothoracic fuison (pedicle screws).

In one patient undergoing atlantoaxial fusion the image-guidance system was used for preoperative planning only because it showed passage of transarticular screws was contraindicated. There have been no intraoperative complications (neural or vascular injury) during the 35 procedures, and accuracy of transarticular screw placement has improved when graded by postoperative 3-D CT and compared with a retrospective cohort of patients whose procedures were performed without image guidance (unpublished data).

■ Conclusions

Cervical anatomy is complex, and operating on the cervical spine that has been distorted by pathology is challenging. Image-guidance systems help the surgeon navigate this difficult region, thereby increasing surgical accuracy and safety, which should improve patient outcomes. Future developments, such as incorporating intraoperative CT, could possibly increase the accuracy of the registration process by allowing insertion of microfiducials directly onto the vertebrae, which can then be imaged during the procedure, or by enabling true autoregistration by detecting the reference frame during the imaging process. With further refinement, fluoroscopically registered image guidance may also potentially advance the usefulness of this exciting technology.

REFERENCES

1. Zeidman SM, Ducker TB. Rheumatoid arthritis: neuroanatomy, compression and grading of deformity. *Spine* 1994;19(20):2259–2266.
2. Ebraheim NA, Klausner T, Rongming X, et al. Safe lateral-mass screw lengths in the Roy-Camille and Magerl techniques. *Spine* 1998;23(16):1739–1742.
3. Foley KT, Silveri CP, Vaccaro AR, et al. Atlantoaxial transarticular screw fixation: risk assessment and bone morphology using an image guidance system. *J Bone Joint Surg* [Br] 1998;80-B(suppl 3):245.
4. Wright NM, Lauryssen C. Vertebral artery injury in C1–2 transarticular screw fixation: results of a survey of the AANS/CNS Section on Disorders of the Spine and Peripheral Nerves. *J Neurosurg* 1998;88:634–640.
5. Barnett GH, Kormos DW, Steiner CP, et al. Intraoperative localization using an armless, frameless stereotactic wand. *J Neurosurg* 1993; 78:510–514.
6. Kalfas IH, Kormos DW, Murphy MA, et al. Application of frameless stereotaxy to pedicle screw fixation of the spine. *J Neurosurg* 1995;83:641–647.
7. Pollack IF, Welch W, Jacobs GB, et al. Frameless stereotactic guidance: an intraoperative adjunct in the transoral approach for ventral cervicomedullary junction decompression. *Spine* 1995;20(2):216–220.
8. Welch WC, Subach BR, Pollack IF, et al. Frameless stereotactic guidance for surgery of the upper cervical spine. *Neurosurgery* 1997;40(5):958–963.
9. Bolger C, Wigfield C. Image-guided surgery: applications to the cervical and thoracic spine and a review of the first 120 procedures. *J Neurosurg* 2000;92(2 suppl):175–180.
10. Bolger C, Wigfield C. Frameless stereotaxy and anterior cervical surgery. *Comput Aided Surg* 1999;4:322–327.
11. Kramer DL, Ludwig SC, Balderston RA, et al. Placement of pedicle screws in the cervical spine: comparative accuracy of cervical pedicle screw placement using three techniques [abstract]. *Orthop Trans* 1997;21:484.
12. Foley KT, Smith MM. Image-guided spine surgery. *Neurosurg Clin North Am* 1996;7(2):171–186.
13. Kim KD, Johnson JP, Masciopinto JE, et al. Universal calibration of surgical instruments for spinal stereotaxy. *Neurosurgery* 1999;44(1):173–177.
14. Klein GR, Ludwig SC, Vaccaro AR, et al. The efficacy of using an image-guided Kerrison punch in performing an anterior cervical foraminotomy. *Spine* 1999;24(13):1358–1362.
15. Albert TJ, Klein GR, Vaccaro AR. Image-guided anterior cervical corporectomy: a feasibility study. *Spine* 1999;24(8):826–830.
16. Slomczykowski M, Roberto M, Schneeberger P, et al. Radiation dose for pedicle screw insertion: fluoroscopic method versus computer-assisted surgery. *Spine* 1999;24(10):975–983.
17. Maciunas RJ. Frameless stereotactic guidance for surgery of the upper cervical spine [comment]. *Neurosurgery* 1997;40(5):963.
18. Fuji T, Oda TO, Kato Y, et al. Accuracy of atlantoaxial transarticular screw insertion. *Spine* 2000;25(14):1760–1764.
19. Xu R, Ebraheim NA, Misson JR, et al. The reliability of the lateral radiograph in determination of the optimal transarticular C1–C2 screw length. *Spine* 1998;23(20):2190–2194.
20. Wadley JP, Thomas DGT. Neuronavigation: accuracy, benefits and pitfalls. *Neurosurgery Quarterly* 2000;10(4):276–310.
21. West JB, Fitzpatrick JM, Toms SA, et al. Fiducial point placement and the accuracy of point-based, rigid body registration. *Neurosurgery* 2001;48(4):810–816.

21

Thoracic Instrumentation
Stereotactic Navigation for Placement of Pedicle Screws in the Thoracic Spine

ANDREW S. YOUKILIS AND STEPHEN M. PAPADOPOULOS

Application of transpedicular screws for posterior fixation in the treatment of spinal instability has undergone continuous evolution and refinement in technique since King attempted the first transfacet screw in 1944.[1] Even before the Food and Drug Administration upgraded them from a Class III to a Class II device in July 1998, pedicle screws in the lumbar spine were considered by many to be the best and most rigid form of posterior spinal fixation. Due to the smaller size and more complex three-dimensional morphology of the thoracic pedicle, transpedicular screw placement in the thoracic spine can be extremely challenging and has not been widely advocated. Anatomic studies have demonstrated a wide degree of variability of pedicular diameter, shape, and angle (Fig. 21–1). Given the proximity of the thoracic pleura, nerve roots, and spinal cord itself, serious morbidity can accompany a less than perfectly placed thoracic pedicle screw.

■ Anatomic Background

Over the past several years, a wealth of data has accumulated regarding the anatomy of the thoracic pedicle.[2–7] Utilizing this data, a variety of techniques have been developed in an effort to decrease the complications associated with thoracic pedicle screw placement.[8,9] In contrast to the lumbar spine, there is considerable variation among thoracic vertebrae, in both the relationship of the transverse process to the axis of the pedicle and the angle of the pedicle to the vertebral body.[5] Due to the variability of these individual parameters, freehand placement of thoracic pedicle screws using anatomic landmarks may be imprecise and may thus lead to errors in screw placement. Clinical and cadaveric studies have shown that 15 to 50% of thoracic screws violate the pedicular cortex when placed using anatomic landmarks and fluoroscopic techniques.[8–11] Analysis of pedicular cortex violations has included direct visualization (cadaveric studies), plain x-ray, and thin-cut computed tomographic (CT) scans (Table 21–1).

Image-guided stereotaxy provides three-dimensional, intraoperative guidance, which is well suited for thoracic pedicle screw size and trajectory. Recently, cadaveric studies have investigated the accuracy of this technology with extremely encouraging results.[12–14] In a recent analysis at our institution, we designed a retrospective study to assess the clinical accuracy and safety of thoracic pedicle screw placement utilizing intraoperative navigational techniques by several surgeons of varying experience and skill.

■ Accuracy of Stereotactic Thoracic Pedicle Screw Placement

Since 1996, 266 thoracic pedicle screws, in 65 patients, were placed using image-guided techniques. All screws were placed by one of four surgeons with a range of experience in posterior spinal fixation and intraoperative navigation. Screw diameter ranged from 4.5 mm in the mid and upper thoracic spine to 6.5 mm in the lower thoracic spine. Screw length varied from 25 to 55 mm and was predetermined by measurement on the stereotactic planning station. The StealthStation (Medtronic SNT, Louisville, CO) stereotactic image-guidance computer platform was utilized in all instances of screw placement. Operating sys-

TABLE 21-2. Overview of Stereotactic Thoracic Pedicle Screw Data

Patient	Surgeon	T1	T2	T3	T4	T5	T6	T7	T8	T9	T10	T11	T12	≤Gr I	Gr II + Gr III
1	1	2												2	
2	1	1	2	2										5	
3	1	2												2	
4	1	2												2	
5	1	2												2	
6	3												2	2	
7	1		2											2	
8	1												2	2	
9	1				2	2		2	2					8	
10	1											2	2	4	
11	1										2	2		4	
12	1									2	2		2	6	
13	1											2	2	3	1
14	1										2	2		3	1
15	1											2	2	4	
16	2		2											1	1
17	1											2	2	4	
18	3										2	2	2	4	2
19	2									2	2		2	5	1
20	2												2	1	1
21	1										2	2		4	
22	2		2											2	
23	1										2	2		4	
24	2											2	2	4	
25	1		2											2	
26	1			2	2			2	2					6	2
27	1											2		2	
28	2												2	2	
29	1											2	2	4	
30	2		2											2	
31	2											2	2	4	
32	1										2	2		4	
33	1			2	2	2	2							7	1
34	1							2	2		2	2		8	
35	1									2	2		2	5	1
36	1									2	2		2	6	
37	1												2	2	
38	1		2											2	
39	1										2	2	1	5	
40	1					2	2	1	2					7	
41	1											2	2	4	
42	1											2	2	4	
43	2		2											2	
44	1		2	2	2									5	1
45	1		2											2	
46	2		2											2	
47	4					2	2		2	2				6	2
48	1									2	2	2	2	8	
49	1				2	2	1	2	2					6	3
50	3					2	2			2	2			6	2
51	1					2	2		2	2				8	
52	4											2	2	4	
TOTALS		29	6	10	12	12	9	11	10	14	30	40	41	205	19

compared with the upper thoracic (T1–T4 = 8.8%) and lower thoracic (T9–T12 = 5.6%) regions (Table 21–3B). After controlling for surgeon difference and accounting for correlation of multiple screws placed within the same patient, a logistic regression analysis demonstrated a statistically significant difference in the rate of pedicular violation in the midthoracic spine [$P = 0.0072$, odds ratio (OR) = 5.66, and 95% confidence interval = 1.6–2.0 from T4 to T9]. Thoracic levels with the highest rates of cortical violation in our series included T4 ($P = 0.0005$, OR = 31.3), followed by T8 ($P = 0.0049$, OR = 21.9) and T2 ($P = 0.0173$, OR = 18.5).

Of the eight Grade III screws, three were placed intentionally through the rib head in the lateral aspect of the pedicle due to thin, scaphoid-shaped, or laterally directed pedicles. Out of a total of 224 screws evaluated,

TABLE 21–3A. Review of Cortical Violations

Patient	Surgeon	Side/Level	Direction	Grade	Comment
13	1	Right T11	Lateral	III	Intentional
14	1	Right T10	Lateral	III	Thin pedicles
16	2	Left T1	Medial	II	
18	3	Right T10	Lateral	III	
18	3	Left T10	Lateral	II	
19	2	Left T9	Lateral	III	Intraop instability
20	2	Left T12	Lateral	II	
26	1	Left T6	Inferior	II	
26	1	Right T6	Inferior	II	
33	1	Right T2	Lateral	II	
35	1	Right T9	Lateral	III	Intentional
44	1	Right T4	Lateral	II	
47	4	Left T4	Medial	III	
47	4	Left T8	Lateral	III	
49	1	Left T4	Medial	II	Thin pedicles
49	1	Left T7	Superior/lateral	II	Thin pedicles
49	1	Left T8	Lateral	III	Intentional
50	3	Right T5	Lateral	II	
50	3	Left T5	Lateral	II	

only five (2.2%) were felt to be structurally significant, inadvertent violations of the pedicular cortex (Fig. 21–4).

■ Thoracic Pedicle Screw Placement: A Unique Challenge

It is well accepted that pedicle screws and rods provide superior stability in comparison to other posterior spinal fixation techniques. Specifically, biomechanical studies have suggested pedicle screws to be superior to other posterior fixation techniques, providing increased rigidity and construct stiffness.[15–17] This increased rigidity allows for shorter construct lengths and decreased time in external orthoses. Although techniques for pedicle screw fixation in the lumbar spine have become quite common, there has been considerable debate over the safety of pedicle screw placement in the thoracic spine.[7,8,11,16]

Pedicle screw placement in the thoracic spine presents a unique challenge. Unlike the lumbar pedicle,

TABLE 21–3B. Subset Analysis of Grade II, Grade III Cortical Violations

	T1	T2	T3	T4	T5	T6	T7	T8	T9	T10	T11	T12
Total screws	29	6	10	12	12	9	11	10	14	30	40	41
Grade II/III violations	1	1	0	3	2	2	1	2	2	3	1	1
Percentage out	0.034	0.167	0.000	0.250	0.167	0.222	0.091	0.200	0.143	0.100	0.025	0.024
	Miss % = 0.088					*Miss % = 0.167*				*Miss % = 0.056*		

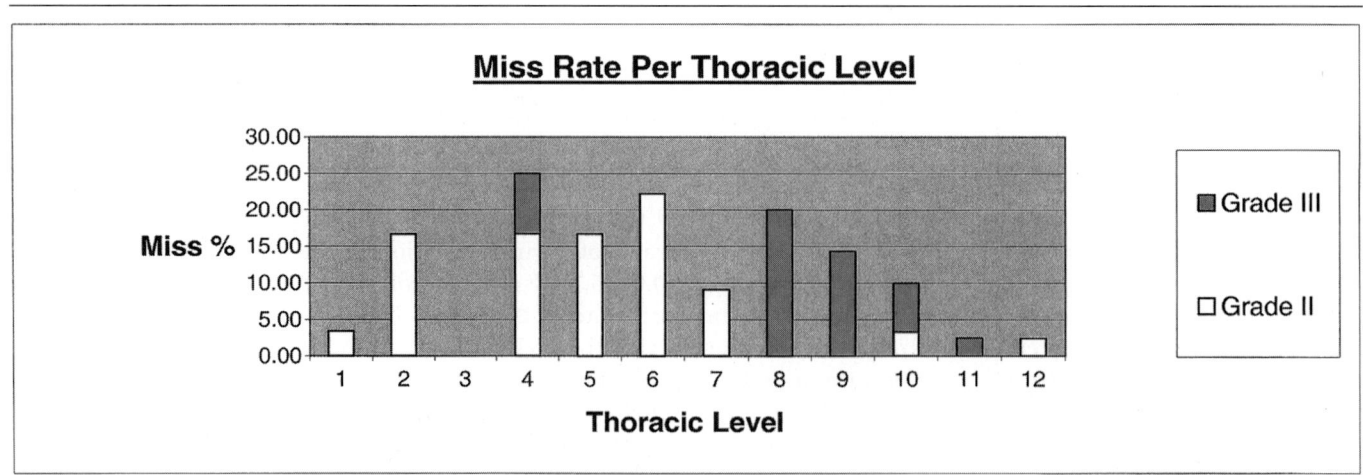

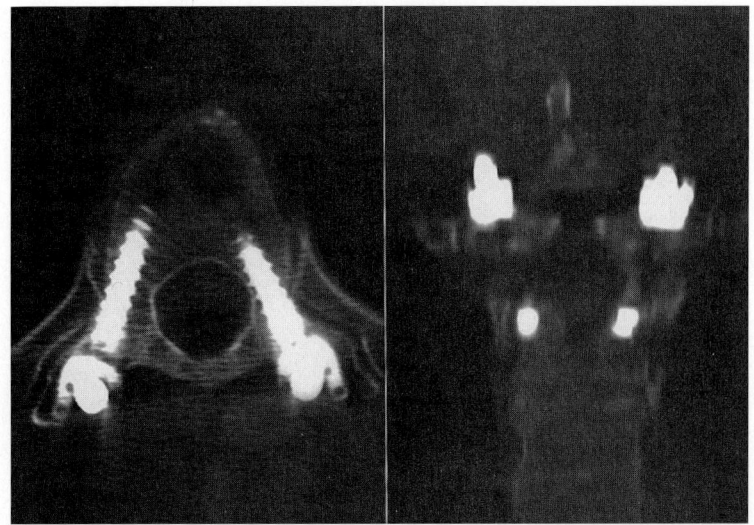
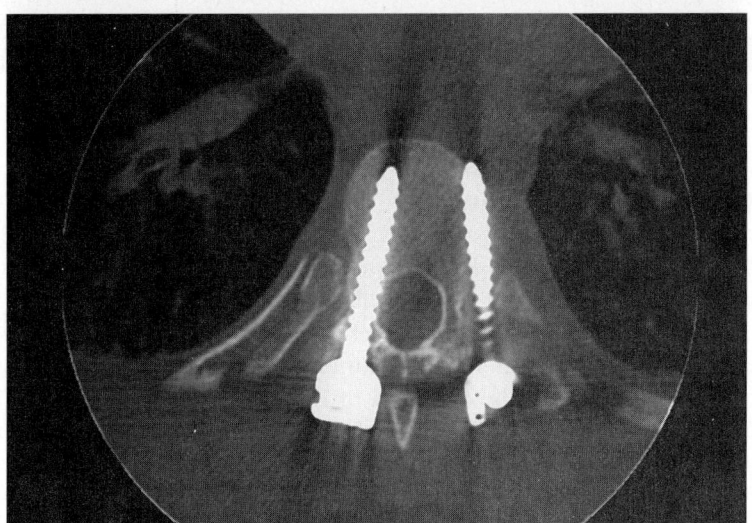

FIGURE 21–4. (A). Axial computed tomographic (CT) scan with coronal reformats demonstrating a Grade II lateral, cortical violation at T3. (B). Axial CT scan demonstrating a Grade III lateral, cortical violation at T8.

there is little room for error in the smaller and more three-dimensionally complex thoracic pedicle. Morphometric studies have shown pedicular size to be widely variable, ranging from a smallest mean transverse diameter of 4.5 mm at T4 to a largest mean transverse diameter of 7.8 mm at TI2.[16] Medial errors are less forgiving in the thoracic spine because there is less mobility of the spinal cord than that of the nerve roots in the cauda equina. Lateral perforations of the pedicular cortex are potential threats to the pleural cavity and great vessel.[18] Although anatomic studies have shown pedicle screw placement to be feasible in the thoracic spine,[7] spine surgeons may be reluctant to attempt thoracic pedicle screws, given the increased technical difficulty and inherent risks associated with their placement.

Considerable debate has arisen concerning the best method for screw placement in the thoracic spine. The specific anatomic location for screw entry is much more difficult to determine compared with the lumbar pedicle. The general rule, which places the rostral-caudal center of the pedicle at the midpoint of the transverse process, does not necessarily hold true in the widely variable thoracic spine.[5] Not only is this location quite variable as one moves from the rostral to the caudal portions of the thoracic spine, there is also segmental variability from left to right. Moreover, unlike the large-ovoid lumbar pedicle, the cross-sectional morphology of a single thoracic pedicle is widely variable in the coronal plane (see Fig. 21–1).[4] Several surgical techniques have evolved to more accurately locate the center of the pedicle in the thoracic spine using anatomic landmarks and in combination with intraoperative fluoroscopy.[8,9] In spite of these techniques, several authors have concluded that some thoracic pedicles may be too complex for safe screw placement, given the accuracy that is required and the limited margin of tolerable error.[7,8]

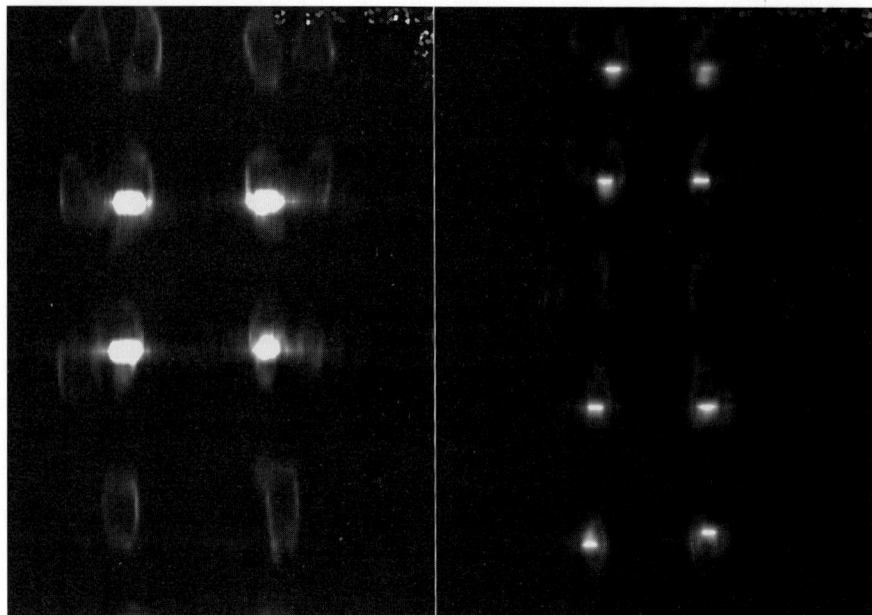

FIGURE 21–5. Coronal computed tomographic reformats demonstrating the utility of this view in assessing cortical integrity.

■ Literature Review

Review of the published literature on thoracic pedicle screw accuracy has revealed an alarmingly high rate of cortical disruptions (see Table 21–1). Cadaveric series using landmarks alone have documented "miss" rates as high as 55%.[9] With the addition of fluoroscopy, the accuracy of screw placement modestly improves but is still unacceptably high, in the range of 15 to 25%. In the largest published clinical series to date, Liljenqvist et al reported their results of 32 patients with idiopathic scoliosis who underwent thoracic pedicle screw fixation.[10] Thoracic screws were placed from T4 to T12 using anatomical landmarks and fluoroscopy. Of the 120 thoracic screws placed, they reported a cortical penetration rate of 25%, evaluated by plain x-rays and thin-cut CT scans. They reported a higher incidence of cortical violation in the upper thoracic spine (T4–T7, 35.3%) than in the lower thoracic spine (T8–T12, 23.3%). Medial penetration occurred in 8.3% of the total thoracic screws placed.

It is important to note that the method of accuracy assessment of pedicle screw placement is a topic of controversy. Although many spine surgeons consider anteroposterior and lateral plain x-rays to be an adequate assessment of screw location, Weinstein et al showed there to be "unacceptably high rates of false-positive and false-negative evaluations."[11] Accordingly, thin-cut CT scans should be considered the gold standard in postoperative evaluation of pedicle screw placement. Coronal reconstructions are especially useful in determining the relationship of the screw to the pedicular cortex (Fig. 21–5).

■ Rationale for Stereotaxy in the Thoracic Spine

Given the three-dimensional complexity of the thoracic pedicle and the low tolerance for error in screw placement, image-guided stereotaxy is well suited to the task of thoracic pedicle screw placement. There has been little data comparing the accuracy of image-guided screw placement with that of the more conventional techniques, however. In 1996, a report by Abitbol et al evaluated 48 thoracic screws placed from T1 to T12 in two separate cadavers, one half using image guidance and the other half using biplanar fluoroscopy and anatomic landmarks.[12] Using visual inspection and CT scans, nearly 50% of screws placed with conventional techniques were noted to perforate the pedicular cortex (16% of all screws with "critical" violations), whereas only one cortical disruption was noted in the group with image guidance (4% of all screws). Others have touted the accuracy of stereotactic pedicle screw placement in the thoracic spine,[13,14,19] yet there have been no large clinical series published in the literature.

Image-guided stereotaxy gives the surgeon an added level of preoperative planning and pedicle assessment not previously available using the more conventional techniques of screw placement. Certain pedicles may simply be too small or scaphoid to make perfect screw

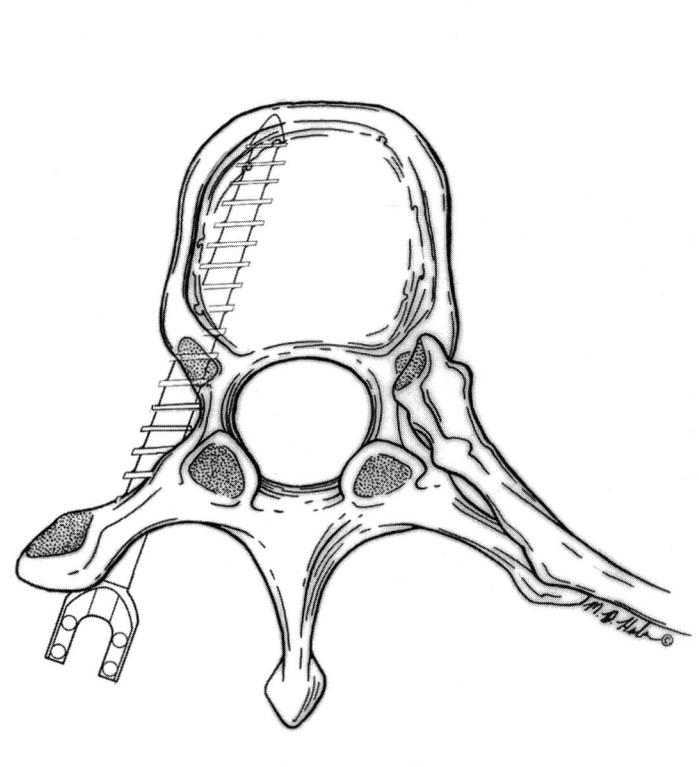
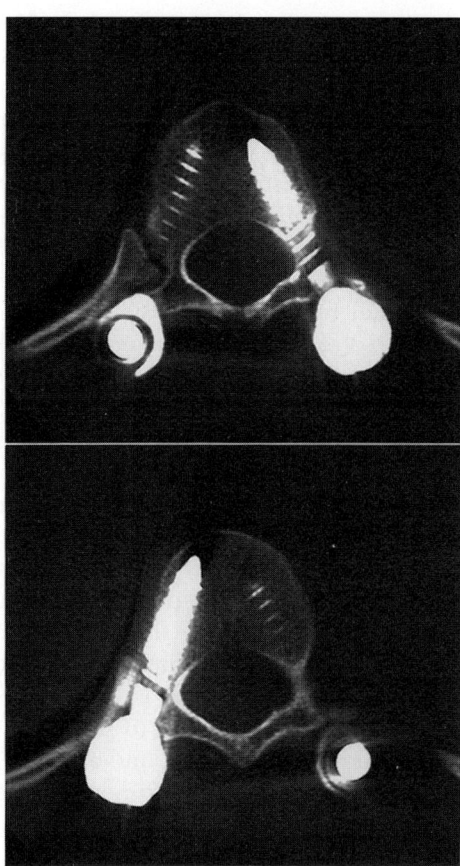

FIGURE 21–6. In cases of thin, scaphoid, or laterally directed pedicles, the surgeon may choose an intentional, lateral trajectory through the rib head to achieve maximum purchase when presented with inadequate-sized pedicles.

placement feasible. In these instances a nontraditional trajectory can be chosen based on the preoperative model, placing the pedicle screw intentionally through the rib head and into the vertebral body (Fig. 21–6). Anecdotal experience indicates that an intentional lateral screw entry is a viable alternative when the pedicle is either laterally directed, scaphoid in shape, or less than 4 mm in its smallest coronal diameter.

In this retrospective series of 224 pedicle screws placed by four surgeons with a wide range of experience with image guidance, there were a total of 19 violations of the pedicular cortex (8.5%). This compares favorably with previously published accuracy rates using standard interoperative landmarks and fluoroscopy (see Table 21–1). Moreover, this high degree of accuracy in this large clinical series is in concordance with smaller cadaveric studies investigating the accuracy of stereotactic techniques in the thoracic spine.[5,12,13] Many of the Grade II violations represented a minor mismatch of pedicular size and contour versus screw diameter. This subset of cortical violations, therefore, may be more dependent on the limit of pedicle screw size from a biomechanical standpoint than the margin of error inherent in stereotactic screw placement. Of the 19 Grade II and Grade III screws, only five were felt to be potential, anatomically significant cortical violations (2.2% of all screws), none of which required subsequent reoperation for change of position. We feel that this figure represents the true anatomic miss rate associated with stereotactic guidance in the thoracic spine and emphasizes the low yet ever present potential for error. Chart review revealed no incidence of postoperative neurological, vascular, or pulmonary injury in any patient in our series.

Some authors suggest that the increased rate of radiographic cortical violations does not necessarily correlate with poorer clinical outcome. In the two largest series of thoracic pedicle screws placed with fluoroscopic guidance alone, the authors touted a low incidence of neurological injury in spite of higher rates of pedicular violations. Gertzbein and Robbins reported two minor neurological complications, which spontaneously resolved in their series of 67 thoracic screws.[20] Although Liljenqvist et al reported no neurological complications, one screw required replacement due to its proximity to the thoracic aorta.[10]

As with any surgical technique, image-guided pedicle screw placement has its limitations. Because the stereotactic image is obtained prior to surgery, gross intrasegmental instability may preclude accurate guidance. Most importantly, stereotactic screw placement is not immune to human error. Interestingly, the majority of screws with unintentional Grade II or Grade III violations occurred in instances of severe traumatic fracture subluxations. This clinical scenario provides two possibilities for error. First, segmental instability in the setting of severe trauma may lead to intraoperative errors in localization from the time interval of CT scan aquisition to navigation and/or registration to navigation. Second, once the pedicle instrumentation is initially applied, it can be moved if vigorous intraoperative forces are applied in an effort to further reduce and align the spine. In fact, one surgeon noted "slippage" of the superior screws on final reduction efforts. Finally, it is important to stress that the ultimate act of screw placement is not image guided but rather intended to follow the path of the image-guided pilot hole. Herein lies the greatest potential for human error. Operative success is based upon careful preoperative planning, attention to the details of accurate registration and navigation, and an understanding of the limitations of specific instrumentation constructs in unique clinical applications.

■ Conclusions

This clinical series provides further evidence that stereotactic placement of pedicle screws may be performed safely and effectively at all levels of the thoracic spine in a variety of clinical scenarios. Although the subset analysis data does show a higher rate of cortical violations in the middle and upper thoracic regions, this rate is still superior to published rates of error using anatomic and fluoroscopic guidance alone. Given the three-dimensional complexity and relatively small size of the thoracic pedicle, careful preoperative planning is required for pedicle evaluation and screw trajectory, especially in the mid to upper thoracic region. When indicated, the utilization of image-guided techniques for the placement of thoracic pedicle screws should be considered the safest and most effective way of stabilizing the thoracic spine.

REFERENCES

1. King D. Internal fixation for lumbosacral fusion. *Am J Surg* 1944;66:357–361.
2. Ebraheim NA, Jabaly G, Xu R, Yeasting RA. Anatomic relations of the thoracic pedicle to the adjacent neural structures. *Spine* 1997;22(14):1553–1556; discussion 1557.
3. Ebraheim NA, Xu R, Ahmad M, Yeasting RA. Projection of the thoracic pedicle and its morphometric analysis. *Spine* 1997;22(3):233–238.
4. Kothe R, O'Holleran JD, Liu W, Panjabi MM. Internal architecture of the thoracic pedicle: an anatomic study. *Spine* 1996;21(3):264–270.
5. McCormack BM, Benzel EC, Adams MS, Baldwin NG, Rupp FW, Maher DJ. Anatomy of the thoracic pedicle. *Neurosurgery* 1995;37(2):303–308.
6. Phillips JH, Kling TF Jr, Cohen MD. The radiographic anatomy of the thoracic pedicle. *Spine* 1994;19(4):446–449.
7. Vaccaro AR, Rizzolo SJ, Balderston RA, et al. Placement of pedicle screws in the thoracic spine, II: An anatomical and radiographic assessment. *JBone Joint Surg* 1995;77(8):1200–1206.
8. Cinotti G, Gumina S, Ripani M, Postacchini F. Pedicle instrumentation in the thoracic spine: a morphometric and cadaveric study for placement of screws. *Spine* 1999;24(2):114–119.
9. Xu R, Ebraheim NA, Ou Y, Yeasting RA. Anatomic considerations of pedicle screw placement in the thoracic spine: Roy-Camille technique versus open-lamina technique. *Spine* 1998;23(9):1065–1068.
10. Liljenqvist UR, Halm HF, Link TM. Pedicle screw instrumentation of the thoracic spine in idiopathic scoliosis. *Spine* 1997;22(19):2239–2245.
11. Weinstein JN, Spratt KF, Spengler D, Brick C, Reid S. Spinal pedicle fixation: reliability and validity of roentgenogram-based assessment and surgical factors on successful screw placement [see comments]. *Spine* 1988;13(9):1012–1018.
12. Abitbol JJ, Smith MM, Foley KT. Thoracic pedicle screw placement accuracy: image-interactive guidance versus conventional techniques. In: *1996 Congress of Neurological Surgeons Annual Meeting*. Montreal, Quebec. September, 1996.
13. Jiang Z, King P, Zamorano L, Holdener H. Interactive image-guided spine surgery. In: *1996 Congress of Neurological Surgeons Annual Meeting*. 1996.
14. McCormack B, McDermott M, Nockels R, Sundaresan S, Weinstein P. Placement of pedicle screws using frameless stereotaxy in a cadaver. In: *1995 Congress of Neurological Surgeons Annual Meeting*. 1995.
15. Ferguson RL, Tencer AF, Woodard P, Allen BL Jr. Biomechanical comparisons of spinal fracture models and the stabilizing effects of posterior instrumentations. *Spine* 1988;13(5):453–460.
16. Vaccaro AR, Rizzolo SJ, Allardyce TJ, et al. Placement of pedicle screws in the thoracic spine, I: Morphometric analysis of the thoracic vertebrae. *J Bone Joint Surg [BR]* 1995;77(8):1193–1199.
17. Wood KB, Wentorf FA, Ogilvie JW, Kim KT. Torsional rigidity of scoliosis constructs. *Spine* 2000;25(15):1893–1898.
18. Mulholland RC. Pedicle screw fixation in the spine [editorial]. *J Bone Joint Surg [BR]* 1994;76(4):517–519.
19. Amiot LP, Lang K, Putzier M, Zippel H, Labelle H. Comparative results between conventional and computer-assisted pedicle screw installation in the thoracic, lumbar, and sacral spine. *Spine* 2000;25(5):606–614.
20. Gertzbein SD, Robbins SE. Accuracy of pedicular screw placement in vivo. *Spine* 1990;15(1):11–14.

22

Image Guidance for Scoliosis

STEPHEN L. ONDRA AND DEAN KARAHALIOS

Image guidance for spinal procedures has been a recent addition to neurosurgery.[1-11] The most common use for stereotactic guidance in the spine is to place pedicle screws.[5,9,11] The ability of image guidance to safely place pedicle instrumentation in rotated, abnormal, or small pedicles has dramatically changed scoliosis surgery.

The complex anatomic relationships and rotation seen in spinal deformities such as scoliosis can place anatomic structures in very different locations than a surgeon might expect based on experience with more routine cases. This has limited the use of pedicle screws, particularly in the thoracic and high lumbar spine where the pedicles are smallest. Unfortunately, these are the most common areas for spinal deformity and the sites of the greatest rotation of the spine.

Although hooks and rods allow segmental control, they provide less corrective power and less stabilization control. This can lead to a partial postoperative loss of the initial surgical correction. Over the years, standard hook patterns and plans for deformity correction were based on such instrumentation.

Pedicle screws constructs provide much more powerful correction and better holding power. The preservation of the ligamentum flavum and interspinal ligament possible with pedicle screws decreases the risk of junctional deformity. The power of correction that screws provide can limit the number of segments involved in the reconstruction. The only segments anatomically required for correction are the rigid portion of the curve.

The rotation seen in spinal deformity, such as scoliosis, not only limits anatomic orientation to screw placement, it makes fluoroscopy virtually useless. The parallax introduced into the fluoroscopic image can lead the surgeon to believe that there is proper orientation when in reality, the screw trajectory is grossly in error. Image guidance allows the surgeon to accurately assess pedicle size and determine screw diameter and length before surgery. This, combined with the inherent accuracy of placement that image guidance offers, allows constructs to be planned using pedicle screws for the majority or all desired fixation points. This has led to a fundamental change in the rules of correction. Constructs can be limited to the rigid portion of the curve. Greater correction is possible, and more segments of control are available.

The planning programs for the image-guidance system also clarify the anatomic relationships of spinal deformity, and the presence of hemivertebrae or severely distorted spinal anatomy can be better understood prior to surgery (Fig. 22–1). Improved understanding of anatomy prior to surgery leads to a safer procedure, even if the system is not used for intraoperative guidance.

Improved preoperative planning also leads to accurate implant size selection, which saves time. Knowing what type, size, and position the implants will be in allows the surgeon to know exactly what construct will be in place after surgery. In spinal deformity, such knowledge leads to more realistic plans by allowing the surgeon to assess what forces can be applied in correction.

This chapter explores in detail the preoperative planning and surgical techniques for image guidance in spinal deformity.

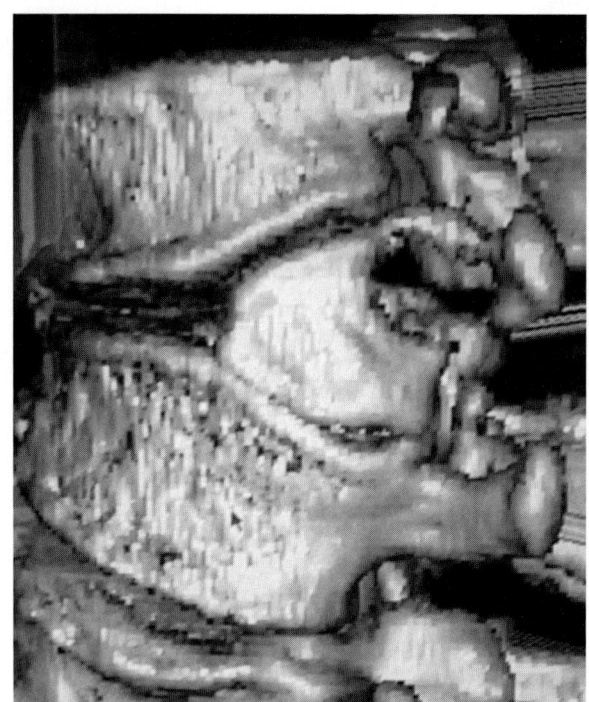 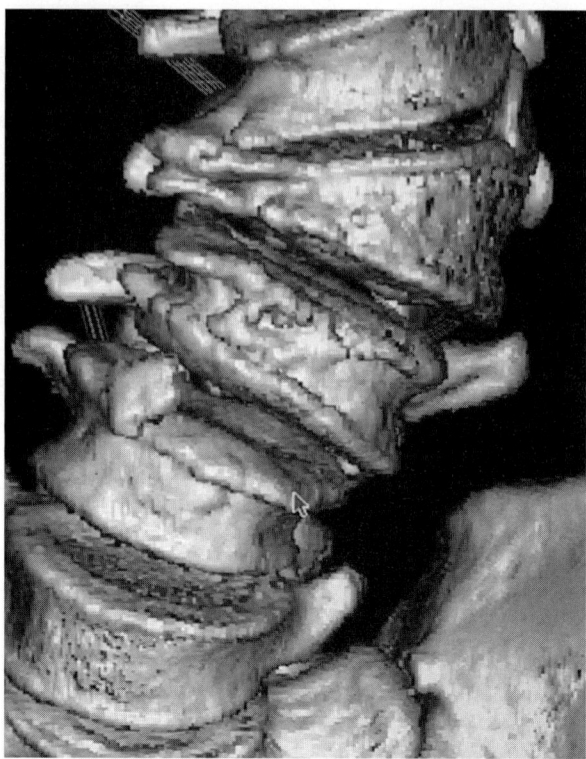

FIGURE 22–1. Anteroposterior and lateral 3-D reconstructed views of the lumbar spine in a patient with a congenital hemivertebrae showing the hemivertebrae and the adjacent segment abnormalities associated with it.

■ Preoperative Planning

Once the patient has been scanned, the data are transferred to the workstation, and the software is used to reconstruct the images. The system software then displays the images in two- or three-dimensional (2-D or 3-D) multiplanar views. The 3-D view can be rotated. The planes of the simultaneous 2-D views can be selected, and areas of interest can be highlighted to improve understanding of a particular anatomy or pathology. This is particularly important in spinal deformity cases. In these situations, anatomic relationships can be distorted, confusing the surgeon and making accurate preoperative planning difficult. Combining a rotatable 3-D image with 2-D reference in multiple planes allows a surgeon to understand even the most complex anatomic distortion. The image sizes can also be manipulated. Some systems provide drop-down menus with tools that enable precise measurement of structures.

Lending even more power to these systems is the capability to superimpose precisely scaled cursors with the same relative dimensions as planned implants. Prior to surgery, we will place virtual screws in each pedicle that we would like to control. This generates a realistic assessment of where screws can go or hooks must be utilized, and accurate preoperative plans that are critical in deformity corrections can be made. The surgeon will know precisely the length and diameter of each implant. The entry point, angle of entry, or dimensions of the screw can be manipulated to obtain an appropriate fit.

This preoperative plan can be stored and used intraoperatively to select the appropriate screw, to find the entry point, and to follow the selected trajectory. Some systems integrate this information into a targeting view so that the multiple images do not need to be simultaneously viewed and processed during the actual placement of the instrumentation. This precise localization and placement allows safe placement of implants. Implants placed in ideal positions offer more powerful control and corrective force. Eliminating maneuvers such as laminotomies to palpate pedicles saves bone surface for grafting and prevents blood loss. With experience, time savings are also realized.

■ Operating Room Setup and Patient Positioning

The patient is positioned on the operating room table as for a conventional spinal procedure. The workstation monitor is placed so that the surgeon has a clear view

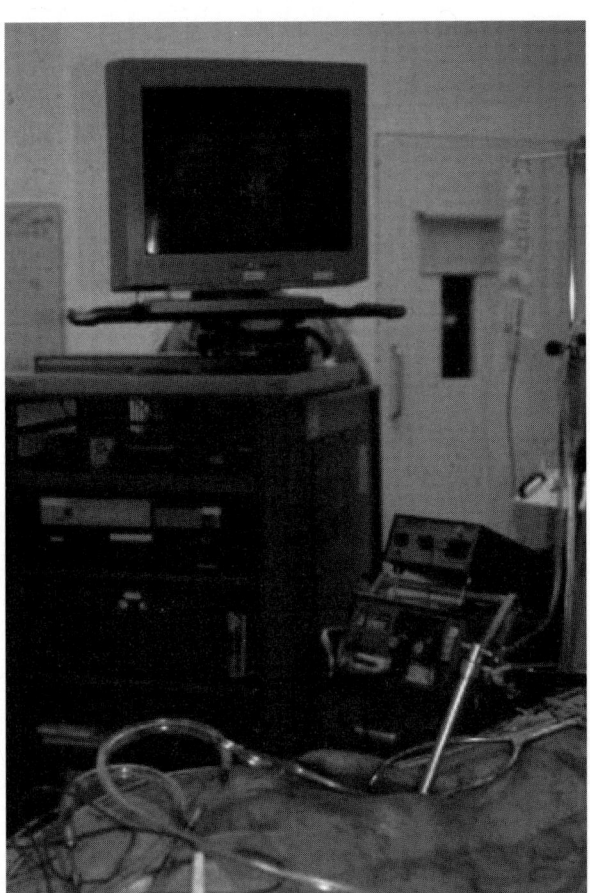

FIGURE 22–2. The reference array affixed to the opened spine and the surrounding setup, including the viewing monitor, for the image-guidance system (StealthStation, Medtronic SNT, Louisville, CO).

(Fig. 22–2). Some systems also have an additional lightweight, flat-color, liquid crystal display (LCD) that can be mounted on a boom over the operative field. These displays may have touch-sensitive screens (covered by a clear, sterile drape) that the surgeon can activate during the procedure.

The infrared camera must be placed in the line of sight of the instruments to be tracked; the best location is usually near the foot or head of the table. The camera can be moved if the line of sight is obstructed during the procedure. During the positioning and preparation of the patient, the line of sight between the camera and the locations of the instruments should be maintained.

■ Registration

Registration involves "matching" the patient's anatomy to the imaging data set in the computer. First a reference frame is placed on the spine (Fig. 22–3). The computer adjusts for the movement accordingly, keeping the patient's anatomy aligned or correlated with the imaging data set. The segmental spine requires the reference frame to be placed at the same level that is to be registered and operated on. If multiple levels are to be operated on, the reference frame should be moved to each of the levels. This process can be very time-consuming and cumbersome. There is no safe way around this in highly mobile segments. In segments that are relatively rigid, a single registration may have overlap to the segment above and below it with sufficient accuracy to allow use. One must always be aware that there is some accuracy degradation in these situations. If the anatomic and visual correlation does not fit with the computer image, the image guidance should be re-registered to that segment rather than using the overlap registration. Another safety check is to confirm anatomic landmarks on each vertebra to be instrumented with a particular plan after registration is complete.

The technical process of registration begins with a point-to-point registration. This process involves finding a point on the patient's anatomy and matching it to the same point on the workstation's display. The target may be viewed in multiple planes and in 3-D to insure the proper point is chosen. In general, the more points that are chosen, the better is the accuracy. We have found that the procedure moves more quickly if the surgeon picks the points on the 3-D model prior to surgery and then finds the same points on the spine during registration. For a typical pedicle screw case, six points are chosen: the superior and inferior aspects of the distal transverse process bilaterally and the superior and inferior aspects of the spinous process. Additional points (e.g., facet, pars interarticularis) can be added to increase accuracy. These secondary points are less distinct and seldom chosen as the primary localizing points.

If greater accuracy is needed or desired, a surface fit algorithm is performed. This process involves touching multiple points over the surface of the dorsal elements to create a 3-D contour of the structure. Usually 30 to 40 points are chosen. Through a mathematical transformation, the computer matches the contour to its own imaging data set for that level.

Both registration techniques can be used together to decrease the error.[8] Point-to-point registration is often accurate alone. Techniques such as fluoroscopic navigation also have little use in deformity. The same limits introduced by the rotational parallax for traditional fluoroscopy are seen in fluoroscopic navigation. This can lead to erroneous and dangerous errors in orientation.

Spinal deformity surgery is often a staged procedure. This is particularly true in adults and revision surgery. The rigidity of adult spines often requires both anterior and posterior mobilization to correct deformity. Additionally, decompression is often needed. It is possible to take advantage of this staging by performing instrument removal, when needed, bone exposure, and osteotomies

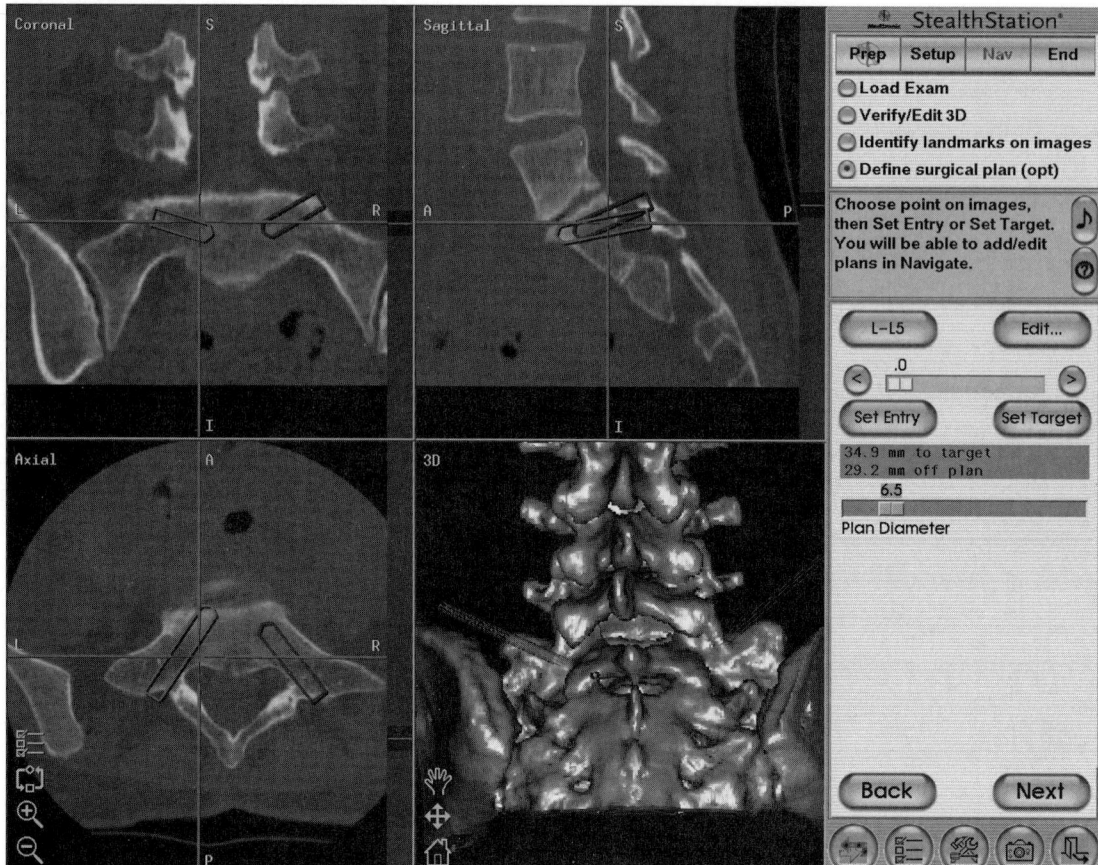

FIGURE 22–3. The intraoperative view of the image-guidance viewing station showing the 3-D reconstructed image of the spine and the multiplanar imaging of the spine. The figures on each image represent the planned trajectories for the screws to be placed with image guidance (StealthStation, Medtronic SNT, Louisville, CO).

as a first step. If the final correction will be done in the second stage, internal fiducials can be placed at each segment to be instrumented later. The image-guidance CT is then performed between surgical stages (Fig. 22–4). This imaging includes the spine and the hard contact fiducials that were placed in the first stage. Such fiducials give reliable points of registration and greater accuracy than traditional anatomic landmarks. Using this technique, we have found accurate registration can be reliably accomplished in less than 90 seconds per level.[12] Because it is essential to register each level independently, rapid registration is an immense time saver.

Great care should be taken to ensure that the same level for the patient and the image-guided surgery (IGS) display are registered because they can easily be confused. Labeling the levels during the reconstruction process can alleviate potential confusion. If the registration error is over 10 mm, a level mismatch should be considered.

Future changes in registration will speed up this process and thereby expand image guidance's role. Ultrasound and multiplane fluoroscopy may lead to the ability to use image guidance with anterior correction systems. At this point, the lack of ability to track and the flat surfaces that limit registration limit image guidance in the anterior spine. Such changes (e.g., multiplane fluoroscopy) could lead to minimally invasive scoliosis correction techniques by using thoracoscopically placed instruments and grafting into the anterior spine.[13–14]

■ Tracking

In placing instrumentation, tools similar to their conventional counterparts have been fitted with light emitting diodes (LEDs) for tracking. For pedicle screw placement, either a spatula-tipped or pointed awl can be used for sounding the pedicle. Guides are available for drilling out the pedicle. These guided tools not only serve as pointers to find the correct entry point, they also demonstrate the best angle or trajectory through the bony structure.

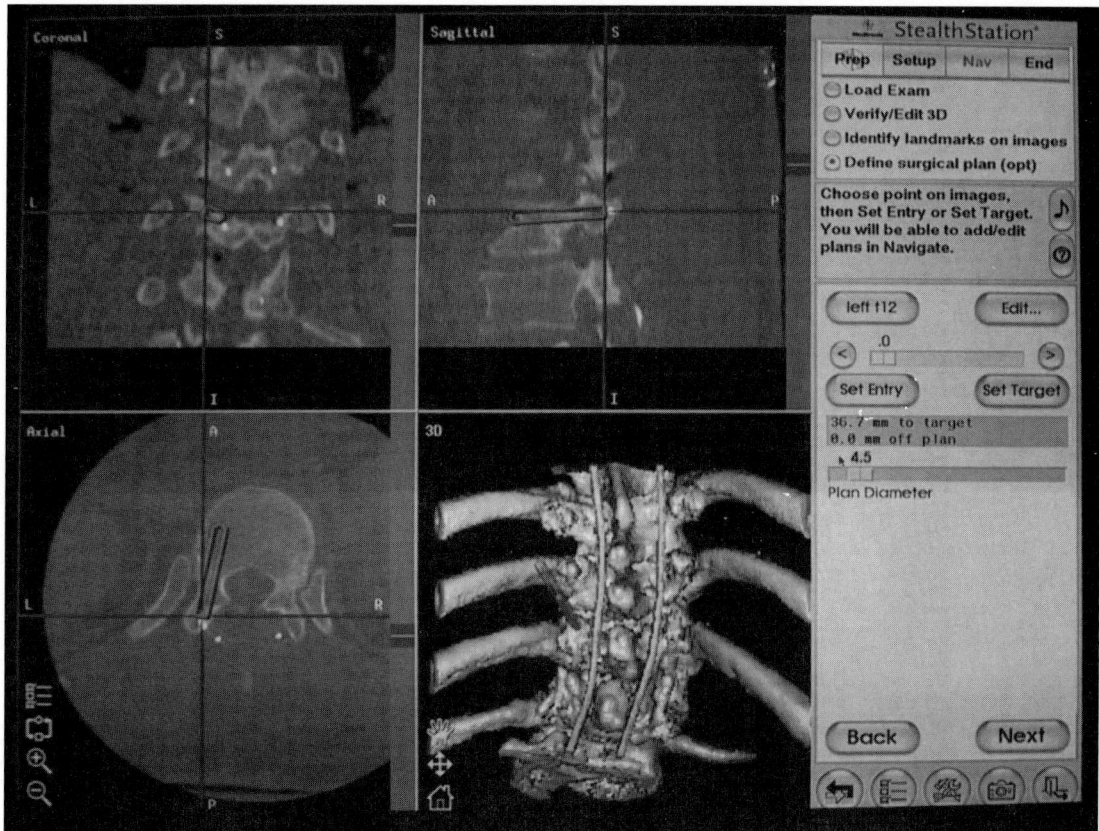

FIGURE 22–4. The intraoperative video of the spine at the image-guidance viewing station with the internal feducials used as reference markers for obtaining accurate registration (Stealth-Station, Medtronic SNT, Louisville, CO).

LEDs can be mounted on the drill, tap, and screwdriver (with screw) so that the tip of the instrument can be tracked as it passes through the bone. Alternatively, once the entry point and the trajectory are chosen, the depth for the drilling can be determined based on measurements made from the workstation images. This depth accuracy is critical in deformity. The rotation of the spine and anatomic variability can lead to surgeon disorientation. This can cause screw penetration into the spinal canal or foramen or anteriorly through the vertebral body, with potentially disastrous consequences. Image guidance allows optimum screw size, position, and depth, resulting in maximum strength and safety.

Viewing the monitor is still a major source of frustration during surgery because the eyes must deviate from the surgical field to view the image-guided information. A preferable image presentation being developed resembles the window of a fighter plane. Targeting information could be displayed on a clear liquid crystal display visor worn by the surgeon; 3-D reconstructions would be superimposed onto the patient's anatomy as viewed through the visor.

■ Conclusions

Image-guided frameless stereotactic techniques have been applied to spinal surgery with success. The potential advantages of this technology include enhanced localizing capability with respect to anatomic structures and pathology and added precision and safety. Additional advantages include less radiation exposure for the patient and operating room staff.

These features have been used in scoliosis and spinal deformity to allow implant placement safely and effectively throughout the spine (Fig. 22–5). This has led to a fundamental change in the way correction is carried out by adding more power to the forces that can be applied. Pedicle screws are also more stable long term and have less late correction loss than hook systems.

Although screw placement is greatly facilitated by image guidance, we have found that the ability to predict what implants can be placed and in which segments, as well as implant size, adds to accurate preoperative planning and better-designed surgery. This aspect of image guidance combines with the ability to better

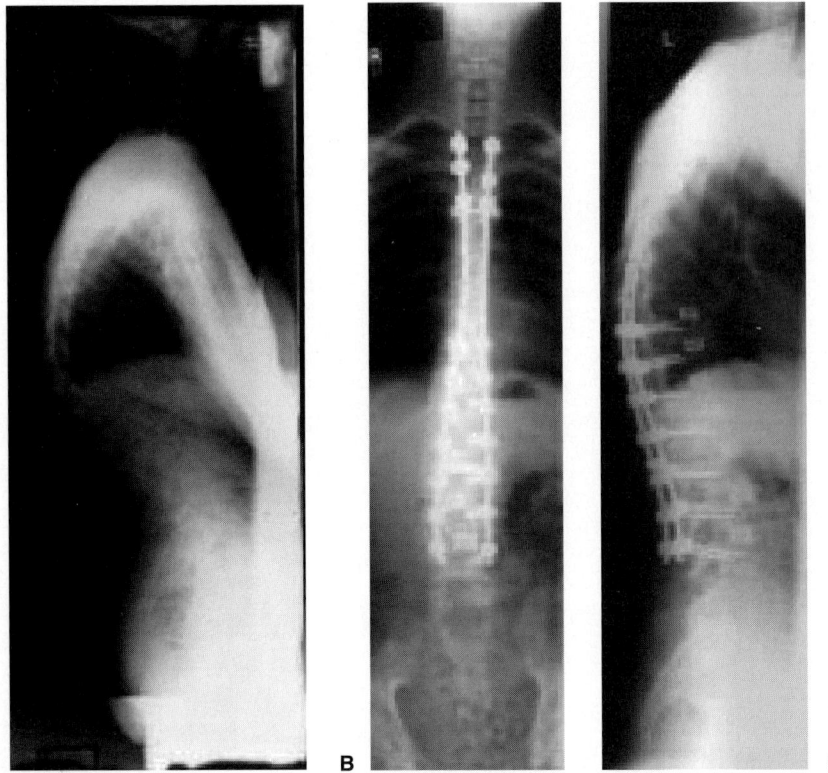

FIGURE 22–5. Preoperative lateral scoliosis film of a patient with a kyphotic abnormality. Postoperative anteroposterior and lateral scoliosis films showing correction of the deformity. Notice the predominant use of pedicle screws.

understand complex anatomic relationships. This is often of equal or greater importance to us than the actual operative use of such systems.

Image guidance has fundamentally changed the way in which we evaluate and treat our patients with spinal deformity. Future developments will undoubtedly continue to have far-reaching impact.

REFERENCES

1. Golfinos JG, Fitzpatrick BC, Smith LR, et al. Clinical use of a frameless stereotactic arm: results of 325 cases. *J Neurosurg* 1995; 83:197–205.
2. Lawton MT, Golfinos JG, Geldmacher T, Spetzler RF. A comparative clinical evaluation of current frameless stereotactic systems: accuracy, performance and surgeon preference. *Perspectives in Neurosurgery* 1998;9(1):47–62.
3. Welch WC, Subach BR, Pollack IF, et al. Frameless stereotactic guidance for surgery of the upper cervical spine. *Neurosurgery* 1997;40:958–964.
4. Patel N, Sandeman DR, Cobby M, et al. Interactive image-guided surgery of the spine: use of the ISG/Elekta Viewing Wand to aid intraoperative localization of a sacral osteoblastoma. *Br J Neurosurg* 1997;11:60–64.
5. Nolte LP, Zamorano LJ, Jiang Z, et al. Image-guided insertion of transpedicular screws: a laboratory set-up. *Spine* 1995;20:497–500.
6. Nolte LP, Zamorano LJ, Arm E, et al. Image-guided computer assisted spine surgery: a pilot study on pedicle screw fixation. *Stereotact Funct Neurosurg* 1996;66:108–117.
7. Kalfas IH, Kormos DW, Murphy MA, et al. Application of frameless stereotaxy to pedicle screw fixation of the spine. *J Neurosurg* 1995;83:641–647.
8. Lossop ND, Hu RW, Randle JA. Computer-aided pedicle screw placement using frameless stereotaxis. *Spine* 1996;21:2026–2034.
9. Foley KT, Smith MM. Image-guided spine surgery. *Neurosurg Clin N Am* 1996;7:171–186.
10. Broadwater BK, Roberts DW, Nakajima T, et al. Extracranial application of the frameless stereotactic operating microscope: experience with lumbar spine. *Neurosurgery* 1993;32:209–213.
11. Lavallee S, Sautot P, Troccaz J, et al. Computer assisted spine surgery: a technique for accurate transpedicular screw fixation using CT data and a 3-D optical localizer. *J Image Guide Surg* 1995;1:65–73.
12. Salehi SA, Ondra SL. Use of internal fiducial markers in frameless stereotactic navigational systems during spinal surgery: technical note. *Neurosurg* 2000;47(6):1460–1462.
13. Trobaugh JW, Richard WD, Smith KR, et al. Frameless stereotactic ultrasonography: method and applications. *Comput Med Imaging Graph* 1994;18:235–246.
14. Hemler PF, Sumanaweera TS, van den Elsen PA, et al. A versatile system for multimodality image fusion. *J Image Guided Surg* 1995; 1:35–45.

23

Image-Guided Lumbar Instrumentation

NARESH P. PATEL, JAE Y. LIM, KEE D. KIM, AND J. PATRICK JOHNSON

Pedicle screw fixation is a widely used method to achieve rigid fixation of the lumbar and sacral spine. It is effective to augment fusion for the treatment of fractures, spondylolisthesis, scoliosis, tumors, and appropriately selected cases of degenerative disk disease with segmental instability.[1-5] Although many surgeons have become adept with placement of lumbar and sacral pedicle screws, considerable knowledge and technical skill are required for accurate screw placement. Screw placement errors may result in either failed fusion or neurovascular injury. The current literature reports pedicle screw placement error rates as high as 30%.[6-8a] Recent advances in stereotactic image-guided surgical techniques may provide spinal surgeons the ability to decrease pedicle screw error rates and maximize safety.[9-13] This chapter reviews the traditional methods and imaging of pedicle screw placement, then focuses on the current state-of-the-art techniques and applications of image-guided lumbar and sacral pedicle screw placement.

■ Traditional Localization Methods

Accurate pedicle screw placement relies on the surgeon's experience and three-dimensional (3-D) conceptualization and understanding of spinal anatomy. Initially spinal surgeons used plain anteroposterior and lateral view standard intraoperative radiographs. However, plain radiographs required significant additional time in obtaining and processing x-ray films, which made plain radiographs an impractical and unpopular method for intraoperative imaging. Also each plain radiograph is acquired independently and cannot be immediately updated as with fluoroscopy. Subsequently, intraoperative C-arm fluoroscopy has been used to assist in accurate pedicle screw placement and still remains a primary method of intraoperative imaging where image guidance is not available. Fluoroscopy can be used to obtain multiple images in rapid sequence, and it allows precise positioning for imaging oblique or other unusual views, particularly if there is any anatomic spinal deformity. This flexibility of fluoroscopy allows intraoperative real-time imaging for accurate "fine-tuning" of pedicle screw trajectories. The disadvantages of fluoroscopy include a potentially higher than acceptable radiation exposure as well as the cumbersome size of the C-arm, which hinders the surgeon's access to the operative field. Regardless of the type of intraoperative radiographic imaging used, successful pedicle screw placement depends upon high-quality imaging that demonstrates pedicle anatomy with each vertebra oriented and aligned anatomically to ensure ideal screw placement.

Despite appropriate intraoperative radiographic techniques or modern image guidance, accurate screw placement cannot be guaranteed, nor is it always feasible. Creating a pilot hole through the pedicle by manual probing requires locating a proper entry point and trajectory with a medial-directed angulation that the surgeon estimates from the preoperative computed tomography (CT) or magnetic resonance imaging (MRI). Screw diameter and length can also be estimated by measuring the preoperative axial CT or MRI. Pedicle screw placement can be extremely difficult when using conventional radiographic imaging technology in patients with altered anatomy due to previous surgery, severe degenerative changes, or deformity. The limitations of plain radiographic and fluoroscopic guidance provided some of the stimuli and indications for computerized image-guided spine surgery to potentially maximize the accuracy of lumbar and sacral screw placement.[9-11] Current image-guided systems are based either on optical imaging [i.e., light emitting diodes (LEDs) or light reflectors], magnetic fields, ultrasound, virtual fluoroscopy, or an articulating arm. This chapter focuses on the optical imaging and virtual fluoroscopy technologies that have applications to the other guidance systems.

■ CT-Guided Frameless Stereotaxy: Anatomy and Preoperative Planning

Image-guided spinal applications were adapted from frameless cranial stereotactic technology that was well established. The lumbar and sacral spinal column is well suited for stereotactic surgical applications because the individual bony vertebral segments are large in size and have distinct and identifiable anatomic prominences on the dorsal surface. Registration requires open surgical exposure of the selected vertebral segment because closed registration with skin fiducials is neither feasible nor accurate for spinal surgery due to mobility of the skin.[14] The spinous processes, facets, and transverse processes are the most frequently used anatomic fiducials that can be identified at surgery and on the 3-D surface rendering images on the workstation, but any other distinct bony prominences are useful. Intersegmental motion between two vertebral segments remains a potential problem and may require registration of each segment intraoperatively to avoid errors. Because preoperative CT scans are obtained in a supine position, the relative position of each vertebra may be significantly different when with the patient is in the prone position for surgery.

A preoperative CT scan of the surgical region must be obtained with a specific protocol that is similar for most image-guided systems using 1 mm contiguous slices over a 10 to 14 cm field of view. Three-millimeter CT slices can also produce acceptable-quality detail for accurate image-guided procedures in the lumbar and sacral spine, but 5 mm scan slices may produce poor-quality imaging for surgery. The scan protocol for the CT technicians can be obtained by the image-guided vendor to assure correct details of the protocol. The CT scan data of the patient are then transferred to the image-guided computer workstation where they are reformatted into axial, coronal, sagittal, and 3-D views.

■ Optical Tracking Image-Guided System Components

Several different optical tracking image-guided surgical systems are now commercially available. Although computer hardware and software profiles may differ somewhat between manufacturers, each system has similar basic components and clinical applications. The main hardware components include a computer workstation, a digitizer, and a camera (Fig. 23-1A). The peripheral components are a dynamic reference frame (DRF) (Fig. 23-1B), a standard pointer probe (Fig. 23-1C), and various instrument arrays that provide universal instrument registration (UIR) (Fig. 23-2). The computer workstation consists of a monitor, optical disc drive or CD-ROM or digital audiotape (DAT) drive, as well as an internal hard drive. The CT scan data is received by an optical disc, CD-ROM, or DAT drive or through a hospital network (ethernet) data transfer system. The computer workstation operating system runs the software needed to produce 3-D reconstructions from the scan data and perform surgical tracking with the images. In addition, the computer will run the software that takes the surgeon through the steps of registration, planning, and navigation (Fig. 23-3).

The optical tracking camera system detects LEDs (or passive, reflective ball-markers) on the instruments in the field and digitally detects their positions in space. The spatial location of the instruments (as defined by Cartesian coordinates) is determined by the computer to provide real-time navigation. The use of several distinctly different LED/passive marker configurations now allows simultaneous tracking of multiple instruments during the image-guided procedure.

The DRF is attached to the spine segment of interest (or the adjacent segment being operated) and has a unique pattern of LED/markers that the computer recognizes (see Fig. 23-1B). The DRF is securely attached to the spinous process with a clamp or a modified screw that is attached to the clamp, which allows the digitizer to track any patient movement and immediately update the computer-generated scan image on the monitor screen. During the registration and image-guided surgical procedure, it is essential that the DRF remain undisturbed and within view of the optical tracking camera.

The standard probe is a pointer with LED/passive markers attached that is tracked with the camera system and the computer workstation (see Fig. 23-1C). The probe is used for registration by touching points on the vertebra that were predetermined on the 3-D computer workstation, or by touching multiple points for a surface-matching algorithm that correlates the "virtual patient space" on the computed images to the "actual patient space." After the registration process is complete, the standard probe can be used during the procedure to

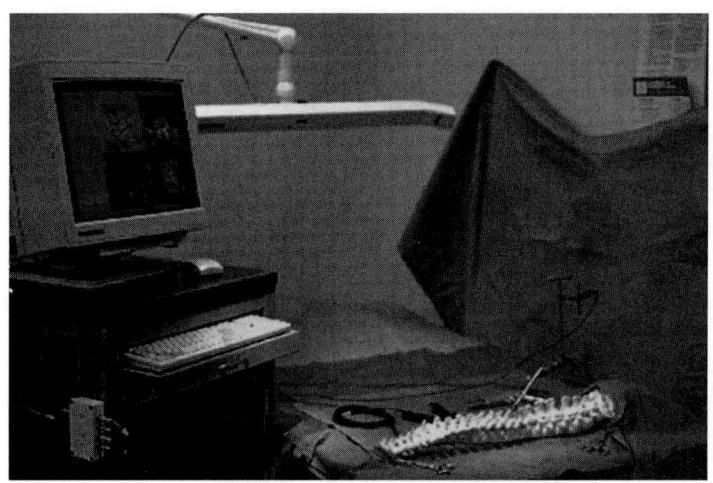
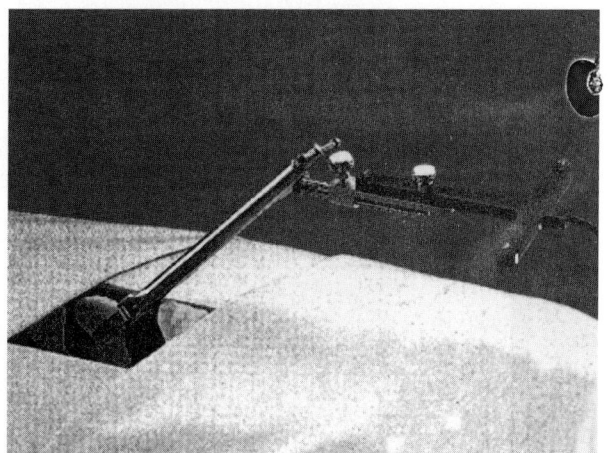
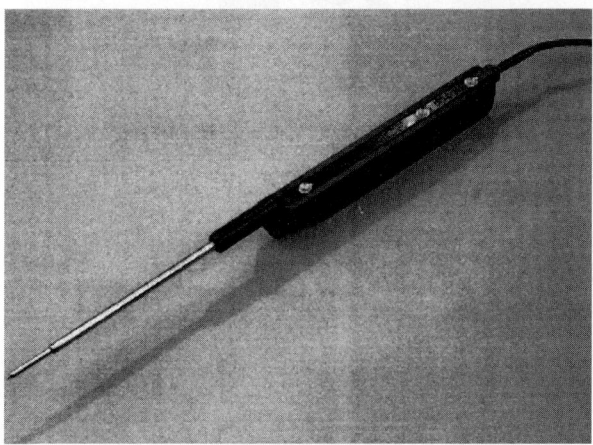

FIGURE 23–1. Stereotactic spine system components. (A). Computer workstation and optical tracking camera system. (B). Dynamic reference frame. (C). Standard probe pointer (Radionics, Burlington, MA).

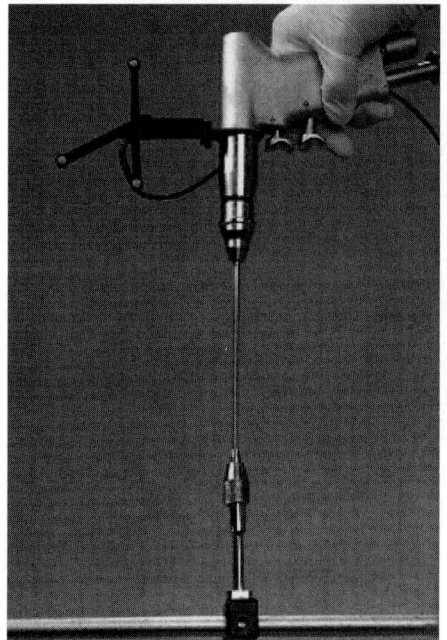
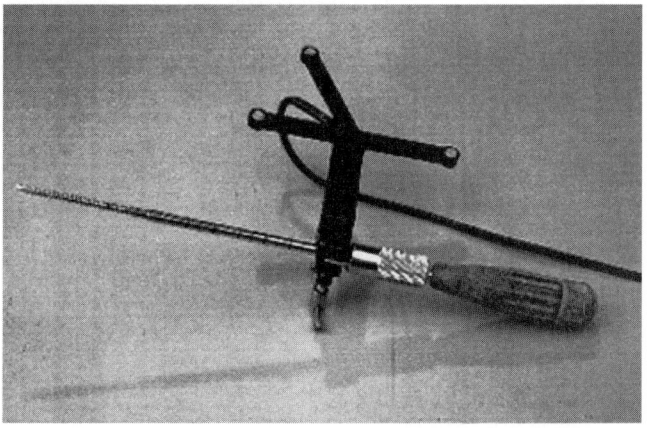

FIGURE 23–2. Universal instrument registration components. (A). Drill with universal instrument registration (UIR) light emitting diode (LED) array attached that is being calibrated in UIR device. (B). Tap with UIR LED array attached.

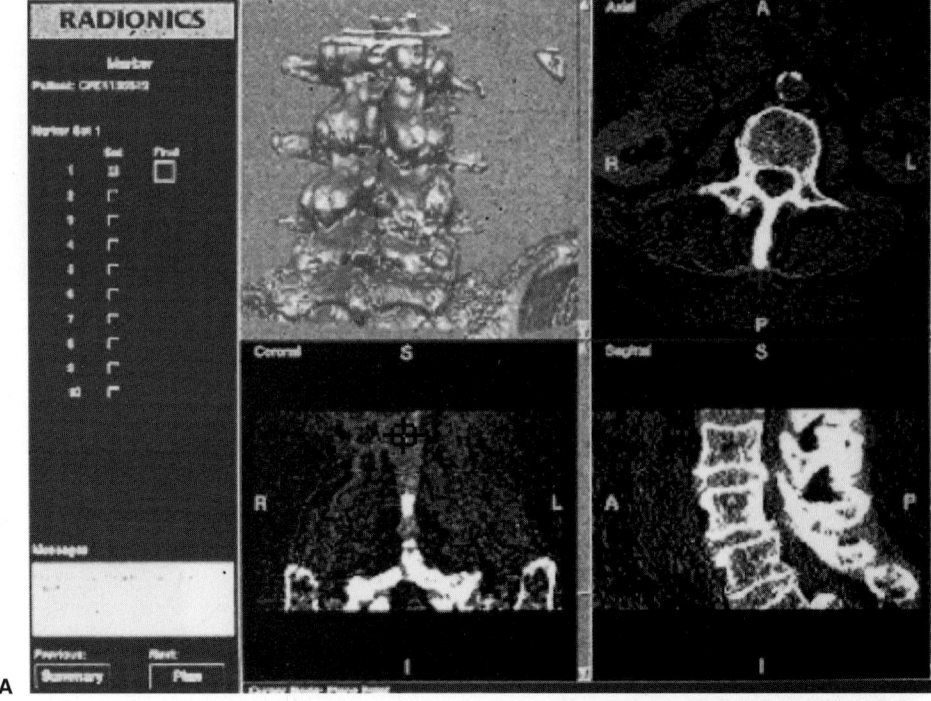
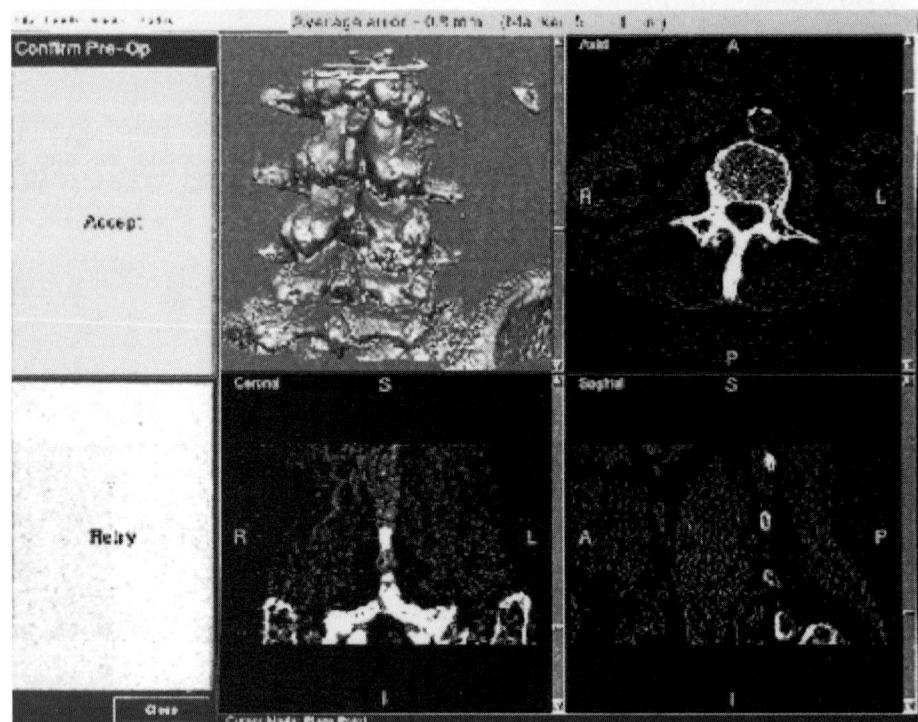

FIGURE 23–3. CT-based image-guided workstation images. (A). Registration process. Bony landmarks are identified on the patient and on the three-dimensional reconstructed images. (B). Mean registration error is calculated and queries to "Accept" or "Retry." (C). Navigation begins; entry points and trajectories are determined, pedicle screws may now be placed in the usual fashion. (Radionics, Burlington, MA)

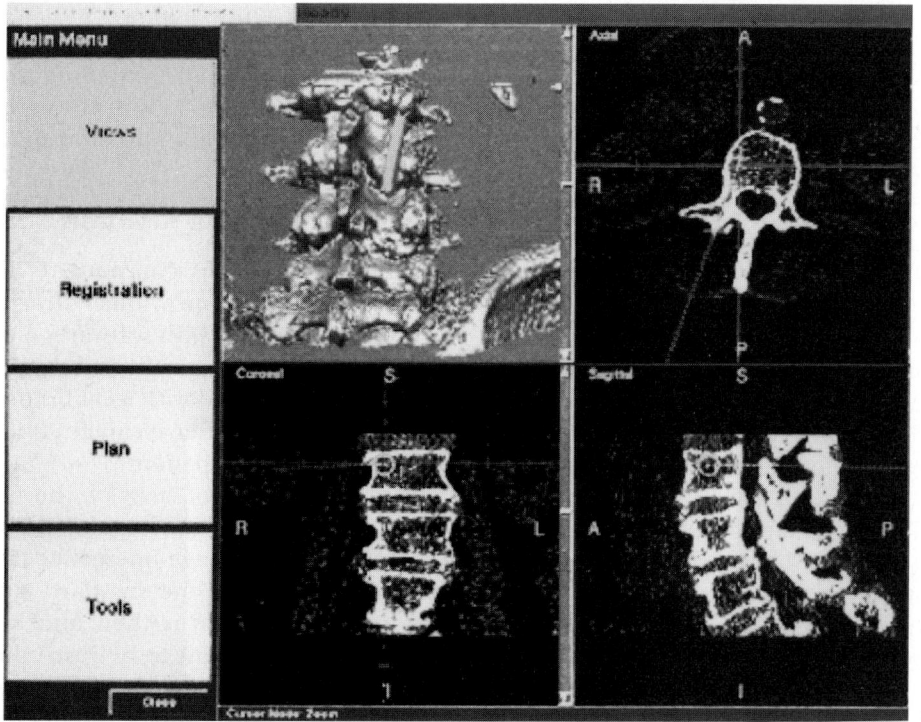

FIGURE 23–3. Continued

determine a screw entry point or plan trajectories for instrumentation placement.

Finally, the UIR technology replaces the standard probe to use standard surgical instruments that are adapted for use during surgery (see Fig. 23–2). Typical instruments that a surgeon may use with an image-guidance system include a tap, pedicle probe, drill guide, drill, or screwdriver, and an awl.

■ Intraoperative Preparation, Registration, and Navigation

Surgical exposure and registration

The operative procedure requires a standard operative exposure of the surgical region with meticulous attention to the removal of soft tissues on bony structures. The DRF is then securely fixed to the spinous process at the level (or adjacent) to be instrumented.

Point-to-point registration requires picking virtual fiducial points on the workstation 3-D image and matching them with anatomic fiducials on the spinal column in the surgical field by touching the anatomic fiducials with the tip of the registration probe to match with points on the workstation image (Fig. 23–3A). A minimum of three fiducials (i.e., x, y, z coordinates) must be selected and four to six generally provide more accurate registration. The computer software then calculates registration accuracy and makes suggestions on how to improve the error, which usually entails re-registering one or more points. The mean error should be less than 2.0 mm (Fig. 23–3B). Surface-matching software improves the registration accuracy slightly by "fine tuning," which is accomplished by touching multiple random anatomic points on the posterior vertebral segment. After registration is completed, a practical confirmation of accuracy is obtained by touching known landmarks (e.g., spinous process) with the probe tip to compare its location with the image on the computer screen. Rapid and accurate registration remains one of the technical limiting difficulties of image-guided spinal navigation procedures.

Intraoperative navigation

After registration is complete, image-guided spinal instrumentation can proceed. Placement of pedicle screws requires establishing the correct entry point and trajectory determined by using the standard probe (Fig. 23–3C). The anatomic entry points are relatively consistent, but image guidance demonstrates any variability. Trajectories of screw angle also have a somewhat constant progression with each level (e.g., 5 degrees medial at L1; 25 degrees medial at L5), but there is sufficient variability that can occur and is demonstrated with image guidance.

■ Lumbar and Sacral Image-Guided Procedures

CT-guided lumbar and sacral image guidance are potentially indicated for any procedure involving pedicle screw placement or resection of mass lesions. The most common and useful applications are for difficult congenital or degenerative scoliosis deformity cases, particularly where the anatomy is variable from each vertebral level to the next. Patients with these complex anatomic alterations need the detailed accuracy of CT data for image-guided screw placement. The multiplanar, orthogonal images with CT-based image guidance can assist in location of the entry point and screw trajectory to guide precision placement that cannot be obtained with fluoroscopic imaging. In addition, the image-guidance virtual pedicle measurements allow the largest-diameter screw to safely fit a given pedicle, and bicortical sacral screws can be placed safely if desired. Resection of mass lesions in the lumbar and sacral spine can benefit from a CT-based image-guidance procedure as shown in Figure 23–4 where neoplasm were resected from the sacrum.

Neurological injuries can occur from violation of the pedicle walls, and injuries to large vessels on the ventral surface of the vertebral column can occur with penetration of the anterior vertebral body cortex. Also, an aberrant middle sacral artery can be injured on the anterior aspect of the sacrum during bicortical screw placement in the sacrum.[8,15]

Screw placement with CT image-guided techniques also has several pitfalls including difficulties with registration, DRF movement from the original site of placement, instrument inaccuracy, and surgical technical errors. The standard axial and sagittal views displayed on image-guidance systems are also not sufficient for accuracy. A trajectory along the plane-of-probe or an in-line trajectory along the long axis of the instrument is needed. This software modification allows projection across several imaging slices that provides optimal accuracy.

Recent studies have provided encouraging preliminary data, with each citing over 100 lumbosacral pedicle screws placed using stereotactic image guidance and having accuracies of placement within the pedicle of greater than 98%.[9–11]

■ Virtual Fluoroscopic Image Guidance

Recently virtual fluoroscopy has been developed and has become increasingly attractive for the more routine lumbar and sacral pedicle screw instrumentation procedures. Stereotactic image-guided technology utilizes standard, pre-acquired, two-dimensional fluoroscopic images to provide real-time intraoperative instrument navigation and instrumentation trajectories.

The system and its function

The necessary system components include an image-guidance system (as previously described in this chapter) that is equipped with software to utilize fluoroscopic images as the image data set, a high-resolution C-arm fluoroscope equipped with a calibration device mounted on the image intensifier, a camera tracking system, and a DRF attached to the patient.

At the beginning of surgery, the fluoroscope is positioned in the usual fashion and the calibration device is attached to the image-intensifier target. The C-arm is sterilely draped and the standard surgical exposure is performed. The DRF is then attached to the spinous process of the segment to be instrumented and anteroposterior (AP) and lateral fluoroscopic images are obtained with the vertebral segments to be instrumented centered in the field to avoid parallax from the fluoroscope image intensifier. The automatic registration technology essentially eliminates the registration process, and multiple surgical instruments can be tracked simultaneously.

The camera tracks the position of the LED/reflectors that are affixed to both the C-arm image intensifier ring and the DRF, which is attached to the patient. The "position sense" of the patient is then generated as the fluoroscopic image is transferred to the image-guidance system at the time of acquisition. The computer workstation then digitizes the acquired fluoroscopic images and calibrates the position of the surgical instruments with the camera system and generates a real-time graphic overlay of the instruments on the acquired images (Fig. 23–5). This usually occurs without the need for further fluoroscopic image acquisition, which drastically reduces the radiation exposure to the surgical team.[16]

Lumbar pedicle screw placement is then carried out with the same techniques as with fluoroscopy; however, both simultaneous AP and lateral images are used without the fluoroscope in place. Conventional fluoroscopy may be used after the instrumentation is placed for documentation purposes; further clinical trials and evaluations are under way to assess the accuracy of this technology.[16]

Advantages and limitations

Virtual fluoroscopy has a number of distinct advantages over conventional fluoroscopy. First, radiation exposure

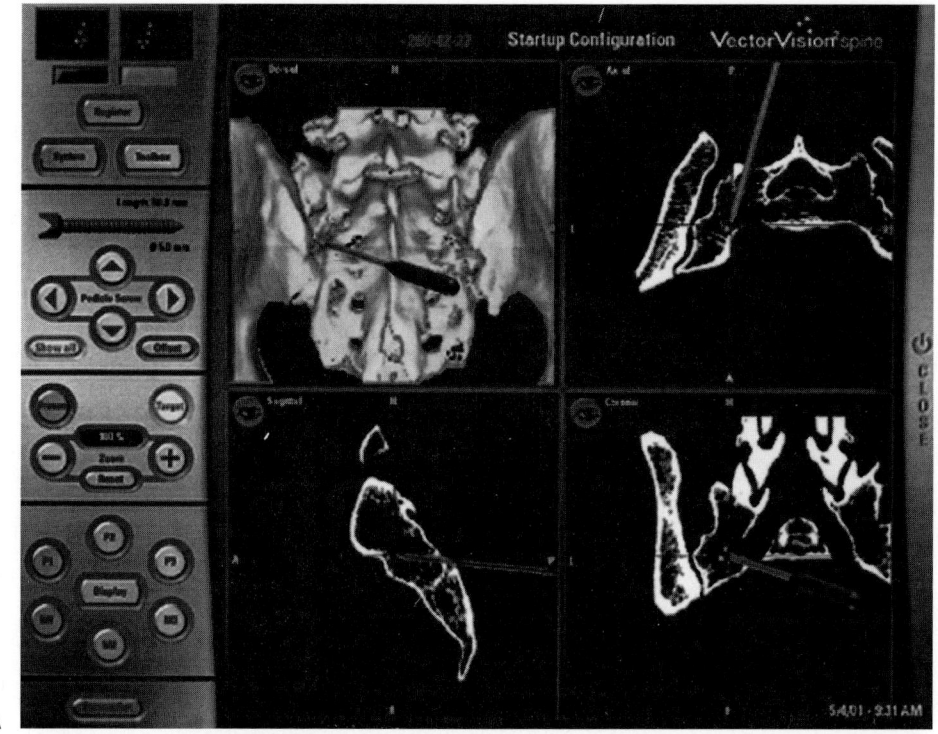

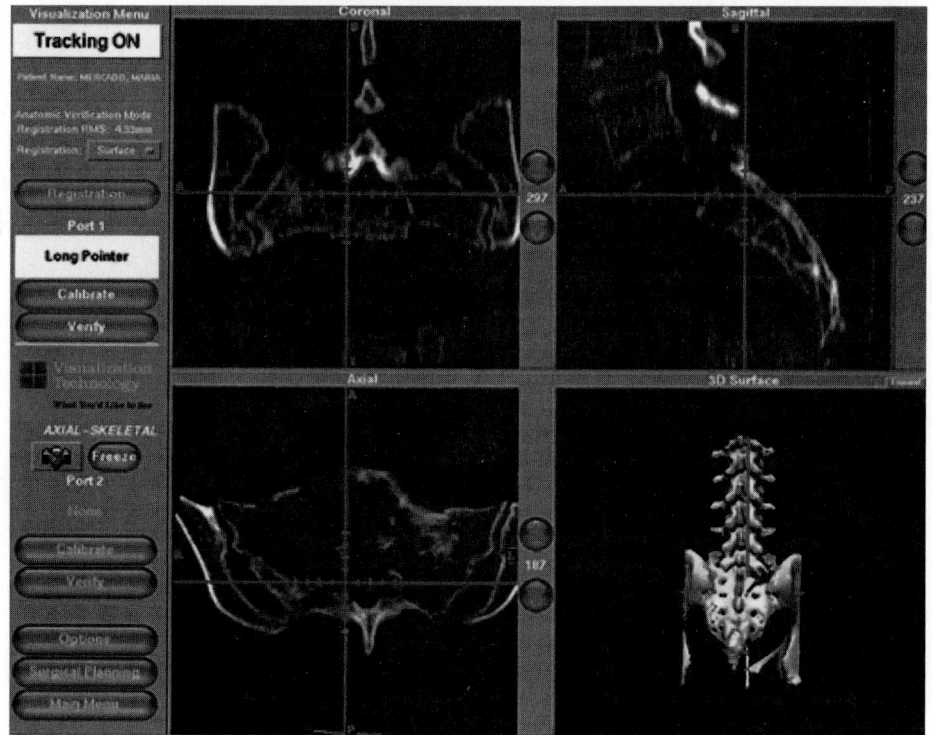

FIGURE 23–4. Image-guided sacral tumor resection of (A) sacral enchrondroma and (B) metastatic carcinoma. (Radionics, Burlington, MA)

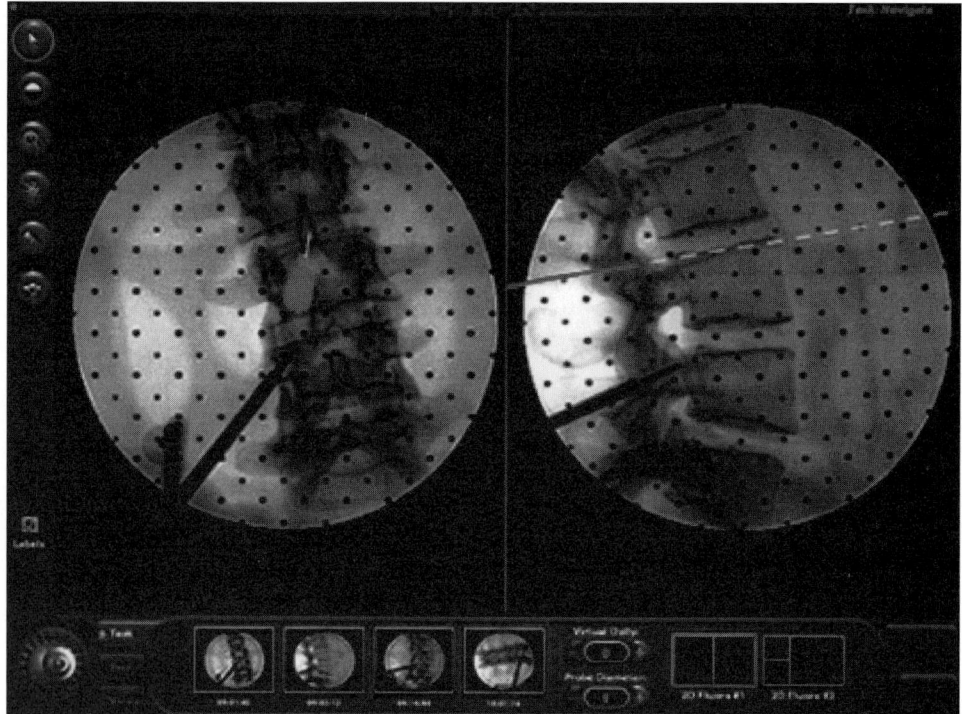

FIGURE 23–5. Virtual fluoroscopic anteroposterior and lateral images during surgical navigation. (Radionics, Burlington, MA)

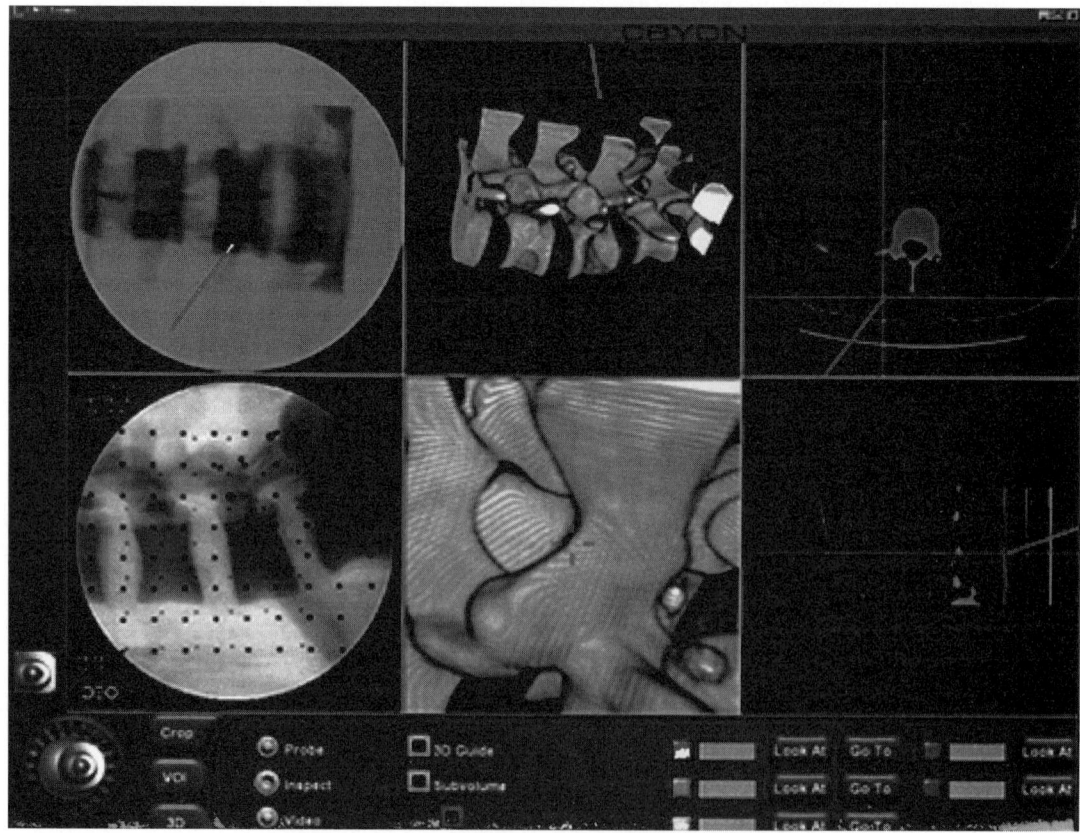

FIGURE 23–6. Endoscopic image-guided spinal procedure combining virtual fluoroscopy, endoscopy, and CT guidance. (Radionics, Burlington, MA)

to all personnel is reduced to only two to four images needed at the beginning of the procedure and acquired in rapid sequence. Second, multiplanar navigation is feasible with up to four views simultaneously. Third, the fluoroscope may be removed from the field after image acquisition, which improves the ergonomics in the crowded surgical field. Fourth, measurement of pedicle screw length and trajectories are easily obtained. Lastly, there is no detailed registration process, which is often the most problematic part of the image-guided procedure.

The most significant limitation of this technology is that two-dimensional navigation does not provide the detailed slice images of CT-based image guidance. As a result, lateral to medial trajectory can be difficult to determine in small pedicles. In addition, obese patients may be difficult to fluoroscopically image adequately and this must be considered during the planning stages of the procedure.

■ Conclusions

Precise knowledge of the lumbosacral anatomy and presurgical planning are prerequisites for a successful spinal instrumentation procedure. Image-guided spinal surgery was an outgrowth of cranial image-guidance applications to improve screw placement accuracy and to decrease the potential complications associated with pedicle screw misplacement errors. However, image-guidance technology is not a substitute for anatomic knowledge, surgical experience, and technical skill. The spine surgeon must also be familiar with conventional pedicle screw placement techniques without image guidance.

In addition, the proper use of the guidance system is essential to avoid additional errors that are specifically related to the technology. The registration process of stereotactic spinal image-guidance systems remains one of the critical steps in achieving successful navigation. Also, if the reference frame position is altered during the procedure, the registration procedure must be repeated.

Image-guided lumbosacral spine surgery has developed from theory to practical use in recent years with both CT-based virtual fluoroscopy procedures, which have been very successful. The future of image-guided technology will continue to improve in regard to registration for both open and closed techniques, including the combination of endoscopy and image guidance with either CT or fluoroscopy (Fig. 23–6). Merging other existing technologies with CT image fusion and fluoroscopy would allow 3-D navigation without the difficult

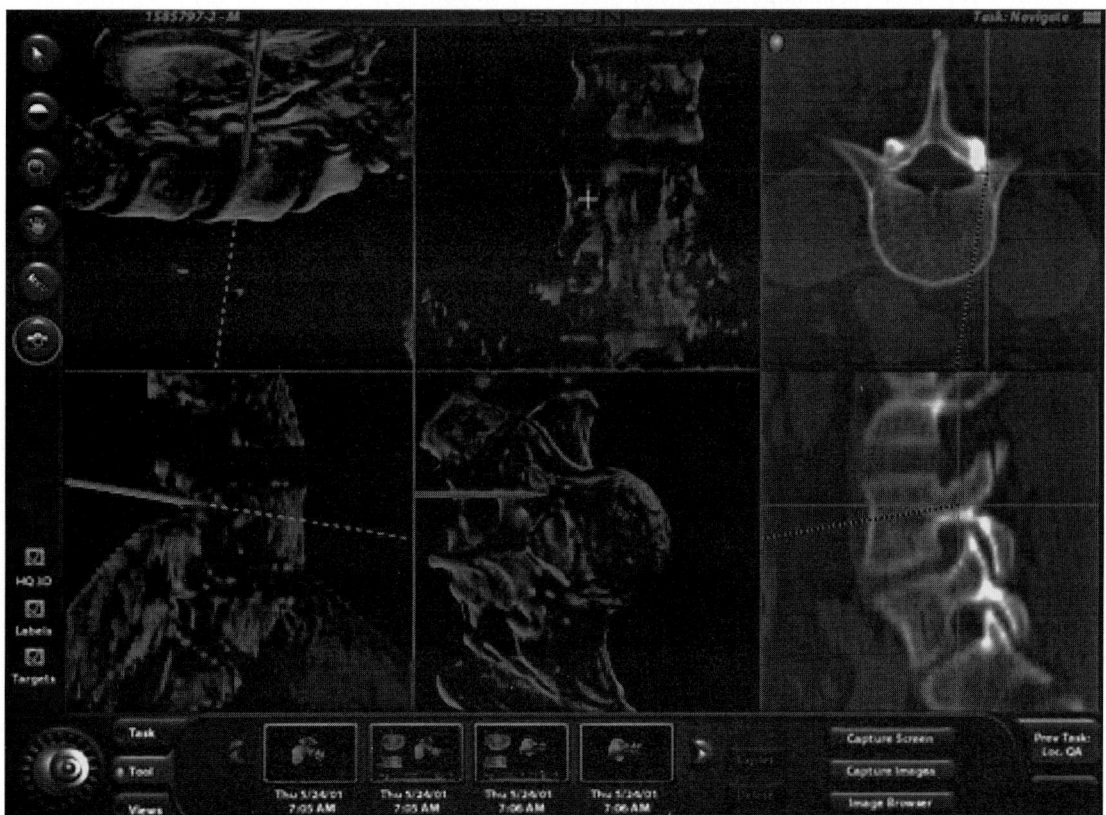

FIGURE 23–7. Three-dimensional volume-rendered CT image guidance that provides transparent, holographic imaging effect to "see through" solid structures. (Radionics, Burlington, MA)

registration process that is inherent with stereotactic systems today. Other developments in volume-rendered 3-D imaging will provide transparent, holographic imaging to visualize the otherwise solid, internal anatomy of spinal structures (Fig. 23–7). The goal is to provide rapid, safe, and efficient lumbar and sacral spinal instrumentation procedures.

■ Acknowledgment

The authors thank Samantha Phu for her assistance in the preparation of this manuscript.

REFERENCES

1. Bridwell KH, Sedgewick TA, O'Brien MF, Lenke LG, Baldus C. The role of fusion and instrumentation in the treatment of degenerative spondylolisthesis with spinal stenosis. *J Spine Disorders* 1993;6(6):461–472.
2. Grubb SA, Lipscomb HJ. Results of lumbosacral fusion for degenerative disc disease with and without instrumentation. *Spine* 1992;17(3):349–355.
3. Stefee AD, Brantigan JW. The variable screw placement spinal fixation system: report of a prospective study of 250 patients enrolled in FDA clinical trials. *Spine* 1993;18(9):1160–1172.
4. Yuan HA, Garfin SR, Dickman CA, Mardjetko SM. A historical cohort study of pedicle screw fixation in thoracic, lumbar, and sacral fusions. *Spine* 1994;19(20 suppl):2279–2296.
5. Zdeblick TA. A prospective randomized study of lumbar fusion. *Spine* 1993;18(8):983–991.
6. Esses SI, Sachs BL, Dreyzin V. Complications associated with the technique of pedicle screw fixation: a selected survey of ABS members. *Spine* 1993;18:2231–2239.
7. Gertzbein SD, Robins S. Accuracy of pedicular screws in vivo. *Spine* 1990;15:11–14.
8. Molitor CJ, Wiltse LL, Dimartino PP. Vascular and neurological anatomy of the lumbosacral spine as it relates to injury by pedicle screw placement [abstract]. Proceedings of the North American Spine Society, 6th Annual Meeting, Keystone Colorado, July 31–August 3 1991.
8a. Weinstein JN, Spratt KF, Spengler D. Spinal pedicle fixation: reliability and validity of roentgenogram-based assessment and surgical factors on successful screw placement. *Spine* 1988;13:1012–1018.
9. Foley KT, Smith MM. Image-guided spine surgery. *Neurosurg Clin North Am* 1996;7:171–186.
10. Kalfas IH, Kormos W, Murphy MA, et al. Application of frameless stereotaxy to pedicle screw fixation of the spine. *J Neurosurg* 1995;83:641–647.
11. Kamimura M, Ebara S, Itoh H, Tateiwa Y, Kinoshita T. Accurate pedicle screw insertion under the control of a computer-assisted image guided system: laboratory test and clinical study. *J Orthopaed Sci* 1999;4:197–206.
12. Kim KD, Johnson JP, Bloch O, Masciopinto JE. Computer-assisted thoracic pedicle screw placement: an in vitro feasibility study. *Spine* 2001;26:360–364.
13. Kim KD, Johnson JP, Masciopinto JE, Bloch O, Saracen MJ, Villablanca JP. Universal calibration of surgical instruments for spinal stereotaxy. *Neurosurgery* 1999;44(1):173–178.
14. Welch WC, Subach BR, Pollack IF, Jacobs JB. Frameless stereotactic guidance for surgery of the upper cervical spine. *Neurosurgery* 1997;40:958–964.
15. Mirkovic S, Abitbol JJ, Steinman J, et al. Anatomic considerations for sacral screw placement. *Spine* 1991;16(6 suppl):289–294.
16. Foley KT, Simon DA, Rampersaud R. Virtual fluoroscopy. *Op Techn Orthopaed* 2000;10(1):77–81.

24

Computer-Assisted Image-Guided Fluoroscopy (Virtual Fluoroscopy)

MICHAEL A. LEFKOWITZ AND KEVIN T. FOLEY

The field of spine surgery has witnessed many advances in recent years. Numerous technological developments, particularly in the areas of imaging, intraoperative navigation, and spinal instrumentation, have expanded the range of disease processes that may be treated.

To surgically manage patients with spine disease, it is necessary to have reliable preoperative and intraoperative imaging. Magnetic resonance imaging (MRI) and computed tomography (CT) have revolutionized the spine surgeon's ability to diagnose and treat spinal pathology. However, technical limitations and cost considerations have hindered the widespread availability of these imaging modalities in the operating room. Nevertheless, accurate visualization of anatomy is essential in the surgical suite, and it has become more important as the complexity of spine surgery has increased. Variations in musculoskeletal anatomy, either as a result of congenital anomaly, degenerative disease, or trauma, can adversely affect a surgical procedure and lead to a suboptimal result or a serious complication.

Fluoroscopy is an imaging technique that is familiar to spinal surgeons. It is routinely employed to improve intraoperative visualization of bony anatomy. By replacing direct visualization with radiographic visualization, it has enabled a reduction in surgical exposure, duration, and blood loss. Its use has facilitated a variety of complex spinal procedures, including pedicle screw insertion, interbody cage placement, odontoid screw insertion, and atlantoaxial transarticular screw fixation. This imaging technology has also been vital in the development of percutaneous spinal procedures, such as vertebroplasty.

Despite the advantages of intraoperative fluoroscopy, the technique has its limitations. The C-arm can be cumbersome to maneuver around a sterile operative field. Because only a single projection can be visualized at one time (without a second fluoroscope), it is necessary to reposition the C-arm during procedures that require multiple planes of visualization. There is also the issue of radiation exposure, which can be considerable for spinal surgeons.[1]

A desire to improve intraoperative visualization led to the development of image-guided surgery systems for spinal surgery. The first such systems were CT based and were an extension of systems used for cranial neurosurgery.[2] Further development of image-guided technology has resulted in a second class of systems that differ in terms of the type of imaging that is used to provide the image guidance. These systems are based upon fluoroscopy itself.[3-6]

A CT-based image-guided system relies upon the acquisition of a preoperative computerized tomogram with a specific protocol. The data from this image is transferred to the image-guidance system prior to surgery. Intraoperatively, patient registration is performed by identifying anatomic landmarks, or fiducial points, that correspond to analogous points in the image data set. The advantage of a CT-based system is that CT provides excellent anatomic detail for common spine regions of interest, such as the pedicle, and it allows for true three-dimensional guidance. The disadvantages of a CT-based system are several.[5] First, there is the need to obtain a preoperative CT scan with a specific protocol. This adds time and cost to the process (typically, even if a preoperative CT scan has been obtained for diagnostic purposes, it does not follow the parameters necessary for image-guided system use). Second, the CT scan is obtained in the supine position on the scanner gantry, whereas most spine procedures that use image guidance are performed in the prone position on an operating table. This changes the relationships between the individual vertebrae (rigid bodies) that exist in the CT image (image space) and those same vertebrae in the patient (surgical space). Thus, each vertebra must be individually registered, adding time to a multilevel procedure. As well, intersegmental trajectories (e.g., for C1–2 transarticular screw fixation) are not accurately depicted by the image-guided computer. Third, the CT-based system's images cannot be refreshed intraoperatively (without an intraoperative CT scanner). If intersegmental relationships change intraoperatively, as with distraction of an interspace or reduction of a deformity, this cannot be depicted by the image-guided computer display. Finally, registration of fiducial landmarks, which can be tedious and time-consuming, is required during surgery when using a CT-based system.

A fluoroscopy-based system employs commonly available C-arms augmented with accessories that allow accurate measurement of the relationship between the C-arm and the patient.[3-6] The system takes patient and C-arm position data for a given projection and relates that data to the fluoroscopic image from that projection. After calibrating the system with positional and fluoroscopic data from one or more projections, the computer generates a mathematical model of the fluoroscopic image that enables the superimposition of tracked surgical instruments onto the saved fluoroscopic images. Thus the real-time position of these instruments is displayed as it relates to one or more previously acquired fluoroscopic images, even in multiple planes, simultaneously. We term this process virtual fluoroscopy.[3,4,6] The advantages of virtual fluoroscopy are that no special preoperative study is required, intraoperative patient registration is automated (for some systems[3,4,6]), the images may be updated as necessary in the operating room, and an imaging modality is employed that many surgeons use routinely in the course of spine procedures. Table 24–1 provides a comparison of the CT-based and fluoroscopy-based image-guided systems.

Fluoroscopy-based systems are available that are either integrated with conventional image-guided surgery systems (FluoroNav Virtual Fluoroscopy System and StealthStation, Medtronic Surgical Navigation Systems, Louisville, CO) or exist as stand-alone devices (StealthStation Ion Fluoroscopic Navigation System, Medtronic Surgical Navigation Systems, Broomfield, CO; Z-Kat, Inc., Miami, FL).

The use of virtual fluoroscopy has not been limited to spine procedures. It has also been used to assist in the navigation of the bony anatomy of the parasellar region for transsphenoidal hypophysectomies.[7] In addition, it has been used extensively for orthopedic procedures such as intramedullary nail or screw insertion, acetabular fracture fixation, iliosacral screw insertion, and hip pinning. A variant of the technology involves the road-mapping utility, which is used during angiography procedures. In this application, the image of a vessel of interest is stored as a digital template and the real-time fluoroscopic image, which includes a catheter or guidewire, is superimposed on the previously stored vessel of interest during device manipulation.

■ Description of Systems

A typical virtual fluoroscopy system (Fig. 24–1) consists of an image-guidance computer system, a commercially available fluoroscopic C-arm, a calibration device that attaches to the C-arm, and specially modified surgical instruments that are capable of being tracked by the image-guidance system. The system may be operated by the surgeon through a sterile interface, or it may be operated by an assistant.

The operation of a virtual fluoroscopy system may be divided into four basic steps: (1) fluoroscopic image acquisition, (2) C-arm and patient position measurement, (3) merging of the fluoroscopic images with their unique C-arm and patient positions to create a mathematical model (mapping) of the image formation process, and (4) measurement of the position of surgical instruments in the operative field so that their likeness may be superimposed upon the virtual fluoroscopic images.[4,6]

In the first step, conventional fluoroscopic images are automatically transferred to the computer for image processing. In the second step, information about the relative position of the C-arm and the patient is acquired. This can be done by cameras that detect the location of light emitting diodes or passive reflectors that have been attached to the C-arm and the patient. The markers that are attached to the patient are in the form of a dynamic reference array (DRA), which rigidly attaches to the portion of the patient's anatomy that is to be imaged. Other means of position sensing (electromagnetic, sonic, mechanical, etc.) can also be used.

In the third step, the computer calibrates the acquired fluoroscopic image by taking into account the positional data acquired in the second step. Based upon the inputted images, a mathematical mapping function is generated that allows a virtual fluoroscopic image to be produced for a unique combination of C-arm and patient position. The calibration process compensates for factors such as gravity-dependent changes in the C-arm

TABLE 24–1. A Comparison of CT-Based and Fluoroscopy-Based Image-Guided Systems

Parameter	CT-Based IGS	FluoroNav (Medtronic Sofamor Danek)	Fluorolab (Z-Kat, Inc.)
Preoperative study necessary	Yes (added radiation exposure)	No	No
Intraoperative image acquisition possible	No	Yes	Yes
Intraoperative patient registration by surgeon	Yes, variable number of fiducials	No (carried out by the software)	Yes, eight fiducials
Potential for intraoperative image updating	No	Yes	Yes
Intraoperative radiation exposure	No	Yes (but less than standard fluoroscopy)	Yes (but less than standard fluoroscopy)

image center, the effect of external electromagnetic fields generated by electrical equipment in the operating room, and the effect of changes in the C-arm's position with respect to the earth's magnetic field. Because of these compensation factors, which are unique to every C-arm position, it is necessary that every acquired image be independently calibrated.[6] This can be accomplished quickly and efficiently through the use of a computerized algorithm.

In the fourth step, the computer determines the position of one or more trackable surgical instruments using a position-measuring camera and then superimposes an

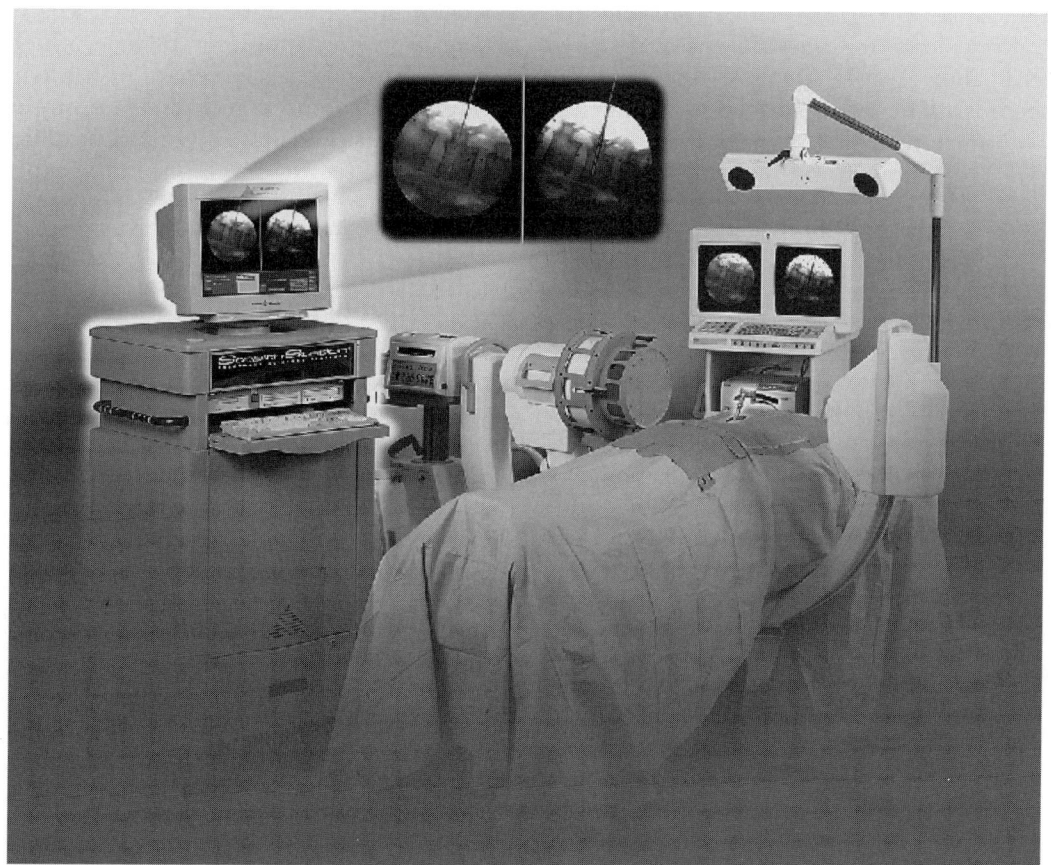

FIGURE 24–1. The FluoroNav (Medtronic SNT, Louisville, CO) virtual fluoroscopy system is shown, consisting of an image-guidance computer system and camera array, a calibration target that is attached to a standard C-arm fluoroscope, and various tracked tools. (From Foley KT, Simon DA, Rampersaud YR. Virtual fluoroscopy: computer-assisted fluoroscopic navigation. *Spine* 2001;26:347–351. With permission.)

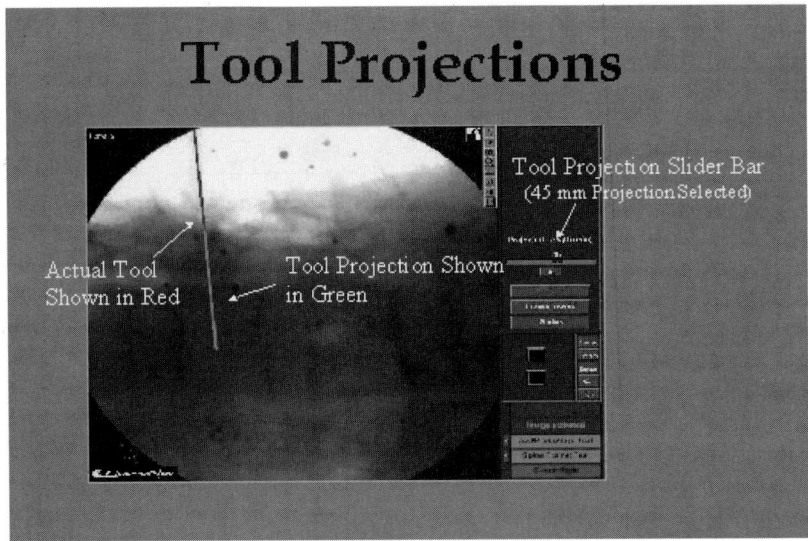

FIGURE 24–2. A lateral virtual fluoroscopic view of the lumbar spine is shown. The pedicle probe (dark line) has been positioned at the pedicle entry point. Its trajectory (light line) has been virtually extended 45 mm into the pedicle and vertebral body.

image of the instrument(s) in the virtual fluoroscopic display. Dedicated tracked awls, probes, taps, and screwdrivers are available, and any rigid surgical instrument may be tracked with the assistance of a universal tool array. The system is capable of correctly displaying the position of the surgical instrument(s) in any of the previously acquired fluoroscopic images, in multiple planes, simultaneously. The system also allows the actual projection of a surgical instrument (in one color) and the simultaneous projection of the linear extension of that instrument's proposed trajectory (in a second color) (Fig. 24–2).

System accuracy

The accuracy of various virtual fluoroscopy systems has been tested experimentally. Foley et al performed a cadaver study comparing live and virtual fluoroscopic images in which a tracked probe was inserted into pedicles from L1 to S1.[3] Differences in positioning of the probe tip and probe trajectory angle were measured for the live and virtual images. The mean error in probe tip localization was 0.97 ± 0.40 mm (99% confidence interval = 2.2 mm, maximum probe tip error = 3 mm). The mean trajectory angle difference between the virtual and actual probe images was 2.7 degrees ± 0.6 degrees (99% confidence interval = 4.6 degrees, maximum trajectory angle difference = 5 degrees).

■ Specific Techniques

Certain general principles apply to all virtual fluoroscopy procedures. Although the acquisition of CT or MRI scans is not necessary for surgical navigation with virtual fluoroscopy, diagnostic three-dimensional images are part of a good preoperative evaluation and they will contain information that will be useful for planning and executing the operation. These preoperative studies should be evaluated for anatomic anomalies, such as a tortuous vertebral artery or a hypoplastic pedicle, which will prevent successful and safe placement of instrumentation.

Good fluoroscopic technique is important during image-guided procedures. One must endeavor to place the anatomic region of interest in the center of the fluoroscopic image to minimize parallax.

Conventional pedicle screw insertion

Pedicle screw insertion begins with an exposure of the desired levels as far lateral as the screw entry site (for the lumbar spine, the junction of the pars, transverse process, and superior articular process). The DRA is rigidly affixed to the spinous process of the vertebra in which pedicle screws are to be placed. For a typical degenerative case (without gross instability), the end vertebra can be utilized for this purpose (e.g., attach the DRA to L4 for screw placement at L4, L5, and S1). The fluoroscopic views normally obtained by the surgeon are then acquired. These may include lateral views, anteroposterior (AP) views, or oblique ("owl's eye") views down the length of the pedicle. The appropriate views for bilateral pedicle screw placement may be obtained and stored at the beginning of the operation, thus reducing the need to manipulate the C-arm throughout the procedure. At this time, the fluoroscopic images may be compared with preoperative CT and MRI scans to determine the optimal entry points in the pedicle for screw insertion. For example, an AP fluoroscopic image could be obtained and compared with preoperative im-

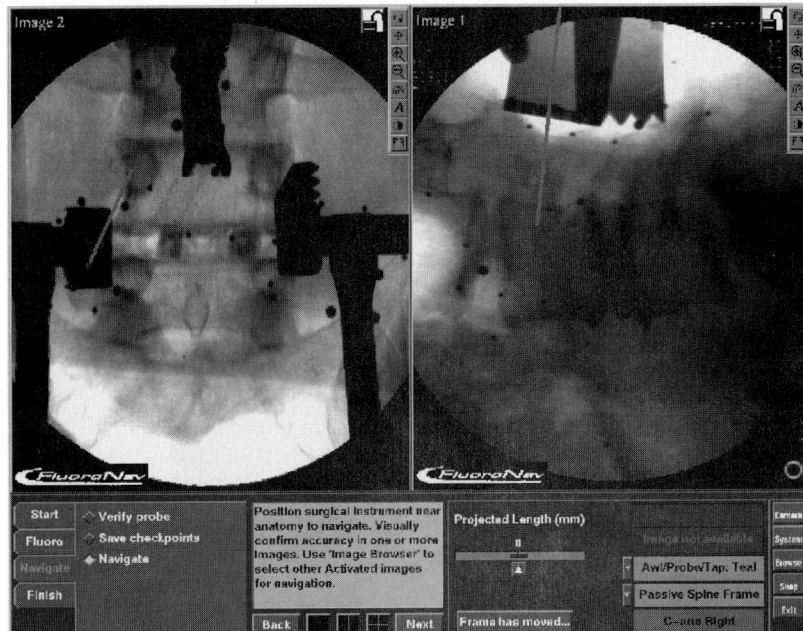

FIGURE 24–3. Open lumbar pedicle screw placement. A pedicle probe is being advanced into the left L4 pedicle. Note that its course and progress can be followed simultaneously in the anteroposterior and lateral planes with the use of virtual fluoroscopy (FluroNav, Medtronic SNT, Louisville, CO).

ages to determine the distance from midline and angle of trajectory that result in the ideal entry point and course of pedicle screw insertion. By positioning the tracked instruments over the pedicle, the anticipated entry point and trajectory of the instruments may be displayed prior to probing the pedicle. The system will also allow the virtual projection of pedicle screws of a selected length and diameter onto the chosen trajectory. The use of tracked awls, probes, and taps permits continuous visualization of the instruments along their course through the pedicle and into the vertebral body (Fig. 24–3). The fluoroscope may be used in the live mode at any time during the procedure for visualization of instrument or screw position.[4]

Percutaneous pedicle screw insertion

Because the virtual fluoroscopy system does not rely on direct exposure of the spine for registration, percutaneous screws may be inserted. After visualizing the spine levels that are to be treated with conventional fluoroscopy, a small incision is made over the spinous process of one of the levels to be instrumented. The DRA is rigidly attached to the spinous process. The desired fluoroscopic projections (AP, lateral, and oblique) are obtained and calibrated. A tracked, sharp-tip probe is placed on the skin surface over the pedicle. The trajectory of the probe may be virtually extended through the pedicle to visualize the anticipated course of the pedicle screw. A stab incision is made at the skin entry point and a K-wire and dilators are used to dissect through the paraspinous muscles to the pedicle surface. The dilators are withdrawn, and a tracked awl and probe are used to form a pilot hole in the pedicle under virtual fluoroscopic guidance.[8]

Prior to probing and tapping the pedicle pilot hole, it is useful to review the preoperative CT and MRI to decide upon the optimal entry point and trajectory for the pedicle screw. As described in the conventional pedicle screw insertion section, the trajectory of the instruments may be virtually extended to visualize the pathway of the screw prior to probing the pedicle (Fig. 24–4).

Posterior lumbar interbody fusion

The initial exposure is performed in the conventional fashion. The DRA is attached to an adjacent spinous process. AP and lateral fluoroscopic images are obtained with the disk space centered in each image. The images are calibrated and true midline is determined from the AP image. A dedicated set of tracked posterior lumbar interbody fusion instruments is available (Medtronic Sofamor Danek, Memphis, TN). The disk is removed with a combination of curettes and pituitary forceps. A tracked distractor is then inserted into the disk space and the distractor tip is fully seated. The depth of the distractor tip in the disk space may be visualized on virtual fluoroscopy in the lateral position. Because the distractor alters the disk space height, it is necessary to obtain new images for virtual fluoroscopy. A tracked box chisel is then inserted so that the disk space may be prepared for graft insertion. Tracked chisels of various heights are available. The depth of the box chisel may be monitored on the lateral virtual images. The disk space is now ready for graft placement, which may be

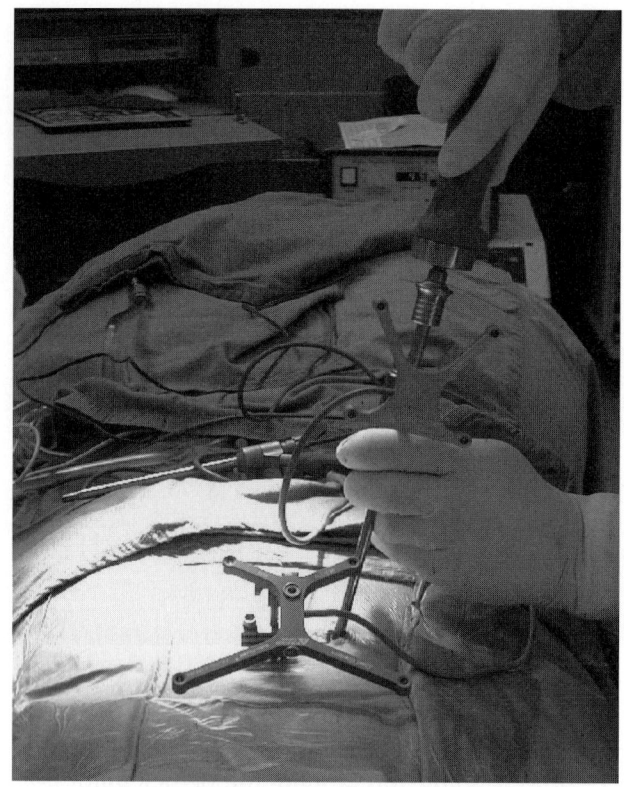

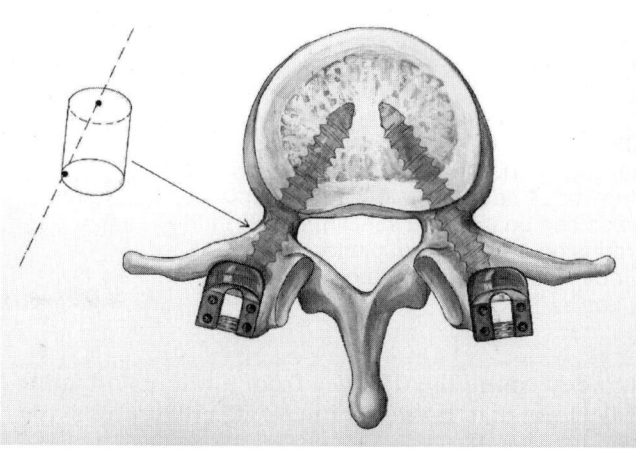

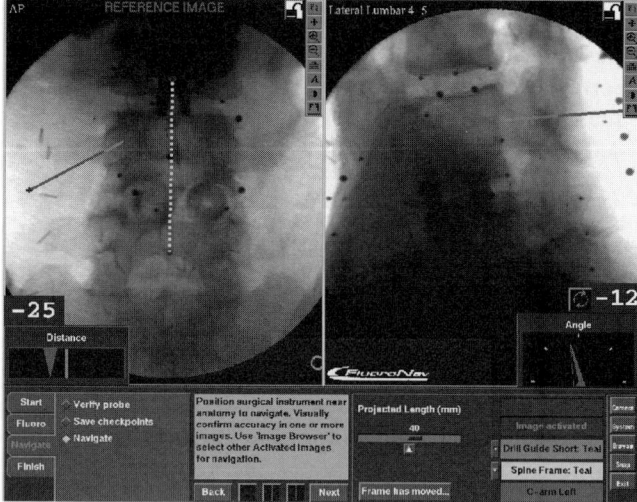

FIGURE 24–4. Percutaneous pedicle screw insertion. A tracked pedicle probe is being inserted into the pedicle through a small skin incision. (A). The pedicle can be pictured as a cylinder (B). The percutaneous pedicle probe is positioned at the pedicle entry point [the "top" of the pedicle cylinder on the lateral view and the lateral edge of the pedicle cylinder on the anteroposterior (AP) view]. Its trajectory is then virtually extended to the "bottom" of the pedicle cylinder (the junction of the pedicle and the vertebral body). As long as this trajectory stays lateral to the medial edge of the pedicle on the AP view (enough to accommodate the anticipated screw diameter), then the pedicle can be safely probed and a screw safely placed percutaneously (C) (Fluro-Nav, Medtronic SNT, Louisville, CO). (From Foley KT, Gupta SK, Justis JR, Sherman MC. Percutaneous pedicle screw fixation of the lumbar spine. *Neurosurg Focus* 2001;10:Article 10. With permission.)

monitored on the AP and lateral virtual images (Fig. 24–5). The process is repeated on the other side for contralateral graft placement.

Atlantoaxial transarticular screw fixation

Preoperative evaluation includes a review of all appropriate images to determine the patient's suitability for surgery. If a preoperative study demonstrates an anomalous vertebral artery or a fracture or destruction of the C1 or C2 lateral mass or the C2 pars interarticularis, then the patient may not be a candidate for transarticular screw fixation on the affected side. Furthermore, if an atlantoaxial subluxation is present and it is determined that it is not reducible, then another stabilization procedure should be considered.[9]

The procedure is performed in the prone position with the head affixed in a Mayfield headrest. It is important to have the Mayfield positioned in such a fashion as to allow AP views of the atlantoaxial complex to

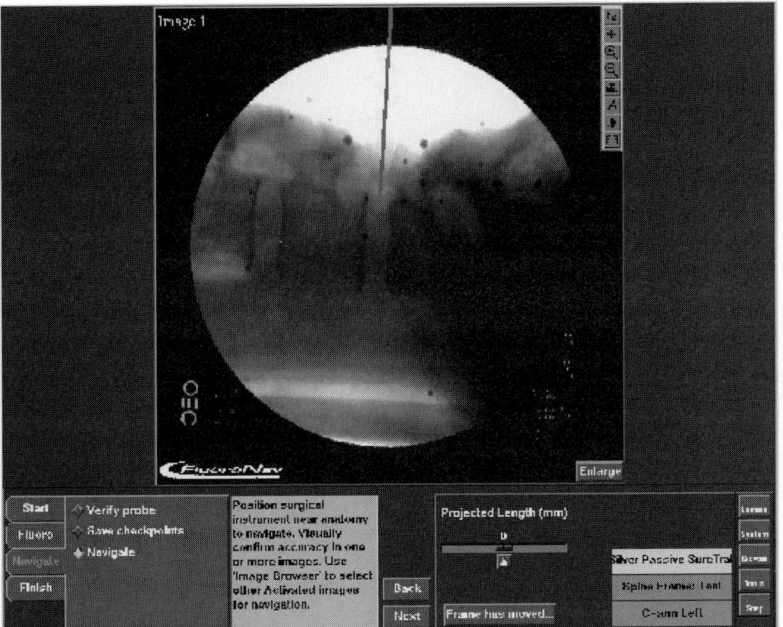 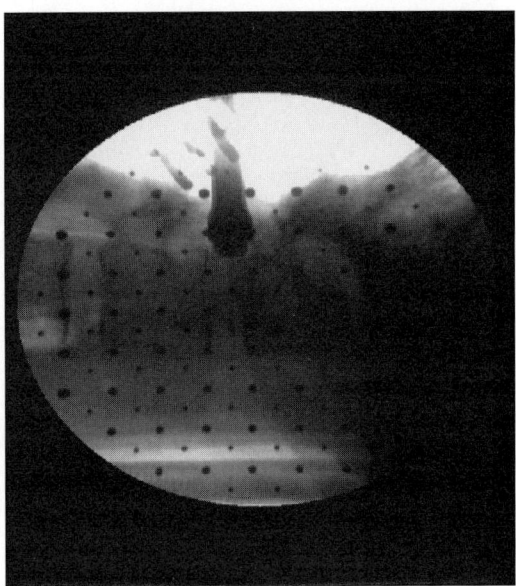

FIGURE 24–5. A lateral virtual fluoroscopic image of a PLIF box chisel is seen. The chisel is at the dorsal margin of the disk space and is aligned with the interspace, (A). A "live" fluoroscopic image of the box chisel corresponding with the virtual fluoroscopic view. Note the calibration grid on this view, (B). (FluorNav, Medtronic SNT, Louisville, CO)

be obtained. Under lateral fluoroscopic guidance, the atlantoaxial subluxation is gently reduced and the head is fixed in place. A conventional midline occiput to C3 exposure is performed so that the C1 and C2 lateral masses and the C1–C2 and C2–C3 facet joints are revealed. The soft tissue is reflected from the C1 and C2 laminae. The DRA is attached to the C2 spinous process. At this point, AP and lateral fluoroscopic images are obtained and calibrated. The preoperative CT and/or MRI are reviewed for information on the optimal screw entry point and trajectory. A typical entry point is approximately 2 to 3 mm above the C2–C3 facet joint line and 2 to 3 mm lateral to the junction of the C2 lamina and lateral mass. A tracked probe is placed on the skin surface at the cervicothoracic junction, 1.5 to 2 cm lateral to the midline. The trajectory of the probe is virtually extended through the C2 inferior facet, the C2 pars, across the C1–C2 joint, into the C1 lateral mass, to the posterior cortex of the C1 anterior arch. The position of the probe is adjusted until a proper trajectory is observed. A paramedian stab incision is then made where the probe contacts the skin, and a tracked drill guide is inserted through this incision and the underlying paraspinous tissues to the C2–C3 facet. The entry point is decorticated. A drill is then passed through the tracked guide and is used to create a pilot hole along the C1–C2 transarticular pathway. The trajectory of the drill and guide is followed using virtual fluoroscopy, simultaneously visualizing this trajectory in the AP and lateral views. Progress of the actual drill tip is followed using live lateral fluoroscopy. An appropriate-length screw is inserted once the pilot hole has been tapped. The process is repeated on the contralateral side.

Odontoid screw insertion

The patient is positioned supine with the neck extended. The odontoid fracture is reduced under live fluoroscopy. The proper position is maintained using a Mayfield apparatus. The DRA is attached to the Mayfield. The Mayfield must be positioned such that an open-mouth fluoroscopic view of the odontoid can be obtained (Fig. 24–6A). Open-mouth and lateral fluoroscopic images of C2 are obtained, calibrated, and saved using a single fluoroscope. The C-arm is returned to the lateral position. The patient is prepped and draped. An incision is made at the level of the C5–C6 interspace and dissection proceeds down to the ventral surface of the cervical spine, as far rostral as the C2–C3 interspace. A handheld retractor is inserted. A shallow, midline trough is created in the ventral surface of the C3 vertebral body and the C2–C3 annulus to facilitate a steep trajectory for the screw. A tracked drill guide is positioned against the anterior, inferior aspect of the C2 vertebral

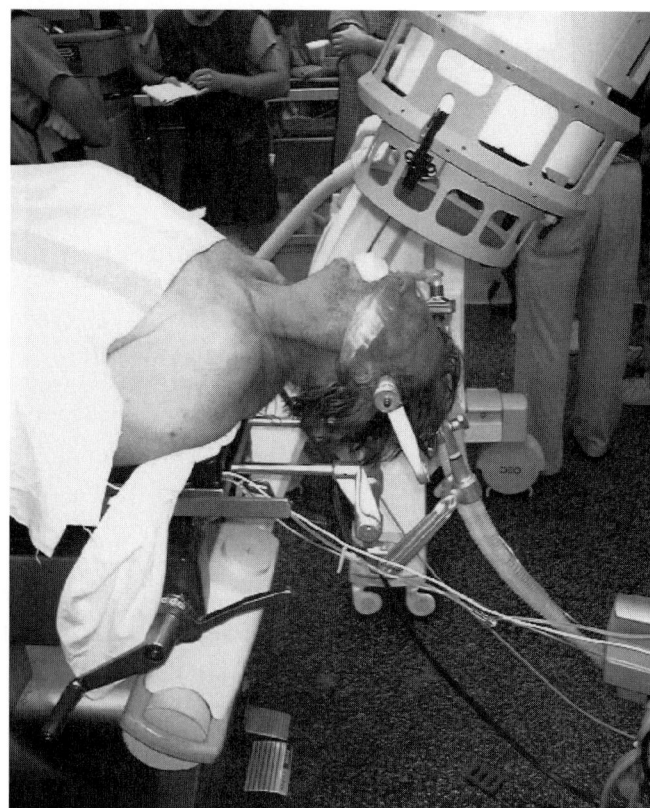

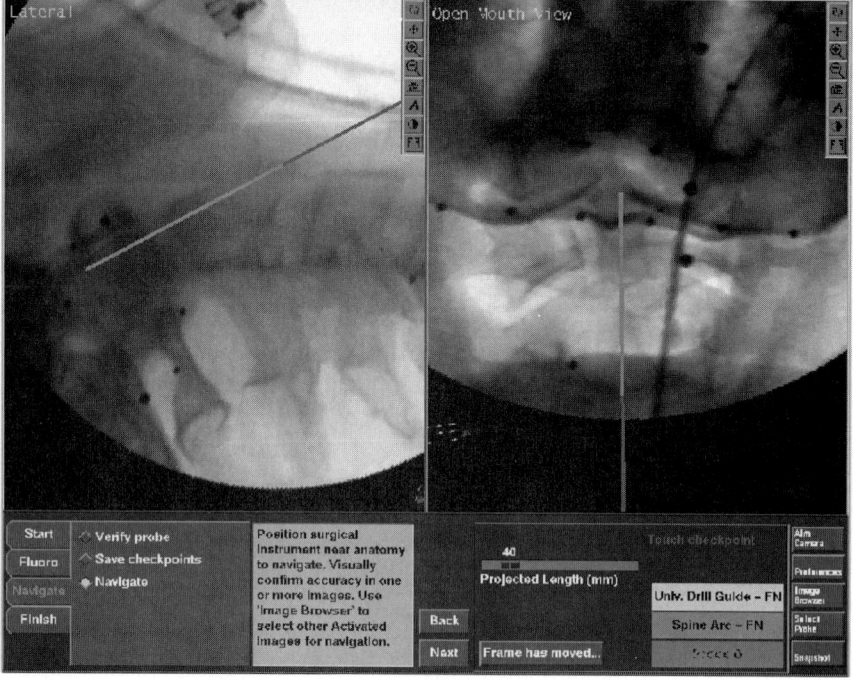

FIGURE 24–6. A patient with a type II odontoid fracture has been positioned for odontoid screw fixation with virtual fluoroscopic guidance. The head is fixed in a Mayfield apparatus, which has been positioned to allow for acquisition of an open-mouth view of the odontoid. (A). Lateral and open-mouth virtual fluoroscopic views of the odontoid. The drill guide is positioned at the anterior inferior aspect of the C2 vertebral body; its virtual trajectory has been extended along a proper path to the apex of the odontoid process. (B). (FluorNav, Medtronic SNT, Louisville, CO)

body in the midline. Proper position is confirmed with the open-mouth and lateral virtual fluoroscopic views (Fig. 24–6B). A K-wire is then inserted through this drill guide to penetrate the anterior aspect of the inferior C2 endplate and directed through the middle of the dens to a point just proximal to its tip (Fig. 24–6B). Progress of the K-wire is monitored with live lateral fluoroscopy. After the K-wire has been appropriately positioned, the screw length is measured using a gauge, and a self-tapping, cannulated lag screw is inserted over the K-wire. The K-wire remains in place while the screw is being inserted to maintain the proper alignment of the dens with the C2 body. After the screw has been fully inserted, the K-wire is removed. To achieve the proper lag effect, the lag screw threads must lie distal to the fracture line.[10]

Transoral decompression of the craniocervical junction

The procedure is performed in the supine position. As for odontoid screw placement, the head is positioned using a Mayfield apparatus and the DRA is fixed to the Mayfield. A transoral retractor is placed so as to open the jaw and retract the tongue caudally. The soft palate is split in the midline and retracted. AP and lateral fluoroscopic images are obtained of the craniocervical junction and calibrated. A posterior pharyngeal incision is made over the anterior tubercle of C1. The longus colli muscles and the anterior longitudinal ligament are separated from the arch of C1. The ventral arch of C1 is removed with a drill to expose the odontoid. However, if the pathology permits, it may be desirable to preserve a portion of the anterior arch of C1. This serves two purposes: it prevents spreading of the C1 lateral masses and subsequent craniocervical instability, and the anterior tubercle of C1 may serve as a landmark for the placement of atlantoaxial transarticular screws, should this be necessary.[11] The limit of lateral exposure is typically 10 mm on either side of the midline. More extensive dissection places the vertebral arteries and the structures of the jugular foramen at risk. The alar and apical ligaments are sectioned prior to removal of the dens. The ventral aspect of the dens is removed until only the dorsal cortical rim remains. This remaining bone is removed in a piecemeal fashion with a Kerrison or pituitary rongeur. There are two principal advantages to the use of virtual fluoroscopy in this procedure. First, the midline may be identified on AP images, and a tracked probe may be used to determine the extent of lateral exposure. Second, a tracked probe may be used to determine the extent of resection of the odontoid as it is being removed so that the drill does not inadvertently breech the dorsal cortical margin of the dens.

■ Published Studies

Several studies have demonstrated the efficacy of virtual fluoroscopy systems for spine procedures. Choi et al performed a cadaver study where they compared pedicle screw insertion using a virtual fluoroscopy system versus a CT-based image-guidance system.[5] The virtual fluoroscopy system employed in this study was a first-generation clinical version that incorporated an electromechanical arm that held the drill guide sleeve in secure alignment so that instruments would be constrained to the correct entry site and angle of trajectory. The measured parameters of the study were the rate of successful pedicle screw placement as well as the average time required to insert a pedicle screw. Pedicle screw placement was unsuccessful in 12.7% of image-guided system attempts (2.9% medial pedicle wall perforations, 9.8% lateral pedicle wall perforations) and unsuccessful in 17.9% of virtual fluoroscopy attempts (6.6% medial pedicle wall perforations, 11.3% lateral pedicle wall perforations). The difference between the rates of success for the two modalities was not statistically significant ($P = 0.34$). For each image-guidance modality, the vast majority of cortical perforations were noted in the upper- and midthoracic pedicles, where the pedicle cross-sectional area is smaller. No nerve root injuries were observed in either group.

The total time required to place a pedicle screw was divided into the registration time and the operating time. The registration time consisted of the time required to locate the appropriate level, select the fiducial points (three for the CT guided system, eight for the fluoroscopically guided system), and identify the same fiducial points on the individual vertebra. For the fluoroscopically guided system, the registration time also included the time required to perform the AP and lateral fluoroscopic images and the time required to position the virtual guidewire to the orientation of the targeted pedicle. The operating time consisted of the time required to place the pedicle screw after registration. For the fluoroscopically guided system, this time segment included the positioning of the electromechanical arm. The mean time to register and operate on one level using the virtual fluoroscopy system was 14.6 minutes (registration time = 9.3 minutes, operating time = 5.2 minutes), compared with 6.8 minutes (registration time = 3.0 minutes, operating time = 3.8 minutes) using the CT-guided system. This difference in time was found to be statistically significant ($P = 0.0006$), with the majority of the time difference being in the registration time. This study suggests that virtual fluoroscopy can be as reliable and accurate as a CT-based image-guided system, but that screw insertion is more time-consuming with a fluoroscopy-based system that requires a surgeon-based registration step. The particular virtual fluoroscopy system used in this study required the registration of eight fiducial markings, a process that was found to prolong the average time of pedicle screw insertion. Manipulation of the electromechanical arm also contributed to the prolonged registration time.

Foley et al performed a study of lumbar pedicle screw fixation using a novel percutaneous technique.[8] A virtual fluoroscopy system was used as the imaging modality (FluoroNav; Medtronic Surgical Navigation Technologies, Louisville, CO). Twelve patients were successfully treated using this technique. The versatility of the imaging system allowed registration of unexposed spine elements for the percutaneous procedure. Registration was completely automated, requiring no surgeon input, and occurred in seconds. All percutaneous pedicle screws were successfuly placed.

■ Conclusions and Future Directions

Computer-assisted virtual fluoroscopy provides a number of benefits over conventional fluoroscopy. Virtual fluoroscopy allows the acquisition of all necessary images at one point during the surgery, rather than requiring intermittent use of the C-arm. Because operating room personnel need not be in the vicinity of the C-arm during image acquisition, there is a significant reduction in radiation exposure to the surgeon and surgical team. The patient benefits from reduced radiation as well because C-arm images don't need to be reacquired each time an instrument is repositioned or a new trajectory is chosen. Virtual fluoroscopy allows the acquisition and simultaneous visualization of multiple image projections in multiple planes with a single C-arm apparatus. This is useful when attempting to position an instrument along a particular trajectory. To achieve similar visualization with a conventional fluoroscopic system, it would be necessary for the surgeon to simultaneously use two C-arms while manipulating the surgical instrument.

Virtual fluoroscopy also offers advantages over CT-based image-guided systems. There is no need for a preoperative CT or MRI that requires special formatting and additional cost. Patient registration is much less complicated with some virtual fluoroscopy systems; in fact, the process is automated when using the FluoroNav system.[6] Finally, real-time updating of the fluoroscopic images is easily performed intraoperatively.

Although the accuracy of virtual fluoroscopy systems is quite good, one must be aware that the margins of error are small in many areas of the spine for common procedures. Foley et al studied the mean probe tip error and the mean trajectory angle difference between virtual and actual fluoroscopic images during pedicle screw placement and found them to be 0.97 ± 0.40 mm and 2.7 degrees ± 0.6 degrees, respectively.[3] These findings compare favorably with the results of Glossop and Hu, who found an average of 2 to 3 mm translational and 4 to 7 degrees rotational clinical utility error for pedicle screw placement using a CT-based image-guided system.[12] However, in their morphologic-mathematical study of accuracy requirements for pedicle screw insertion, Rampersaud et al reported that a maximal permissible translational error of less than 1 mm and rotational error of less than 5 degrees were allowable at the midcervical spine, the midthoracic spine, and the thoracolumbar junction.[13] How can image guidance be of use when its error tolerances, in some cases, are less precise than those required for a given procedure? It is postulated that image guidance is useful because it initially directs the surgeon to the optimal screw entry point and trajectory; surgeon haptic feedback likely refines the trajectory during the course of the procedure. These findings emphasize that image guidance is a tool that can be of considerable assistance to a surgeon, but it is not a substitute for surgical skill and vigilance.

Technology is currently being developed that may ultimately allow intraoperative registration of the spine with fluoroscopic imaging. This may eliminate the need for time-consuming tactile anatomic registration. Two-dimensional fluoroscopic registration could then be used as an adjunct to CT or MRI to allow for three-dimensional real-time navigation.[14] In fact, the recent development of isocentric C-arm fluoroscopy, which generates CT images using an intraoperative fluoroscope, may offer another means of three-dimensional navigation using a two-dimensional intraoperative imaging source. Finally, it is quite likely that virtual fluoroscopy technology will be routinely integrated into C-arm fluoroscopes, allowing the surgeon to use a single device in either a "live" or virtual mode, as navigational needs dictate.

REFERENCES

1. Rampersaud YR, Foley KT, Shen AC, et al. Radiation exposure to the spine surgeon during fluoroscopically assisted pedicle screw insertion. *Spine* 2000;25:2637–2645.
2. Foley KT, Smith MM. Image-guided spine surgery. *Neurosurg Clin N Am* 1996;7(2):171–186.
3. Foley KT, Rampersaud YR, Simon DA. Virtual fluoroscopy: multiplanar x-ray guidance with minimal radiation exposure. *European Spine Journal* 1999;8(suppl 1):S36.
4. Foley KT, Simon DA, Rampersaud YR. Virtual fluoroscopy. *OpTech Orthoped* 2000;10(1):77–81.
5. Choi WW, Green BA, Levi ADO. Computer-assisted fluoroscopic targeting system for pedicle screw insertion. *Neurosurgery* 2000;47(4):872–878.
6. Foley KT, Simon DA, Rampersaud YR. Virtual fluoroscopy: computer-assisted fluoroscopic navigation. *Spine* 2001;26(4):347–351.

7. Jane JA, Thapar K, Alden TD, Laws ER Jr. Fluoroscopic frameless stereotaxy for transsphenoidal surgery. *Neurosurgery* 2001;48(6): 1302–1308.
8. Foley KT, Gupta SK, Justis JR, Sherman MC. Percutaneous pedicle screw fixation of the lumbar spine. *Neurosurgical Focus* 2001;10 (4):1–8.
9. Madawi AA, Casey AH, Solanki GA, Tuite G, Veres R, Crockard HA. Radiological and anatomical evaluation of the atlantoaxial transarticular screw fixation technique. *J Neurosurg* 1997;86: 961–968.
10. Dickman CA, Foley KT, Sonntag VKH, Smith MM. Cannulated screws for odontoid screw fixation and atlantoaxial transarticular screw fixation: technical note. *J Neurosurg* 1995;83:1095–1100.
11. Bhangoo RS, Crockard HA. Transoral exposures. In: Kaye AH, Black PM, eds. *Operative Neurosurgery*. New York: Churchill-Livingstone; 2000:1399–1415.
12. Glossop ND, Hu RW. Practical accuracy assessment of image-guided spine surgery. Presented at the 2nd Annual North American Program on Computer Assisted Orthopedic Surgery, Pittsburgh, Pennsylvania, June 1998.
13. Rampersaud YR, Simon DA, Foley KT. Accuracy requirements for image-guided spinal pedicle screw placement. *Spine* 2001;26(4): 352–359.
14. Theodore N, Sonntag VKH. Spinal surgery: the past century and the next. *Neurosurgery* 2000;46(4):767–776.

25

Controversies in Image-Guided Spine Surgery

CHRISTOPHER J. BARRY, TIMOTHY C. RYKEN, AND VINCENT C. TRAYNELIS

Traditionally, stereotaxy utilized a fixed reference or fiducial system to create reference marks on the image that have known positions with respect to the frame. The advent of computed tomography (CT) in the late 1970s sparked a rapid evolution of stereotactic neurosurgery. The inherent two-dimensional aspect of the axial CT scan allowed for accurate identification of the x and y coordinates; however, determination of z-axis coordinates remained problematic. This was solved in 1980 with the development of a fiducial system known as the N bar configuration of the modern stereotactic frame. Each bar is seen in cross section on every axial slice. The distance between the center bar and the adjacent bars is used to calculate the z-axis coordinates. Kelly introduced volumetric stereotactic guidance for tumor resection in the early 1980s.[1] CT data were transferred to a computer workstation to create a three-dimensional (3-D) rendering, thus defining the target as a volume rather than a point in space. These advances allowed the rigid framed system with its restrictive, complex, and nonintuitive nature to evolve into the field of frameless stereotaxy.

Frameless stereotaxy utilizes 3-D reconstruction of digital images obtained from CT or magnetic resonance (MR) scans and complex algorithms to create a fixed relationship between the image space and the physical space. This process is known as registration and is based upon a fiducial system. Through registration there is a complete mapping of each point in the reconstructed images to the physical space of the patient. Once localization is accomplished, the 3-D anatomy of the patient can be viewed and intraoperative interactive 3-D targeting can be performed.

Frameless stereotactic neurosurgery has been effectively applied to cranial applications, reducing morbidity involved in resection of tumors and vascular lesions, and for precise cannulation of the ventricular system.[2–5] Given the successful application of frameless stereotactic image-guided surgery for cranial lesions, there has been increased interest in applying this technology to the spinal axis.[6–12] Currently, frameless stereotaxy has found its greatest utility in the spine as an aid in instrumentation procedures.[6,13–17] Prior to frameless guidance, experienced surgeons relied on their understanding of anatomy based on two-dimensional preoperative and intraoperative images, anatomical landmarks, and tactile feedback during surgery to ensure accurate and safe placement of instrumentation. Lack of proper anatomical landmarks, significant deformation, and poor intraoperative imaging can increase morbidity in spinal reconstructive procedures. Frameless stereotactic guidance appears to provide increased accuracy in placement of spinal instrumentation and thus should decrease the morbidity associated with these operations.

Several frameless stereotactic systems are currently available to the spine surgeon, including the VectorVision[2] Spine (BrainLAB USA, Redwood City, CA), the Optical Tracking System (Radionics, Burlington, MA), and StealthStation (Medtronic, Louisville, CO). At our institution, we have used the StealthStation for spinal applications. The chief components of the system include a computer workstation onto which the digital images of the spine are transferred either via optical disc or network interface. Once loaded onto the station, complex mathematical registration algorithms are performed to enable preoperative and intraoperative planning. Movement of the vertebral segment is tracked in real time with a dynamic reference arc and various customized spinal surgical instruments equipped with light emitting diodes (LEDs). The spatial position of the arc and instruments is tracked via an optical camera array (Figs. 25–1 and 25–2).[18]

The general steps required to use frameless spinal stereotaxis are relatively similar for all systems. Prior to surgery, a CT scan of the spinal levels of interest is obtained using a standard protocol. The scan is transferred to the computer workstation either via a network interface or optical media. The images are reformatted by the workstation into a 3-D reconstruction. Using this 3-D model, preoperative planning may be performed at the surgeon's convenience. Several different views are created: axial, sagittal, and coronal, as well as axial and orthogonal views in relation to probe trajectory. During the planning, various trajectories, screw diameters, and depths may be tested on the model, and relationships to soft tissues are identified (Fig. 25–3).

The next step is registration. Registration begins with the selection of fiducials on the image set. These must be precise points that will be easily identified intraoperatively. This is in contrast to the "mobile markers" that are affixed to the patient's scalp prior to scanning in cranial operations. The fiducials selected on the image set will be identified intraoperatively and mapped to the coordinate system of the image set. This process, known as paired-point registration, is the most common type of registration. A minimum of four points are necessary; however, increasing the number of points and the distance between the points will increase the registration accuracy.

In the operating room, the optical camera array is placed such that it will have an unobstructed view of the surgical field. The spine is exposed, taking care to preserve the bony landmarks yet exposing the anatomy sufficiently to identify the previously chosen fiducials. The first level of interest (vertebral segment) is identified, and the dynamic reference arc is rigidly fixed to the spinous process (Fig. 25–4). Every segment must be addressed individually because each level moves freely in relationship to the adjacent levels. The purpose of the arc is to track the motion of the individual segment as well as to track the instruments in a fixed relationship to that segment. At this point the fiducials are touched with a probe that is tracked by the optical array in relation to the dynamic reference arc. In doing so, the x, y, and z coordinates of each fiducial are computed. Via complex computer graphic algorithms, the spatial cross-registration of the separate coordinate systems completes the process of paired-point registration. At this time, any point on the image can be mapped to a corresponding point on the vertebral segment of interest. Improved accuracy can be obtained by supplementing paired-point registration with surface-point registration. This is achieved by touching multiple points (usually 30–40) on the exposed vertebral segment with the tracked wand, which allows a 3-D contour of the segment to be established. These surface points in the physical space are mapped to the surface of the image set. The combined paired-point and surface-point registrations allow for reduced registration error and improved accuracy. Obviously registration must take place prior to distortion of the segment anatomy. Once registration is complete, it is verified by touching several identifiable points on the

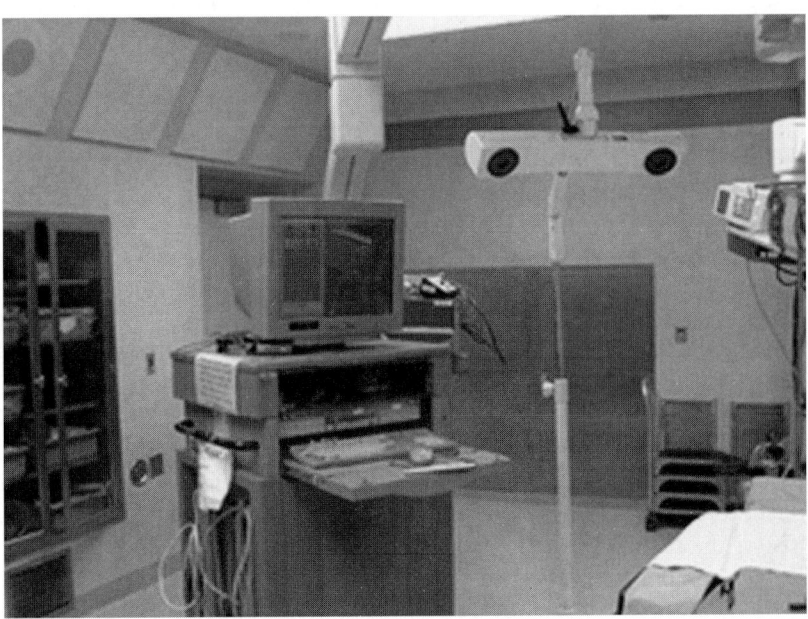

FIGURE 25–1. Computer workstation and optical camera array in the operating room. (StealthStation, Medtronic SNT, Louisville, CO)

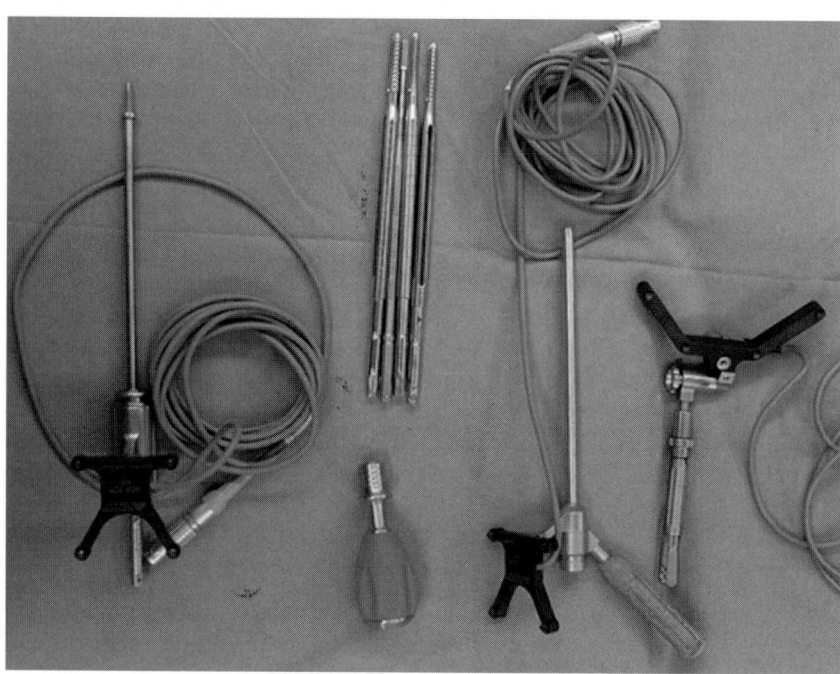

FIGURE 25–2. Various spinal instruments adapted for use with image-guided system.

segment, ensuring that these points correspond to the identical points displayed on the image set on the workstation. At this point, the spinal procedure is performed using the stereotaxic system and custom instruments.

In addition to standard application of frameless stereotactic image-guided surgery to the spine, a new technique has been developed using registration based on intraoperative fluoroscopy.[19] Digitized fluoroscopic images are obtained in the operating room utilizing a special registration grid. This technique allows the surgeon to view virtual lateral and anteroposterior views simultaneously during the procedure, thereby limiting the need for repeated exposure of the patient and surgeon to radiation.[20]

Several applications have been identified for frameless spinal stereotaxy. Pedicle screw placement in the cervical, thoracic, and lumbar spine under frameless guidance has been described.[9,21–23] These reports indicate improved accuracy and decreased morbidity as compared with conventional placement. Stereotactic guidance for C1–C2 transarticular screw placement has been demonstrated to be a useful adjunct.[13] In particular, the ability to plan the screw length, diameter, and trajectory relationship to adjacent critical structures (e.g., vertebral artery) has been reported to be of use.[10,17] Resection of spinal tumors is another potentially useful application for frameless stereotaxis. It may be particularly valuable when the normal landmarks are lost or distorted.[10]

The major controversies regarding image guidance involve accuracy, ease of use, and influence on operative time. Accuracy depends upon several factors: the inherent properties of the scan, marker selection, registration technique, and software algorithms. In regard to scan limitations, the spatial resolution of the image is limited by the slice thickness. The best accuracy that can be achieved is half the slice thickness; therefore, 1 mm acquisitions should be standard.[24] Increasing the number of fiducials and the distance between them will improve accuracy. Error is lowest when the target is in the center of the registered fiducials. Meticulous registration technique is required of the surgeon because inaccurate identification of the fiducials can lead to error. This last point is of greatest concern in the spinal application, given that registration relies on visual identification of landmarks on the exposed anatomy in contrast to the cranial application where fixed fiducials are placed on the patient prior to surgery.[25]

Registration error occurs when there is discrepancy between the virtual image space and the actual physical space. Ideally this would be an exact fit. The conventional indicator of accuracy, known as the mean fiducial error (MFE), describes how closely the points in the image space correlate with the points on the physical space. A low MFE indicates that the computer workstation calculates a close match between these sets; however, this does not give true application accuracy. All errors can be cumulative; thus, meticulous anatomic verification by the surgeon is absolutely necessary throughout the procedure.

Although more data are available on cranial applications and many of the same principles apply to image-

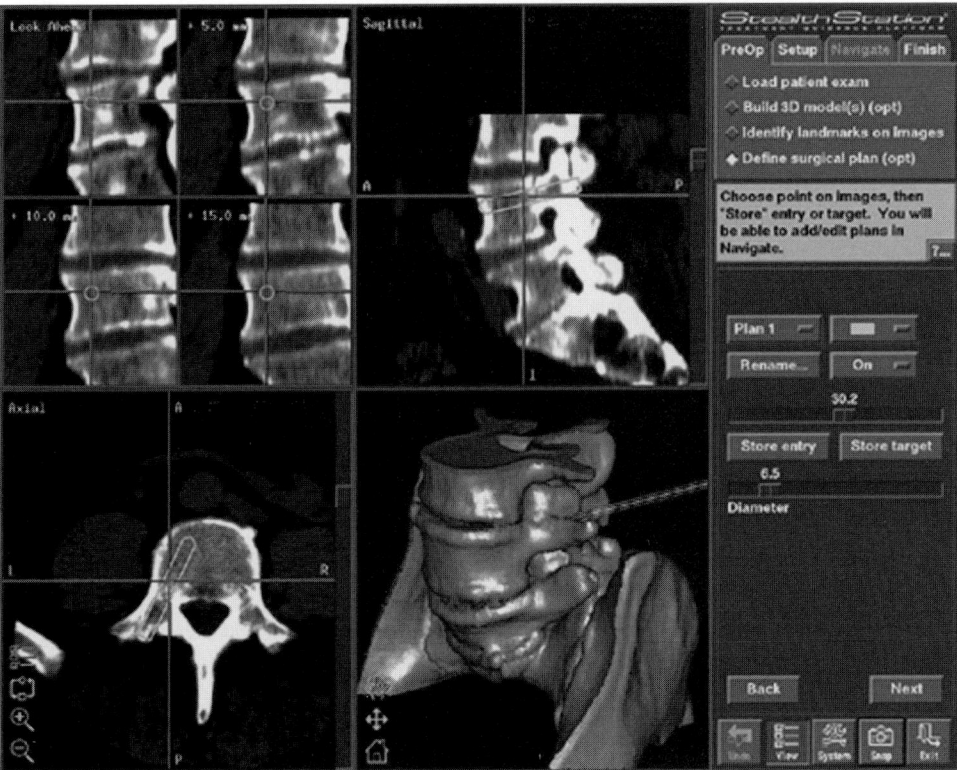

Figure 25–3. Snapshot from computer workstation screen demonstrating preoperative plan prior to placement of lumbar pedicle screws (StealthStation, Medtronic SNT, Louisville, CO).

guided spinal surgery, several key differences exist. The first is that fiducial markers are placed preoperatively and incorporated into the preoperative image set in the cranial application. In the spinal application, however, registration is carried out using intraoperative landmarks identified by the surgeon. A novel approach using internal fiducials has been described.[26] In addition, whereas the head remains in a fixed position in cranial procedures, the spine is a mobile structure with movement between individual segments and across multiple levels as compared with the preoperative scan due to patient positioning, intraoperative manipulations, and respiration. The resultant error is addressed by using the dynamic reference arc, which tracks intraoperative motion of the segment of interest. Because of this, only one vertebral level may be addressed at a time, with each level requiring a separate registration. This makes utilization of the systems in multilevel procedures cumbersome and time-consuming.

One key limitation of frameless image-guided surgery is the reliance on preoperative imaging. It has been demonstrated that significant changes can occur in anatomy intraoperatively that may change anatomical relationships. "Brain shift" during intracranial procedures is well described, and this phenomenon is associated with decreased accuracy. In the spinal application, specifically in instrumentation cases, this does not occur for any individual target (e.g., the vertebral body) because bone is rigid; however, the relationships of each vertebra to the remainder of the spine can be altered. This is particularly true with deformity correction. Frameless stereotaxis cannot adjust to such global changes.

Ease of use is another concern. Although each system strives to be user-friendly, these are highly technological computer applications that can be daunting for the novice user. Each system requires intensive training of the surgeon, the nursing staff, and support persons in the operative suite. In addition, the radiology staff must be trained on appropriate image acquisition and transfer protocols. Each application has unique functions that require patience to master.

The effect of image guidance on operative time is directly related to the surgeon's experience and comfort level with the application. Although we have found a significant learning curve with each new application, leading to increased time per case, there is a predictable reduction in operative times with continued

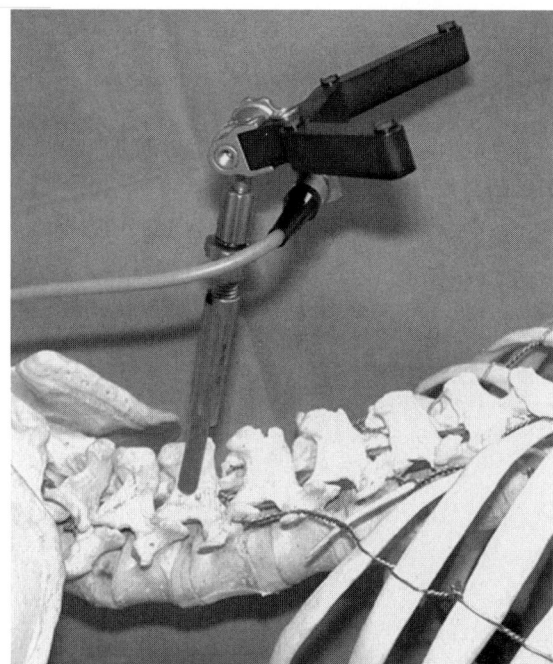

FIGURE 25–4. Demonstration of spinal reference arc rigidly fixed to lumbar spinous process.

use. Although it stands to reason that adding image guidance would increase operative time, this has not been the case when using image-guided techniques for selected cranial applications.[4,27] In one study, the actual "skin to skin" times were significantly shorter for patients who underwent image-guided surgical resection, although there was no significant difference in total operating room time.[4] One also needs to take into account the preoperative planning time that the surgeon must spend at the planning station prior to entering the operative suite.

Another important factor to consider is the cost-effectiveness of image guidance.[28] The average price for a fully operational image-guidance platform ranges between $250,000 and $950,000. In addition to the initial capital purchase, maintenance contacts and platform upgrades increase the overall expenditure. Although we are unaware of any published studies comparing the cost of traditional spinal surgical technique to image-guided technique, comparison of cranial techniques suggests that image guidance is cost effective.[4] It appears that in selected procedures, preoperative planning can reduce operating time and complication rates, thereby justifying the expense.

Finally, it should be stressed that traditional knowledge of the anatomic relationships of the spine must never be replaced by reliance on image-guidance technology. Although this may not be of concern for experienced spine surgeons who choose to add image guidance to their repertoire, it can become important for the spine surgeon in training.

REFERENCES

1. Kelly PJ. Stereotactic surgery: what is past is prologue. *Neurosurgery* 1986;46:16–27.
2. Eljamel MS. Frameless stereotactic neurosurgery: two steps towards the Holy Grail of surgical navigation. *Stereotact Funct Neurosurg* 1999;72:125–128.
3. Rohde V, Reinges MH, Krombach GA, Gilsbach JM. The combined use of image-guided frameless stereotaxy and neuroendoscopy for the surgical management of occlusive hydrocephalus and intracranial cysts. *Br J Neurosurg* 1998;12:531–538.
4. Paleologos TS, Wadley JP, Kitchen ND, Thomas DGT. Clinical utility and cost-effectiveness of interactive image-guided craniotomy: clinical comparison between conventional and image-guided meningioma surgery. *Neurosurgery* 2000;47:40–48.
5. Wadley J, Dorward N, Kitchen N, Thomas D. Pre-operative planning and intra-operative guidance in modern neurosurgery: a review of 300 cases. *Ann R Coll Surg Engl* 1999;81:217–225.
6. Bolger C, Wigfield C. Image-guided surgery: applications to the cervical and thoracic spine and a review of the first 120 procedures. *J Neurosurg* 2000;92(2 suppl):175–180.
7. Foley KT, Smith MM. Image-guided spine surgery. *Neurosurg Clin N Am* 1996;7:171–186.
8. Hurlbert RJ. Frameless stereotactic guidance for surgery of the upper cervical spine [letter]. *Neurosurgery* 1997;41:1448–1449.
9. Kalfas IH, Kormos DW, Murphy MA, et al. Application of frameless stereotaxy to pedicle screw fixation of the spine. *J Neurosurg* 1995;83:641–647.
10. Welch WC, Subach BR, Pollack IF, Jacobs GB. Frameless stereotactic guidance for surgery of the upper cervical spine. *Neurosurgery* 1997;40:958–964.
11. Pollack IF, Welch W, Jacobs GB, Janecka IP. Frameless stereotactic guidance: an intraoperative adjunct in the transoral approach for ventral cervicomedullary junction decompression. *Spine* 1995;20:216–220.
12. Girardi FP, Cammisa FP Jr, Sandhu HS, Alvarez L. The placement of lumbar pedicle screws using computerised stereotactic guidance. *J Bone Joint Surg* 1999;81B:825–829.
13. Weidner A, Wahler M, Chiu ST, Ullrich CG. Modification of C1–C2 transarticular screw fixation by image-guided surgery. *Spine* 2000;25:2668–2674.
14. Dickman CA. Modification of C1-C2 transarticular screw fixation by image-guided surgery [point of view]. *Spine* 2000;25:2674.
15. Albert TJ, Klein GR, Vaccaro AR. Image-guided anterior cervical corpectomy: a feasibility study. *Spine* 1999;24:826–830.
16. Nolte L-P, Zamorano LJ, Jiang Z, Wang Q, Langlotz F, Berlemann U. Image-guided insertion of transpedicular screws: a laboratory setup. *Spine* 1995;20:497–500.
17. Berlemann U, Monin D, Arm E, Nolte L-P, Ozdoba C. Planning and insertion of pedicle screws with computer assistance. *J Spinal Disord* 1997;10:117–124.
18. Klein GR, Ludwig SC, Vaccaro AR, Rushton SA, Lazar RD, Albert TJ. The efficacy of using an image-guided Kerrison punch in performing an anterior cervical foraminotomy: an anatomic analysis. *Spine* 1999;24:1358–1362.
19. Foley KT, Simon DA, Rampersaud YR. Virtual fluoroscopy: computer-assisted fluoroscopic navigation. *Spine* 2001;26:347–351.
20. Slomczykowski M, Roberto M, Schneeberger P, Ozdoba C, Vock P. Radiation dose for pedicle screw insertion: fluoroscopic method versus computer-assisted surgery. *Spine* 1999;24:975–983.

21. Cammisa FP Jr, Parvataneni HK, Girardi FP, Khan SN, Sandhu HS. Computerized frameless stereotactic image-guided spinal surgery [review]. *Bull Hosp Joint Dis* 2000;59:17–26.
22. Choi WW, Green BA, Levi ADO. Computer-assisted fluoroscopic targeting system for pedicle screw insertion. *Neurosurgery* 2000;47:872–878.
23. Kim KD, Johnson JP, Masciopinto JE, Bloch O, Saracen MJ, Villablanca JP. Universal calibration of surgical instruments for spinal stereotaxy. *Neurosurgery* 1999;44:173–178.
24. Schulder M, Fontana P, Lavenhar MA, Carmel PW. The relationship of imaging techniques to the accuracy of frameless stereotaxy. *Stereotact Funct Neurosurg* 1999;72:136–141.
25. Rampersaud YR, Simon DA, Foley KT. Accuracy requirements for image-guided spinal pedicle screw placement. *Spine* 2001;26:352–359.
26. Salehi SA, Ondra SL. Use of internal fiducial markers in frameless stereotactic navigational systems during spinal surgery: technical note. *Neurosurgery* 2000;47:1460–1462.
27. Alberti O, Dorward NL, Kitchen ND, Thomas DG. Neuronavigation: impact on operating time. *Stereotact Funct Neurosurg* 1997;68:44–48.
28. Jolesz FA, Kettenbach J, Grundfest WS. Cost-effectiveness of image-guided surgery. *Acad Radiol* 1998;5(suppl 2):S428–S431.

Index

Note: Page numbers followed by f or t indicate figures and tables respectively.

AccuPoint sphere, 75, 75f
Acoustic neuroma, neuroendoscopy for, 92–93
Adjuvant therapy, after brain tumor resection, 139
Amygdalohippocampectomy, selective, in epilepsy surgery, 157
Aneurysms. *See also* Intracranial aneurysms
    frameless stereotactic surgery for, 66–67, 66f
    neuroendoscopy for, 93, 94f, 95f
Angiomas, cavernous, frameless stereotactic surgery for, 66–67
Arachnoid cysts, neuroendoscopy for, 90–91
    middle fossa, 90–91
    posterior fossa, 91
    suprasellar, 91
Arteriovenous malformations, frameless stereotactic surgery for, 66
Articulated arm, intraoperative use of, 7
    in cervical spine surgery, 178, 179f
Artifacts, 15
Atlantoaxial transarticular screw fixation, virtual fluoroscopy for, 212–213
Atlas-assisted stereotactic functional neurosurgery, 162–173
    brain atlas applications in
        Cerefy atlas, 165–166, 167f, 168f
        in commercial systems, 166–168, 169f–171f
        electronic brain atlas database for, 162, 163f, 164f
        Internet portal for, 171–173
        probabilistic functional atlas in, 169–171, 172f
Atlas-enhanced targeting, 168f
AtlasPlan module, 168, 171f

Beam hardening artifacts, 15
Biopsies
    of brain. *See* Brain biopsy
    frameless navigation for, 52

Bipolar suction-coagulator, for resection in exoscope procedure, 86f
Bone-implanted fiducial markers, 20f, 25–26, 27
Brain atlas, stereotactic. *See* Stereotactic brain atlas
Brain Atlas Geometrical Models library, 166
Brain biopsy
    image-guided stereotactic, 116–119
        frame, 116–117, 117f
        frameless, 117–118, 118f
        freehand, 116
        intraoperative MRI in, 118, 119f
    needle biopsy
        frameless image-guided surgery for, 132–133
        for malignant gliomas, 133
        PET and MR spectroscopy for, 133
Brain deformation, intraoperative, 30, 32–34, 33f
    factors inducing, 30, 32–33
Brain shift
    and intraoperative MRI updating, 151–152, 152f
    mechanical arm system and, 58
    during tumor resection, 135–137
        strategies to minimize, 137t
Brain tumor, resection of. *See* Tumor resection, brain tumor
BrainLAB VectorVision neuronavigation system
    components of, 68, 68f
    fiducial placement for, 68–69
    image acquisition by, 69–70, 69f
    intraoperative three-dimensional guidance and, 71–72
    operating room positioning and setup for, 70–71
        patient draping, 71
        pointer, 71
        reference frame instrumentation, 70, 71f
        registration, 71

patients and, 72
surgical planning and, 70
Brown-Roberts-Wells stereotactic localizer, 5
in brain biopsy, 116, 117f

Calculated accuracy, in image guidance, 62, 64f
Callosotomy, in computer-assisted image-guided epilepsy surgery, 157
Carcinoma, metastatic, in sacral spine, 202, 203f
Carotid angiogram, 127, 128f
Carotid bypass vein graft, preoperative evaluation of postoperative patency in, 127, 129f
Cartesian coordinate system, 5, 39
CASS system, 167
Catheter cerebral angiography, pretreatment evaluation for intracranial aneurysms, 121
Catheter placement, frameless stereotaxis for, 67
Cavernous angiomas, frameless stereotactic surgery for, 66
Cavernous malformation, preoperative evaluation for intraoperative navigation in, 127, 130f
CCD camera. *See* Charge-couple device camera
Cerebrospinal fluid, brain deformation and, 31, 32
Cervical instrumentation, image-guided, 176–181
  clinical experience with, 179–180
  indications for, 177, 177t
  technique with, 177–179, 178f–180f
Cervical spine disorders, surgical treatment of, 176–181
  clinical experience in, 179–180
  indications for image guidance in, 177, 177t
  technique of, 177–179, 178f–180f
Charge-couple device camera
  in image-guided brain biopsy, 117
  in radiosurgery system, 108
Chronic subdural monitoring grids, in epilepsy surgery, 159, 159f, 160f
Colloid cysts, neuroendoscopy for, 88–90, 89f
Color Doppler ultrasonography, arterial, 143, 145f
Commercial stereotactic functional neurosurgery systems
  StealthStation. *See* StealthStation
  StereoPlan 2.1, 168, 171f
  Stryker Navigation System Neuro, 167–168, 170f
COMPASS system, 167
Computed tomographic angiography, for intracranial aneurysm pretreatment evaluation, 121
Computed tomography
  versus fluoroscopy, 207–208, 209t
  geometrical distortion in, 15
  image correlation with MRI, 61, 63, 63f
  image fusion with, 11–12, 13f
  image registration with, 11, 11f, 12
    image-to-physical, 12, 14f
  image volume, 15
  intensity-based registration in, 29–30, 31f–32f
  intraoperative image updating with, versus MRI image updating, 153
  intraoperative use of, 4
  in lumbar spine stereotaxy, 198
  postoperative, image-guided cervical instrumentation and, 179f, 180f
  in spinal surface mapping registration, 41, 42f

surgical planning and, 54
Computer-assisted image-guided epilepsy surgery, 156–160
  callosotomy in, 157
  depth electrode placement in, 157, 158f
  lesional, 156–157
  multimodality imaging and, 158–160, 159f, 160f
  radiosurgery, 157–158
  selective amygdalohippocampectomy, 157
Computer-assisted image-guided fluoroscopy. *See* Virtual fluoroscopy
Computer-assisted stereotaxis, 4
Computer workstation. *See* Workstation
Cortical violations, in thoracic pedicle screw placement, 183, 185, 186t, 187f, 188f
Cosman-Robert-Wells stereotactic frame, 5
  in exoscope procedure, 82, 82f, 83–84
Craniocervical junction, virtual fluoroscopy for transoral decompression of, 215
Craniotomy
  exoscope procedure in, 84
  minimally invasive, and open tumor resection, 133–135, 134f–137f
CRW frame. *See* Cosman-Robert-Wells stereotactic frame
CT. *See* Computed tomography
Cyberknife (robotic radiosurgery system), 108–109, 108f
  accuracy of dose placement with, 110
  for intracranial lesions, 111
  for spinal lesions, 111–112, 111f, 112f
  target localization with, 109
  treatment with
    methodology using, 109–110
    planning for, 110–111
Cygnus-PFS image-guidance system
  advantages of, 60–61
  applications of, 63–64
  data acquisition by, 61
  features of, 61, 61f, 62f
  image display on, 62, 65f
  registration readout on, 62, 64f
  setup of, 60–61, 61f
Cysts, neuroendoscopy for
  arachnoid, 90–91
  colloid, 88–90, 90f

Data display, intraoperative, in brain tumor resection, 139
Data transfer, in image-guided neurosurgery, 47–49
Decompression, transoral, of craniocervical junction, 215
Degree-of-freedom transformation, in image registration, 19
Depth electrode placement, in computer-assisted image-guided epilepsy surgery, 157, 158f
Descartes, René, 5, 39
DOF (degree-of-freedom) transformation, in image registration, 19
Dose placement, accuracy with Cyberknife radiosurgical system, 110
DRF (dynamic reference frame), 198, 199f

Ear, magnetic system and, 67
Electrocorticography, intraoperative, in lesional epilepsy surgery, 156–157

Electrodes, in computer-assisted image-guided epilepsy surgery
   chronic subdural monitoring grids, 159, 159f, 160f
   placement of, 157
Electronic brain atlas database, 162–163, 163f–165f
Electronic Brain Atlas Library, 166
The Electronic Clinical Brain Atlas, 165
Enchondroma, sacral spine, 202, 203f
Endoscopy, in image-guided surgery, 87–95. *See also* Neuroendoscopy
   intraoperative use of, 4
Entropy, information theory and, 29, 30f
Epilepsy surgery
   computer-assisted image-guided, 156–160
      callosotomy, 157
      depth electrode placement in, 157, 158f
      in lesional epilepsy, 156–157
      multimodality imaging and, 158–160, 159f, 160f
      radiosurgery, 157–158
      selective amygdalohippocampectomy, 157
   frameless stereotaxis for, 67
   image-guided neurosurgery and, 52
   intraoperative MRI in, 147
   mechanical arm system in, 57f, 58f
   SPECT in, 57, 58f
Erlangen concept, 146
Error
   fiducial localization, 21, 21f
   in image registration. *See* Registration error
   mean fiducial, 220
   in point-based registration, 19–26
      theory, 34
      types, 21, 21f
   scaling, in MR images, 19
Exoscope procedure, in videotactic surgery, 83–84, 85f, 86f
   equipment for, 82, 82f
   incorporation into StealthStation, 84–86
   modules in, 84
   planning for, 83
   scanning and, 83–84

Feedback, intraoperative real-time, in neuronavigation, 50
Fiducial localization error, 21, 21f
Fiducial markers
   bone-implanted, 20f, 25–26, 27
   effect of configuration on TRE distribution, 22, 23f–25f
   optical digitizer and, 48–49
   placement guidelines, 22
      for passive navigation system, 68–69
   in point-based registration, 20–21, 20f, 25, 26
      errors associated with, 21, 21f
   skin-affixed, 20, 20f, 24, 27
Fiducial registration error, 21, 21f
   available feedback on, 24–25
   mean, 220
Flair attenuated inversion recovery MRI, in lesional epilepsy surgery, 156–157
FluoroNav virtual fluoroscopy system, 209f
Fluoroscopy
   CT-based systems versus, 207–208, 209t
   intraoperative, in spinal surgery, 220
   virtual. *See* Virtual fluoroscopy
fMRI (functional magnetic resonance imaging), surgical planning and, 54
Fourth ventricular tumors, neuroendoscopy for, 92
Frame-based stereotaxis
   in endoscopic surgery, 93, 95
   equipment and imaging modalities for, 4
   frameless image-guidance versus, 5
      for needle biopsy, 132–133
   versus image-guided neurosurgery, 45
   limitations of, overcoming, 6
Frameless image-guided surgery
   for brain needle biopsy, 132–133
   magnetic field generator for. *See* Magnetic system, for frameless image-guided surgery
   methods of, 60
   nonmicroscope-based tool for, 7
   stereotactic, 220
      accuracy of, 142
      cranial applications of, 218
      intraoperative fluoroscopy with, 220
      limitations of, 221
Frameless stereotaxis, 73, 218
   concept of, 73, 74–76
   in endoscopic surgery, 95
   Mayfield ACCISS system, 73–78. *See also* Mayfield ACCISS system
   mechanical arm system, 54–59. *See also* Mechanical arm system
   spinal, steps in, 219
   system components in, 76
"Free-form" surface matching problem, 27
Frequency encoding, and geometrical distortion in MRI, 16
   minimizing problem of, 17
Functional magnetic resonance imaging, surgical planning and, 54
Functional neurosurgery, atlas-based stereotactic. *See* Atlas-assisted stereotactic functional neurosurgery
Fusion
   image, 11–12, 13f, 21
   interbody, in postoperative lumbar spine, 211–212

Gamma knife radiosurgery, 107
Gene therapy, after brain tumor resection, 139
Geometrical distortion, in preoperative images, 15–19
   CT images, 15
   methods for correcting, 17
   MRI images, 15–19, 18f
   scaling error, 19
Glioblastoma, right frontal, and intraoperative MRI, 150, 150f
Glioma
   brain needle biopsy for, 133
   surgery for, intraoperative MRI in, 148–151, 150f
Global shimming, in MRI, 17
Gradient-pulse echo sequence, in MRI, 17

Heads-up display, in Zeiss MKM system, 99–100
Helical CT image acquisition, 15
Hemivertebrae abnormality, 191, 192f

High field magnetic resonance systems, for intraoperative imaging, 153
Hydrocephalus, neuroendoscopy in, 87–88
    multiloculated, 87–88
    for shunt placement, 87
    for third ventriculostomy, 88, 89f
Hydrogen protons, in MRI, 15, 17

ICP (intracranial pressure), brain deformation and, 31, 32
IGS. *See* Image-guided surgery
IIR. *See* Image-to-image registration
Image
    correlation of MRI with CT, 61, 63f
    intensity histograms, 29, 30f
    intraoperative updating of. *See* Intraoperative image updating
    registration. *See* Registration
    voxel values of, and intensity-based registration, 28
Image acquisition
    optical digitizer and, 48
    and surgical planning, 76–77, 76f
    with Z-touch registration instrument, 69, 69f
Image fusion, 11–12, 13f, 21
Image guidance
    accuracy in, 62–63, 64f, 66f
    for brain biopsy. *See* Brain biopsy, image-guided stereotactic
    for scoliosis, 191–196. *See also* Scoliosis
    in spinal surgery, 37. *See also* Spinal surgery
    workstations and. *See* Workstation
Image-guided surgery, 10. *See also* Information-guided therapy; *specific surgeries*
    for biopsy. *See* Brain biopsy, image-guided stereotactic
    cerebrovascular applications of, 121–130. *See also* Intracranial aneurysms
    defined, 3
    endoscopic. *See* Neuroendoscopy
    frameless. *See* Frameless image-guided surgery; Magnetic system, for frameless image-guided surgery
    historical perspective on, 2–8
    spinal
        cervical spine, 176–181. *See also* Cervical instrumentation, image-guided
        lumbar spine, 197–206. *See also* Lumbar instrumentation
    stereotactic, 10
Image-to-image registration, 10
    point-based, 20
    surface-based, 26, 27f, 28
Image-to-physical registration, 10, 12, 14f, 21
    point-based, 20
    surface-based, 26, 27f, 28
Imaging protocols, for robotic microscopes, 100
Information acquisition, periprocedural, 3–4
Information-guided therapy
    defined, 3
    future of, 7–8
    intraprocedural tracking in, 5–7
    periprocedural information acquisition for, 3–4
    telesurgery with, 8, 8f
Information registration, 4–5
Information theory, entropy and, 29, 30f

Infratentorial lesions, frameless stereotactic surgery for, 65–66
Intensity, definition, 28
Intensity-based registration
    algorithms for, 29
    error in, 28–30
Interbody fusion, posterior lumbar spine, 211–212
Interference, surgical light, in image-guided neurosurgery, 52
Internet portal, for stereotactic functional neurosurgery, 171–173
    combined PFA and/or datasets, 173
    data loading and editing, 172–173
    parameter setting, 173
    PFA display and, 172f, 173
Intracranial aneurysms, pretreatment evaluation of, 121–127
    and intraoperative navigation for cavernous malformation, 127, 130f
    middle cerebral artery, 122, 124f
    paraclinoid, 122, 125, 125f, 126f, 127, 128f
    posterior communicating artery, 121–122, 123f
    for postoperative patency in carotid bypass vein graft, 127, 129f
Intracranial lesions, Cyberknife radiosurgery for, 111
Intracranial pressure, brain deformation and, 31, 32
Intraoperative image updating
    during brain tumor resection, 136–137
    by high-field magnetic resonance, 153
    by MRI, 146–153
        and brain shift, 151–152, 152f
        in glioma surgery, 148–151, 150f
        operating room setup for, 147–148, 147f
        in transsphenoidal surgery, 148, 149f
    by other modalities, 152–153
    by ultrasound, 141–145
        color Doppler, 143, 145f
        neuronavigation systems and, 141–142
        sononavigation systems and, 142–144, 142f–145f
Intraoperative period
    brain deformation in, 30–34
    localization methods in
        for accurate pedicle screw placement, 197–198
        articulate arm for, 7
    navigation during
        for brain tumor resection, 137f
        lumbar instrumentation and, 201–202, 201f
    real-time feedback and navigation in, 51f
    3-D guidance during, 71–72
    tracking system in, 5–7, 5f, 7f
Intraventricular tumors, neuroendoscopy for, 91–92
    fourth ventricle, 92
    lateral ventricle, 91
    third ventricle, 91–92

Joint probability distribution functions, 29, 30f

Kyphotic abnormality, surgical correction of, 196f

Lateral ventricular tumors, neuroendoscopy for, 91
LEDs. *See* Light-emitting diodes
Leksell system, 5

Lesional epilepsy, computer-assisted image-guided surgery for, 156–157
Light detector array, in navigation system, 45, 46, 46f
Light-emitting diodes
  neuronavigation systems and, 142
  and optical digitizers, 46, 73
  in optical tracking systems, 198, 199f
  for reference frame, 46
    positioning and registration of, 46f, 50, 51f
    in spinal surgery, 38–39, 39f
    in scoliosis surgery, 194–195
Light interference, in image-guided neurosurgery, 52
LINACs (linear accelerators), 107, 108–110, 108f
Line-of-sight problems, in image-guided neurosurgery, 52
Lumbar instrumentation, image-guided, 197–206
  anatomical considerations in, 198
  CT frameless stereotaxy for, 198
  intraoperative navigation and, 201–202, 201f
  for lumbar and sacral spine procedures, 202, 203f
  optical tracking components in, 198, 199f–201f, 201
  preoperative planning in, 198
  surgical exposure and registration for, 200f, 201
  traditional localization methods in, 197–198
  virtual fluoroscopic, 202–205
Lumbar spine
  surgery for. *See* Lumbar instrumentation, image-guided
  virtual fluoroscopic view of, 210f

Magnetic field referencing, of stereotactic space
  applications and setup of, 60–61, 61f, 62f, 63f
  features of, 61–62, 63f, 64f, 65f
Magnetic resonance angiography, for intracranial aneurysm pretreatment evaluation, 121
Magnetic resonance imaging
  in brain tumor resection, 133, 134f–136f, 137, 138f
  cervical spine compression due to pseudoarthrosis, 177, 178f
  coronal, of colloid cysts, 90f
  geometrical distortion in, 15–19, 18f
  image correlation with CT, 61, 63, 63f
  image fusion with, 11–12, 13f
  image registration with, 11, 11f, 12
    image-to-physical, 12, 14f
  intensity-based registration in, 29–30, 31f–32f
  for intracranial aneurysm pretreatment evaluation, 121
  intraoperative image updating by, 4, 146–153
    during brain biopsy, 118, 119f
    and brain shift, 151–152, 152f
    in glioma surgery, 148–151, 150f
    high-field MR, 153
    operating room setup for, 147–148, 147f
    in transsphenoidal surgery, 148, 149f
    versus other imaging modalities, 148
  surgical planning and, 54
Magnetic resonance spectroscopy, and PET, for brain needle biopsy, 133
Magnetic system, for frameless image-guided surgery, 60–67
  accuracy in, 62–63
  applications of, 63–64
  catheter placement and, 67
  comparison with optic systems, 63
  Cygnus-PFS image-guidance. *See* Cygnus-PFS image-guidance system
  epilepsy surgery and, 67
  neurosurgery and, 64–67
  ophthalmology and, 67
  of sphenoid and maxillary sinuses, 67
  stereotactic space and, 60–62
  of tumors, 64–66
  of vascular system, 66–67
Magnetization, spatial modulation of, 17, 19
Magnetoencephalographs
  mechanical arm system combined with, 55, 56f, 57f
    in monoparesis of right hand, 57, 57f
    in right parietal tumor, 56–57, 56f
  surgical planning and, 54
Mayfield ACCISS system, 75–76, 75f, 76f
  AccuPoint sphere in, 75, 75f
  applications for, 74
  clinical experience with, 73–78
  development of, 73–74
  frameless stereotaxis concept and, 73, 74–76
  image acquisition and surgical planning in, 76–77, 76f
  postoperative image sequence in, evaluation of, 77–78, 77f, 78
  stereotactic components of, 76
  stereotactic experience with, 78
  workstation in, 75–76, 75f, 76f
Mayfield clamp, in passive navigation system, 70, 71f
Mechanical arm system, 54–58, 55f
  applications in neurosurgery, 55–56
  brain shift and, 58
  clinical experience with, 56–57
    in epileptic patient, 57, 58f
    in monoparesis of right hand, 57, 57f
    in right parietal tumor, 56–57, 56f
  magnetoencephalographs combined with, 55, 56f, 57f
  navigation method with, 54–55
  near infrared spectroscopic topography combined with, 55–56
  and optical digitizer combined. *See* Mayfield ACCISS system
  virtual tip in, 55, 55f
MEGs. *See* Magnetoencephalographs
Mesial temporal lobe epilepsy, radiosurgery for, 158
Metastatic carcinoma, sacral spine, 202, 203f
MFE (mean fiducial error), 220
Microscope
  operating, 6
  robotic, 98–105. *See also* Robotic microscopes
Middle cerebral artery aneurysm, pretreatment evaluation of, 122, 124f
Middle fossa arachnoid cysts, neuroendoscopy for, 90–91
Minimally invasive crainiectomy, 133–135, 134f–136f
MKM (multicoordinate manipulator) robotic microscope. *See* Zeiss MKM system
Monoparesis, of right hand, clinical experience with, 57, 57f
MRA (magnetic resonance angiography), for intracranial aneurysm pretreatment evaluation, 121
MRI. *See* Magnetic resonance imaging

MRS (magnetic resonance spectroscopy), and PET, for brain needle biopsy, 133
MTLE (mesial temporal lobe epilepsy), radiosurgery for, 158
Multicoordinate manipulator robotic microscope. *See* Zeiss MKM system
Multimodality imaging, in epilepsy surgery, 158–160, 159f, 160f
Mussen's stereotactic frame, 5, 6f

Navigation
   intracranial, optical digitizer for. *See* Neuronavigation; Optical digitizer
   intraoperative
      for brain tumor resection, 137f, 139
      lumbar instrumentation and, 201–202
   in spinal surgery
      principles, 41, 43
      technique, 38–39, 38f, 39f
   stereotactic
      for pedicle screw placement in thoracic spine. *See* Thoracic instrumentation, for pedicle screw placement
      robotic microscopes and, 104–105
   systems for. *See specific systems*
   passive. *See* Passive navigational system
Navigus guidance device, in intraoperative magnetic resonance imaging, 119f
Near infrared spectroscopic topography
   mechanical arm system combined with, 55–56
      in epileptic patient, 57, 58f
   surgical planning and, 54
Neuroendoscopy, 87–95
   for acoustic neuroma, 92–93
   for aneurysm, 93, 95f
   for arachnoid cysts, 90–91
   for colloid cysts, 88–90, 90f
   for hydrocephalus, 87–88
   for intraventricular lesions, 91–92
   stereotactic techniques in
      frame-based, 93, 95
      frameless, 95
   for transsphenoidal surgery, 92
Neuroma, acoustic, neuroendoscopy for, 92–93
Neuronavigation. *See also specific systems*
   advances in. *See* Virtual fluoroscopy
   clinical applications of, 50–52
   first adjustable device for, 6
   intraoperative
      for image updating, 141–142
      real-time feedback in, 50
   mechanical. *See* Mechanical arm system
   passive system for, 68–72. *See also* BrainLAB VectorVision neuronavigation system
   procedure for, 47
   robotic microscopes and, 100
   system development in, 141
"Neuronavigator." *See* Mechanical arm system
Neuroplanner atlas, 166
   user interface of, 167f, 168f

Neurosurgery
   image-guided
      benefits and limitations of, 52
      clinical applications of, 50–52
      in epilepsy, 52
      versus frame-based stereotaxy, 45
      magnetic system and, 60–67
      optical digitizer for. *See* Optical digitizer
      planning for, 49, 49f
      preoperative imaging and data transfer in, 47–49
   image registration error in, 10–34
   intraoperative ultrasound image updating in, 141–145
   magnetic system and, 64–66
   mechanical arm system applications in, 55–56
   orientation in, 54
   skin-affixed fiducial markers in, 20, 20f, 24
   stereotactic frameless, cranial applications of, 218
   stereotactic functional, atlas-assisted. *See* Atlas-assisted stereotactic functional neurosurgery
NIRS (near infrared spectroscopic) topography, mechanical arm system combined with, 55–56
Nose, magnetic system and, 67

Object-induced static field inhomogeneity, 16–17, 18f
Odontoid screw insertion, virtual fluoroscopy for, 213–215, 214f
Open lumbar pedicle screw placement, 211f
Open resection, of brain tumor, minimally invasive craniotomy and, 133–135, 134f–136f
Operating microscope, 6
Operating room setup
   for image-guided cervical surgery, 178, 179f
   for intraoperative magnetic resonance imaging, 147–148, 147f
   passive navigational system in, 68–72. *See also* BrainLAB VectorVision neuronavigation system
   for scoliosis surgery, 192–193, 193f
   for stereotactic spinal surgery, 219, 219f
Ophthalmology, frameless stereotaxis in, 67
Optical digitizer, 45–46
   clinical applications of frameless navigation, 51f
   development of, 73–74
   history of, for image-guided surgery, 73
   image-guided neurosurgery using, benefits and limitations, 52
   for intracranial navigation, 45–53
      clinical applications, 50–52
   mechanical arm combined with. *See* Mayfield ACCISS system
   navigation systems utilizing, 45–46, 46f
   workstation for, 45, 46f
      early version, 7, 7f
      examples of, 47, 47f, 48f
      image processing by, 47, 47f
Optical Tracking System
   in image-guided lumbar instrumentation, 198, 199f–201f, 201
   in spinal surgery, 218–219
Orientation, in intracranial surgery, 54
Oula neuronavigator system, 143

Paired point registration plan, in spinal surgery, 40, 40f
Paraclinoid aneurysm, pretreatment evaluation of, 122, 125, 125f, 126f, 127, 128f
Parietal tumor, clinical experience with, 56–57, 56f
Passive navigational system, 68–72. *See also* BrainLAB VectorVision neuronavigation system
Patient
   and passive navigational system, 72
      draping of, 71
   positioning, image guidance for scoliosis surgery and, 192–193, 193f
   robotic microscopes and, 101–102
Patient space, virtual versus actual, 198
Pedicle screw placement
   lumbar spine
      instrumentation for, 197–206
         open technique, 211f
      in scoliosis surgery, 191, 195, 196f
   thoracic spine, instrumentation for. *See* Thoracic instrumentation, for pedicle screw placement
   virtual fluoroscopy for, 210–211
      conventional, 210–211, 211f
      percutaneous, 211
Percutaneous pedicle screw insertion, virtual fluoroscopy for, 211, 212f
PET. *See* Positron emission tomography
Phantom (test) object, scaling error and, 19
Phase encoding, 16
Pituitary adenoma, and intraoperative magnetic resonance imaging, 149, 149f
Pituitary surgery. *See* Transsphenoidal surgery
Point-based registration
   error in, 19–26
      theory, 34
      types, 21, 21f
   fiducial markers for
      bone-implanted, 20, 20f, 25–26, 27
      skin-affixed, 20, 20f, 24, 27
   lumbar instrumentation and, 200f, 201
   surface-based registration versus, 27
Point-in-space targeting, in videotactic surgery, 80–81
Pointer, freehand, for passive navigational system, 71
Positron emission tomography
   in epilepsy surgery, 52
   intensity-based registration in, 29–30
   and MR spectroscopy, for brain needle biopsy, 133
Posterior communicating artery aneurysm, pretreatment evaluation of, 121–122, 123f
Posterior fossa cysts, neuroendoscopy for, 91
Posterior lumbar interbody fusion, virtual fluoroscopy and, 211–212, 213f
Preoperative images
   and data transfer, in neurosurgery, 48–49
   geometrical distortion in, 15–19
Probabilistic functional atlas, 162, 169–171, 172f
   datasets combined with, 173
   display of, 172f, 173
   reconstructed, 172f
   for subthalamic nucleus, 172f
Probability distribution functions, joint, 29, 30f

Probe
   in Cygnus-PFS system, 62
   navigational, with drill guide, in spinal surgery, 38, 38f

Radiography, versus CT and MRI for accurate pedicle screw placement, 200f
Radiosurgery
   computer-assisted image-guided epilepsy surgery and, 157–158
   robotic. *See* Robotic radiosurgery
Radiosurgery systems
   constraints of, 107–108
   defined, 107
   robotic. *See* Cyberknife (robotic radiosurgery system)
   schematic of, 108f
Reconstruction, three-dimensional, of cervical spine, 178, 178f
Reference frame
   dynamic, 198, 199f
   in navigational system, 45, 46, 46f
      passive, 70, 71f
   in spinal surgery, 39, 39f
Registration, 11–14
   accuracy in. *See* Registration accuracy
   for brain tumor resection, 137f, 139
   in brain tumor resection, 137f, 139
   concept of, 11, 11f
   for cranial image-guided neurosurgery, error in, 10–34
   definition of, 10
   degree-of freedom transformation in, 19
   error in. *See* Registration error
   in frameless spinal stereotaxy, 219
   for image-guided lumbar instrumentation, 200f, 201
   image-to-image. *See* Image-to-image registration
   image-to-physical. *See* Image-to-physical registration
   passive navigational system and, 71
   readout from Cygnus-PFS image-guidance system, 62, 64f
   robotic microscopes and, 101, 102f
   in scoliosis surgery, 193–194, 194f, 195f
   in spinal surgery. *See* Spinal registration
   universal instrument, 198, 199f–201f, 201
Registration accuracy, 30, 31f–32f
   and intraoperative updating with ultrasound, 143, 143f
   mechanical arm combined with optical digitizer, 76, 76f
   in spinal surgery, 39–40, 219
   verification of, 41, 42f
   visual assessment of, 30, 31f–32f
Registration error, 19–30
   geometrical distortions effects on, 17, 18f
   in intensity-based registration, 28–30
   in point-based registration, 19–26
   in spinal surgery, 39–40, 219
   in surface-based registration, 26–28
   target and. *See* Target registration error
Robot, defined, 98
Robotic microscopes, 98–105
   accuracy of, 102–103
   advantages and disadvantages of, 104–105
   clinical utility of, 103–104
   imaging protocols for, 100

neuronavigation procedure with, 100
patient setup with, 101–102, 101f, 102f
technical features of, 98–100, 99f
Robotic radiosurgery, 107–113, 108f
accuracy of dose placement, 110
for intracranial lesions, 111
for spinal lesions, 111–112, 111f, 112f
target localization in, 109
treatment with
methodology for, 109–110
planning for, 110–111
Rotational three-dimensional catheter angiography (3-DA), pretreatment evaluation for intracranial aneurysms, 121

Sacral spine procedures, 202, 203f
Scaling error, in MR images, 19
Scanning, in exoscope procedure, 83
Schaltebrand-Wahren brain atlas, 163f
3-D version of, 163, 165f
Scoliosis surgery, image guidance in, 191–196
for kyphotic abnormality correction, 196f
lumbar spine views, 192f
operating room setup for, 192–193, 193f
patient positioning for, 192–193, 193f
preoperative planning for, 192
registration for, 193–194, 194f, 195f
tracking in, 194
Screw fixation
atlantoaxial transarticular, virtual fluoroscopy for, 212–213
odontoid, virtual fluoroscopy for, 213–215
pedicle. See Pedicle screw placement
Selective amygdalohippocampectomy, in computer-assisted image-guided epilepsy surgery, 157
Shimming, global, in MRI, 17
Shunt placement, in hydrocephalus, neuroendoscopy for, 87
Single photon emission computed tomography, in epilepsy surgery, 52, 57, 58f
Skin-affixed fiducial markers, 20, 20f, 24, 27
Skull base lesions, frameless stereotactic surgery for, 66
Sononavigation systems, for intraoperative image updating, 142–143, 142f–145f
SPAMM (spatial modulation of magnetization), 17, 19
Spatial encoding methods, 15–16
Spatial modulation of magnetization, 17, 19
Spatial position, encoding of, 16
SPECT. See Single photon emission computed tomography
Spiegel-Wycis apparatus, 5
Spinal lesions, Cyberknife radiosurgery for, 111–112, 111f, 112f
Spinal registration
accuracy and error in, 37–43
principles of, clinical application for, 41–43
reference frame for, 39
techniques in, 40–41, 40f, 41f
Spinal surgery, 218–222
anatomical considerations in, 198
cervical spine, 176–181. See also Cervical instrumentation, image-guided
cost-effectiveness of, 222

instruments used in, 220f
limitation of, 221
lumbar spine, 197–206. See also Lumbar instrumentation
navigational techniques in, 38–39, 38f, 39f
operating room setup for, 219f
preoperative planning for, 221f
registration principles in
accuracy and error in, 37–43. See also Spinal registration
clinical application of, 41–43
spinal reference arc in, 219, 222f
stereotactic technology applied to, 37
systems available for, 218
workstation for, 38, 38f
screen display, 41, 42f
Static field inhomogeneity, object-induced, 16–17, 18f
StealthStation
in brain tumor resection, 137, 138f
electronic brain atlases available in, 166–167, 48f
for neuronavigation, 142, 142f
for spinal applications, 218–219
optical digitizer, and, 45–50, 46f, 47f
ultrasound probe for use by, 142–143, 143f
user interface of, 167, 169f
videotactic surgery module in, 84–86
StereoPlan, user interface of, 171f
Stereotactic apparatus
Brown-Roberts-Wells frame. See Brown-Roberts-Wells stereotactic localizer
Cosman-Robert-Wells frame. See Cosman-Robert-Wells stereotactic frame
first linear (Horsley and Clarke), 5
frame-based, 4. See also Frame-based stereotaxy
Leksell system, 5
Mechanically based, 6
Mussen's frame, 5, 6f
Spiegel-Wycis, 5
Talairach system, 5
Todd-Wells, 5
Stereotactic brain atlas, 163, 163f
applications for, 165–168
in commercial systems, 166–168, 169f, 170f, 171f
development of, 4
electronic database form of, 162–163, 163f–165f, 164f
functional neurosurgery assisted by. See Atlas-assisted stereotactic functional neurosurgery
Internet portal for, 171–173
interventions based on, history of, 4
labeling in, 163, 163f
printed form of, 162
probabilistic functional atlas, 169–171, 172f
targeting enhanced by, 168f
Stereotactic endoscopic surgery
frame-based techniques, 93, 95
frameless techniques, 95
Stereotactic frames. See Stereotactic apparatus
Stereotactic functional neurosurgery, atlas-assisted, 162–173. See also Atlas-assisted stereotactic functional neurosurgery
applications, 165–168
electronic brain atlas database, 163f, 164f

Stereotactic functional neurosurgery, atlas-assisted *(continued)*
  Internet portal for, 171–173
  probabilistic functional atlas, 169–171, 172f
Stereotactic space, magnetic field referencing of, 60–62, 63f. *See also* Cygnus-PFS image-guidance system
Stereotactic systems
  equipment for. *See* Stereotactic apparatus
  frame-based. *See* Frame-based stereotaxy
  mechanically based, advantages of, 6
  techniques in neuroendoscopy
    frame-based, 93, 95
    frameless, 95
Stereotactic technology, interactive frameless, in spinal surgery, 37
Stereotaxis. *See also* Stereotactic *entries*
  of thoracic spine, 183t, 188–190, 189f
    pedicle screw placement and. *See* Thoracic instrumentation, for pedicle screw placement
  traditional use of, 218
Streak artifacts, 15
Stryker Navigation System Neuro
  features of, 167–168
  user interface of, 170f
Subdural monitoring grids, in epilepsy surgery, 159, 159f, 160f
Subthalamic nucleus, probabilistic functional atlas for, 172f
Suprasellar arachnoid cysts, neuroendoscopy for, 91
Supratentorial lesions, frameless stereotactic surgery for, 64–65
Surface-based registration
  algorithms for, 27
  error in, 26–28, 27f
  versus point-based registration, 27
  in spinal surgery, 37–38, 40, 41f, 42f
Surgical instrumentation
  cervical, 176–181. *See also* Cervical instrumentation, image-guided
  lumbar, 197–206. *See also* Lumbar instrumentation, image-guided
  in navigation system, 45, 46
    real-time visualization, 51, 51f
  thoracic, 182–190. *See also* Thoracic instrumentation, for pedicle screw placement
Surgical navigation systems, 12
  image-to-physical registration in, 14f
  intraoperative real-time feedback in, 50, 51f
  mechanical arm system, 54–59
Surgical planning
  for brain tumor resection, 139
  for exoscope procedure, 83
  image acquisition and, 76, 76f
  for intracranial aneurysms, case studies, 121–127
  passive navigation system and, 70
  robotic microscopes and, 101, 101f, 102f
SW brain atlas. *See* Schaltebrand-Wahren brain atlas

Talairach system, 5
Talairach-Tournoux brain atlas, 163, 164f
  3-D version of, 163, 165f
Target localization
  atlas-enhanced, 168f
  in Cyberknife radiosurgery, 109
Target registration error, 21–22, 21f
  feedback available on, 24–25
  fiducial configuration and, 23f–25f, 26, 26t
Telesurgery, 8, 8f
Test object, scaling error and, 19
Thoracic instrumentation, for pedicle screw placement, 182–190, 183f, 183t
  accuracy of, 182–186, 184f, 185t, 186t, 187f
  anatomical considerations in, 182, 183f
  challenge in, 186–187
  cortical violations in, 183, 185, 186t, 187f, 188f
  literature review of, 183t, 187–188, 188f
  and stereotaxy in thoracic spine, 183t, 188–190, 189f
Thoracic pedicle
  anatomy of, 182, 183f
  stereotactic screw placement. *See* Thoracic instrumentation, for pedicle screw placement
Three-dimensional atlases, 165f
Three-dimensional reconstruction, cervical spine, paired-point anatomical fiducials in, 178, 178f
Throat, magnetic system and, 67
Todd-Wells apparatus, 5
Tracking
  intraprocedural, systems for, 5–7, 5f, 7f
  in scoliosis surgery, 194
Transformation applications. *See specific registration techniques*
Transoral decompression, of craniocervical junction, virtual fluoroscopy for, 215
Transsphenoidal surgery
  endoscopic, 94f
  intraoperative MRI in, 148, 149f
  neuroendoscopy for, 92
TRE (target registration error), 21, 21f, 22, 23f–25f, 26, 26t
True accuracy, in image guidance, 62, 66f
TT brain atlas. *See* Talairach-Tournoux brain atlas
Tumor
  intraventricular, neuroendoscopy for. *See* Intraventricular tumors, neuroendoscopy for
  right parietal, mechanical arm experience with, 57, 57f
  surgery for. *See* Tumor resection; Tumor surgery
  ventricular. *See* Ventricular tumors
Tumor resection
  brain tumor, 134–136
    adjuvant therapy after, 139
    brain shift and, strategies minimizing, 137t
    caveats for, 135–137, 137t, 138f
    gene therapy after, 139
    intraoperative procedure for, 139
    minimally invasive craniotomy and, 133–135, 134f–137f
    needle biopsy prior to, 132–133
    planning for, 139
  exoscope procedure in, 84
  intraoperative magnetic resonance imaging and, 146–155
  sacral spine, 202, 203f
Tumor surgery, frameless stereotaxis for, 64–66
  infratentorial, 65–66
  of skull base, 66
  supratentorial, 64–65

Ultrasound
  in brain tumor resection, 137, 138f
  intraoperative use of, 4
    for image updating, 141–145
      versus MRI image updating, 152–153
      neuronavigation systems, 141–142
      sononavigation systems, 142–144, 142f–145f
Ultrasound probe, for neuronavigation, 142–143, 143f
Universal instrument registration, 198, 199f–201f, 201
Updating, intraoperative. *See* Intraoperative image updating

Vascular surgery, frameless stereotaxis for, 66–67
  aneurysms, 66–67, 66f
  arteriovenous malformations, 66
  cavernous angiomas, 66
Vector-Vision Spine system, 218–219. *See also* BrainLAB
  VectorVision neuronavigation system
Ventricular tumors
  intraoperative MRI in, 147
  intraventricular. *See* Intraventricular tumors,
    neuroendoscopy for
  of third ventricle, neuroendoscopy for, 91–92
Ventriculostomy
  in hydrocephalus, neuroendoscopy for, 88, 89f
  third ventricle, neuroendoscopy for, 88, 89f
Videotactic surgery, 80–86
  exoscope procedure in. *See* Exoscope procedure
  future of, 86
  history of, 81–82, 82f
  point-in-space targeting in, 80–81
  StealthStation and, 84–86
  3-D information in, 8
  volume-in-space targeting in, 81
Virtual fluoroscopy, 207–216
  accuracy in, 210
  definition of, 207
  future directions in, 216
  lumbar instrumentation and, 202–205
    advantages and limitations of, 202, 205
    system and function in, 202, 204f
  operational steps in, 208–210
  published studies on, 215–216
  systems of, described, 208–209, 209f, 209t, 210f

  techniques in, 210–215
    atlantoaxial transarticular screw fixation, 212–213
    odontoid screw insertion, 213–215, 214f
    percutaneous pedicle screw insertion, 211, 212f
    posterior lumbar interbody fusion, 211–212, 213f
    transoral decompression of the craniocervical junction, 215
Virtual reality simulation, neurosurgical, 49, 49f
Virtual surgery, 49, 49f
  for brain tumor resection, 137f, 139
Virtual tip, in mechanical arm system, 55, 55f
Volume, as image-guided target. *See* Videotactic surgery
Volume-in-space targeting, in videotactic surgery, 81
Voxels
  geometric image distortion and, 15
  in intensity-based registration, 28

Workstation
  for image guidance, 38f
  in Mayfield ACCISS image-guided system, 75–76, 75f, 76f
  for navigation in spinal surgery, 38, 38f
  for optical digitizer, 45, 46f
    early version, 7, 7f
    examples of, 47
    image processing by, 47, 47f
  optical tracking displays, 198, 200f–201f
  screen display
    in cervical surgery, 179, 180f
    in scoliosis surgery, 195f
  for spinal surgery, 219f
    display screen, 221f
  virtual surgery and, 49, 49f

Z-touch registration instrument, 69, 69f
Zeiss MKM system, 82, 98–105, 98–106
  accuracy of, 102–103
  advantages and disadvantages of, 104–105
  clinical utility of, 103–104
  imaging protocols for, 100
  neuronavigation procedure with, 100
  patient setup with, 101–102, 101f, 102f
  technical features of, 98–100, 99f